MW00365992

Yin Yoga Master Class: A Memoir

Marcy Tropin

Printed in the United States of America

First Printing, 2017

ISBN: 978-0-692-88276-4
e-book ISBN: 978-0-692-05285-3

Marcy Tropin
www.marcytropin.com

For Coady

Monday, April 11, 2016

Just after 4 pm.

There were five officers standing in my living room, in a circle, talking. Their hands on their belts. It felt like I was interrupting. In my own home. I stopped there, looking at them. They hadn't noticed me. I'd relive this moment often. It's the moment when my apartment stopped being mine, where I felt like the intruder, an interloper. It's the moment when my bathroom to the left becomes the bathroom to my left, the bedroom to my right, the closet behind me. My apartment and I separate. It's the moment right before they arrest me.

8

Begin

← dont turn your head

✗ no playing with the phone

← feet relaxed out

TER. NOTES

Lying down, on the floor, ten minutes.

Knees to chest, couple of breaths, keep butt on ground.

Exhale legs to the left

5 min

head to right, or center

5 min

— other side, legs to the right.

- finish by rolling to the right and sitting up.

February, 2016

A family moves into the apartment across the air shaft and one flight up from mine. The building is comprised of five floors, with four apartments to a floor. The front and back of the building on my side share the air shaft—an area that is completely enclosed within five brick walls and has a concrete cement bottom. Sound waves bounce, and on the five brick walls I imagine they bounce like the little dot in the arcade game Breakout, pounding each side up and down. Any noise near a window carries through the shaft, a conduit of urban living. When the movie is funny. When the movie is scary. When the beloved team loses or wins. When the neighbor watches X-Files reruns with the distinctive synth-whistling theme song while eating dinner after work. When a pan is being slowly removed from a wire-shelf oven. When a glass is clinking the side of the sink while water runs. When the first-floor college kids, drunk and full of ideas about life, politics and music, have loud, bizarre conversations in the wee hours...we all hear it.

Telephone calls can be stenographed. If I am on the phone and have to give out an account number or tell a personal story, I hustle to the back of the apartment to my bedroom, to the one room that doesn't face the shaft. A delivery person only needs to push a single apartment bell, to any apartment, to get in. Anyone who's home hears it, or my dog hears it and he goes into trigger mode, doing a crazy whining noise. None of this seems to bother any of us. It's city living. As somewhat of a homebody, I kind of like the noises. Long ago, I had developed the ability to hear them and not hear them. More than once the building's fire alarm has rung its warning sirens to deafening decibels, before it occurred to me to acknowledge the noise, asking my dog, "Do you think the building is on fire and how long has that thing been going?" The alarm and the chorus of other city noises rankle me less than the solitary, sudden sounds of the suburbs: settling house noises, trees aching to the wind, crickets, lawn mowers, a car door closing and the ruffling of packages to a doorway. Those were the sounds of my interminable suburban childhood, a jail sentence in and of itself. Give me cars honking at the turn of a green light and wacky sidewalk outbursts. Give me bus brakes, yappy small dogs behind large doors, the film crew truck generators at 6 am, the metal pushcart with the one bad wheel, noises, noises about living, any day. For the most part, my neighbors are respectful when it comes to sound. It seems like there is a "silent" agreement about noise.

I'd been living in the building just over a year. I found my apartment through a tip from a yoga student, then talked my way into the office of the head honcho at the management company, insulting a photo of his dog (to be fair, it was a terrible example of the breed) and asking for an apartment. My budget was tight, my time frame was less than three weeks, and I had a dog myself. By going straight to the offices, I found out about an apartment before it was vacant and listed for rent. I took it sight unseen, as is. I didn't have the time to wait for the place to be renovated. Also, had I been able to wait, the "renovation" would have been a slapdash paint job and maybe added a new cabinet to the kitchen. But the cost of that "renovation" would have increased the rent base. In other words, I'd be paying for it for the rest of my lease. I decided on the spot to do my own renovations and hire someone for the projects that were out of my league. All I knew about the place was the building's location, that it was a one bedroom, and very affordable.

The apartment was located in the Manhattan neighborhood of Washington Heights, fondly called Upper Manhattan or Northern Manhattan by some of the locals. Above 59th Street on the west side you had the Upper West Side, ending at 110th. From there heading north, it was Morningside Heights up to 125th, Hamilton Heights to 145th, and Sugar Hill from 145th to 155th. From 155th to about the George Washington Bridge was Washington Heights. Above that was Hudson Heights and then Inwood. Washington Heights was up there, but it was also beautiful, quiet and near five train lines, two of which were express. I signed the lease on December 18, 2014. Even though I wasn't able to see the inside of the apartment until December 31, I headed up to the building, wanting to check out the neighborhood. Also, I had the front door key.

Getting out at the C train at 155th Street, I was in an area I had never visited in nearly two decades of living in New York City. The first thing I noticed was sky. The sky. Few buildings rose above six stories. Then there was the architecture of wide town houses, brownstones, and incredible old houses, like the Morris–Jumel Mansion. My new street flows alongside a park, with apartments only on one side of the street. Next door to my new building was a catering company that opened as an adorable cafe on the weekends. A hiking trail entrance started right across the street from the building and wove through Highbridge Park, rambling over the just re-opened High Bridge with views of lower Manhattan and fresh cool air. It felt a little bit like a small country town. People said "good morning" or "good evening." They made eye contact. Neighbors knew one another. I would be able to stroll around with my little dog, sometimes the only person on the sidewalk.

Looking at my new building, I liked the glass and the wrought-iron front doors. The apartments Uptown were known for being large and somewhat soundproof, with plaster walls. While the area was predominantly Dominican, for this reason it often attracted musicians, and some mornings while walking around, you could hear warm-ups of voices and instruments. Like many buildings, mine had two entrances: the first with double-glass doors and then a second, just up a couple of stairs, made of glass with thick black metal doorframes.

The building's foyer was painted a light pink in probably the 39th layer of its color career. The walls were a little dirty. Security cameras were placed in some ceiling corners. The stairs, near the back left corner, had marble steps and painted brown metal railings. Directly across from them was a brown wood table (with three drawers in a row, no knobs) where tenants put the mail they didn't want, possessions they didn't want, or packages that delivery people didn't feel like hauling up flights of stairs. The entrance floor was an old tan tiled affair with cracks that had been filled in with cement. Mailboxes lined one lobby wall, with some boxes broken, and doors hanging off hinges. It wasn't an ideal introduction.

Feeling a little bit as though I were trespassing, I quietly went up the two flights to apartment 23. I liked the number as it was Don Mattingly's while he played first base for the Yankees. Each apartment door was painted the same brown as the railings. Doors were numbered with hardware housing numbers meant to be used outside, as they reflected light. Each door had its own version of size and typeface. At the back wall of each floor was a no-smoking sign, sometimes with something in Spanish handwritten underneath it. I stood looking at the door to 23. The knob looked original, while other apartments' knobs had been replaced. In between apartment doors were the original doorbells, painted over. I guessed that people used to just freely walk through the double glass doors at the entrance and then buzz when outside the apartment of choice. Standing there, I desperately wanted to see what was on the other side. Was it really a one-bedroom apartment? Mostly, I'd lived alone in studio apartments or lofts. It would be nice to have a separate room for sleeping. A room for a bed, a bedroom. What else was in there? As I poked around, the building was silent. After a couple of minutes, I left. Walking out of the building, facing the park and the Bronx, I noticed for the first time how Yankee Stadium was just across the East River. It was kind of across the street. As a lifelong, diehard fan, I took this as a good omen.

My move-in date was January 2. I wouldn't see the apartment until December 31. This gave me only two days to get it ready. How bad could it be?

Late in the morning on December 31, I met my new superintendent, who handed me the keys and did a walk-through viewing. The place was not just a "before" picture, it was a "before the before" picture. The front door led to a small vestibule area. To the hard right was the entrance to the kitchen. To the soft right lay the entrance to the living room. It was dark in there. Not dark from lack of light, but dark like hiding something, dark energetically, dark like a bad feeling. The walls were painted "I stepped in dog poop" brown. This wasn't a chocolate cake yummy dark brown. It wasn't a soft mustard brown with hints of creamy yellow. It wasn't the deep brown of an inviting mountainside. It was, instead, a sidewalk-crap brown. If you went into a paint store and said, "What's the color to feel like you accidentally ran over your dog while pulling out of the driveway, only the dog survived long enough to be rushed to the vet for a $5,000 bill, but died the next morning, before you could say goodbye?" It would be this color brown.

My super walked ahead of me while I stood at the entrance, taking it in. He flicked on the living room light switch. Then, a ceiling fan with five long black blades attached to a large black base with a dome light began rumbling to life. It was the sound you'd hear if a garbage truck with a bad air filter were idling outside your home. As the fan worked itself into a spin, dust shot off the blades and onto the walls. There the dust stuck. It didn't drop down, float along, or sway to the ground with the moving air. The dust attached itself to the walls where it had built up into a thick layer. At the base of the original picture frame moldings you could see large piles of it from across the room. On the wall opposite me was a large black stain and above it, near the ceiling, grey-brown stains from water damage. It was hard to believe someone had inhabited the place just yesterday.

I walked over to the fan's chains hanging in the middle of the room and found the one that stopped the fan blades. I pulled three times for the blades to go from fast, slow, to please stop.

Each time, they made a clinking noise, like Morse code for WTF. My face felt slack. On the one hand, I didn't want to seem unimpressed with my new digs while in the company of my new super. At the time, I didn't know if he believed what we were seeing was normal or not. On the other hand, I was wondering if I needed a hazmat suit to get the walls cleaned. They needed painting, obviously—white paint to be specific, so the place had more light and felt lighter, larger. You can't paint filthy walls, though. You're just painting on top of the filth. Walls have to be cleaned. Just how they were going to get clean baffled me. I'm not shy about tackling projects or hard work, but this dust thing made me worry about my precious and hard to replace lungs. Messiness happens. We get busy. Filth though, you have to work at filth. You really have to let things go to get to what I was seeing. It had to be earned over the course of many, many years. This wasn't the product of "the so-and-so was heavy, so I never vacuumed behind it." This was neglect. My personal comfort level of how clean my apartment should be revolves around one fear: if something should happen to me—gawd forbid, as they say—and friends had to get into my place, I wouldn't want them to think, "This is how she lived?" I keep my home tidy, in case of an emergency.

　　　　Proceeding in with caution, I walked towards the far right corner of the living room to the apartment's double windows, looking at my new view of the building's air shaft. Then I followed my super deeper into the apartment. Towards the far right corner of the living room was an entrance to a small hall with three doors. To the right lay the bathroom. Its floors had three-inch square white tiles surrounded by blackened grout, which was covered in various stains from unknown substances and what looked like sticky tape marks. There wasn't a shower curtain, so I could see the bathtub window, also facing the air shaft. There were a couple of missing tiles and a small patch of the wall near the window where plaster and grout were crumbling. The window itself didn't stay open from the bottom, you had to slide it open from the top while standing on the tub's edge. Someone had done this, maybe a decade ago, leaving a three inch opening where it was glopped-up by something dark and overflowing, so much so it looked like whatever was there was trying to sinisterly sneak in over the window's edge.

I looked down to the tub as a reflex. While it was original cast iron, the bottom had been stripped of its white glazing. It was now a shade of red-rimmed blue. The previous tenant was showering in a rusted tub. Did she do this barefoot or with flip-flops? Either unnerved me. The tub unnerved me. As I stared into the bottom there was a dowp dowp dowp of constant drips coming from a hole the size of a softball in the ceiling between the tub and sink. What didn't drip out from the hole flowed through the ceiling from the bathroom to the living room, joining the grey-brown water stains that were already there.

Despite all her neglect of the place, the previous tenant went to the trouble of taking the shower head when she vacated, leaving just a pipe sticking out of a dirty, white tiled wall. I wondered about the incongruity of someone caring enough about the way water came out of a pipe, but not caring at all about it coming from the ceiling, or traveling above the ceiling into living spaces. The tub was rusted because the building was leaning away from the drain. Bathwater flowed naturally towards the back end of the tub and stayed there. Later, I reasoned that the shifting of the building may all have started with the apartment two stories below mine, on the first floor, where a tenant had removed the load-bearing wall between the kitchen and living room. After the tub was reglazed, I'd make sure not to repeat the previous issue by sponging excess water towards the drain.

Thus far, I wasn't particularly enjoying the tour. My super and I left the bathroom, and were back in the hallway together. There were two doors left to pursue in this little nook, and I wasn't excited about either of them. I pointed to the door closest to the bathroom and asked my super, "What's this?" It must have seemed

17

like I'd never been in an apartment before, or was new to planet earth. "A closet," my super replied. *Wow, a closet!* You never get proper closets in New York City apartments. The closet door had two doorknobs: one beautiful original glass with the original brass keyhole painted over 17 times and another doorknob above it that was new and cheap and brass colored. Instead of replacing the original knob that didn't close perfectly, someone problem solved by simply adding another knob. Eventually I'd remove the cheap doorknob and patch the hole. The original glass one worked fine enough for me. The apartment doors were original, solid oak probably, and nearly eight feet tall. Drilling a hole into a solid wood door for a doorknob is a big deal. If you're not going to take the door off its hinges, then it's even harder to make sure the hole is perfectly level.

Of all the home improvement projects deemed important, this one should have been at the bottom of the list, or not on a list at all. Out of all things that could have bothered the previous tenant, was the closet not closing perfectly more important than an active bathroom leak, or any cleaning? Inside the closet were the usual suspects: a bar for hanging clothes and two shelves above it. In the near right corner were two pipes that came from the apartment below and disappeared into the apartment above. I used my cell phone light to make sure they weren't leaking. This is where my things would be stored. Would they be safe? Would anything be safe in this place? Myself? My dog? The joy of having a closet felt muted by the overwhelming terrible condition of the place.

The last door led to the bedroom. To open this door, my super had to lift the doorknob, walk the door open to the right, then let it rest down on the floor. The door's bottom hinge was attached to the door, but not to the doorframe. Though I was aghast at all the other neglect, this really annoyed me. The hinge wasn't even broken. Its holes weren't stripped. It just wasn't screwed in. The tenant chose to drag the heavy door on its one top hinge along the floor. She could have chosen to either reattach it herself or ask for help from the super, who didn't seem at all put off by his job, judging by how chill he was during this apartment showing. *C'mon lady, that's only four screws!* There was a half moon black circle on the tile floors from all the door dragging. The floor tiles were like those at public school: 12 inches square and light brown, with grey and white confetti-shaped speckles. It was the kind of tile that said, "Throw up on me, no one will notice." To get into the bedroom, there was about a four-inch step up. The original floor was under there, just sagging. Something terrible had happened to it. I went through a brief moment of mourning for what was probably once gorgeous old tongue-and-groove and a longer moment of mourning for what they had replaced it with.

While the dragging door initially brought my gaze downward, when I looked up it was like seeing the photo of a 1950s murder scene. Directly across the room was a singular window with an accordion-style metal security gate that was supposed to track along channels placed on the bottom and tops of the window frame. Only someone had bent the security gate out from the bottom, in all likelihood to position an air conditioner in the window and use the gate at the same time. Without the air conditioner for context, it looked as though something had tried to escape and didn't quite make it out. Behind the security gate was a yellowed, dried-out rolling shade, the right side of which was missing, and it was no longer attached on the left side. It hung at a falling angle, covering a little bit of the window on the left. Wow, did this room have bad mojo. To the left of the window was a steam pipe with two layers of rotting cardboard insulation. Where the air conditioner had probably been, there was water damage that affected the floor; two tiles lay next to where they were supposed to be. The exposed plywood baseboard showed warping from where excess water had probably pooled and began to rot the wood.

The bedroom was painted the same brown as the rest of the apartment and had the same huge heavy black ceiling fan as the living room. As with the rest of the place, there was leftover cable wiring, and lots of it. The whole apartment was spider-webbed with white cables. In one corner of the bedroom sat a coil of about 15 feet of wire, a hole drilled into the wall where the cable was fed in from the living room, and black burnt dust marks on the wall from where a television set had probably been. Some floor tiles had dug-out marks. My super told me the previous tenant was heavyset, and I imagine the years of her getting into and out of bed carved holes into the flooring. This wasn't a bedroom where you went to rest, snuggle with the dog, or read after a long day. It looked more like a place where someone was held captive for decades.

Eventually, I would throw every improvement I could think of at it: putting down an inexpensive but nice wood-looking floor, scraping the cardboard off the pipe and repainting it silver, screwing the hinge on so the door opened and closed without dragging, cleaning the window and screens for an entire afternoon, patching up holes, vacuuming, washing and repainting the walls white, removing the ceiling fan, and getting rid of all those wires. Still, the bedroom didn't feel right until I took down the zombie apocalypse preventative security gate. Once the gate was off, sun shined into the room and whatever bad energy was in there promptly fled.

Walking back through the living room with my super, I noticed a door on the opposite wall, nearer the front door, that the dust-spewing ceiling fan had distracted me from. Turning the door's handle with careful enthusiasm, I found a clean and empty walk-in closet. *Wow, two closets!* It was now time to see the kitchen, which tied all the other rooms in merit points for filth and shock. If each room had the vibe of a clown, the bathroom would be the type of clown who clumsily trips over his large shoes and goofily messes up tricks, the bedroom would be the clown that plays tricks, and the kitchen would be the sad clown. The saddest clown of them all, with a painted white head, red upside-down frown, tufts of red air above the ears, but a bald head, lumpy in the middle, and wearing an ill-fitting onesie.

The kitchen had the same tile floors as the bedroom and the same brown paint as the rest of the apartment, so there was definitely a closeout sale somewhere. The stove appeared thankfully unused, but everything else was sticky. The paint on the walls was thin, showing the previous color underneath. The refrigerator was about 15 years old and no longer stayed cold inside. This is really the only purpose of a refrigerator, to keep cold inside. Otherwise, it's just a big white box with a large exterior betraying a small interior. Inside there were dead flies and hair.

I'm a yoga teacher, and if you asked me what's something I don't like about teaching yoga, a little tidbit no one outside of the profession would know, an insider's view, a behind-the-scenes nugget, I would say it's other people's hair. No matter how much I brush off my bottom and my socks before heading home, a student's hair, a long brown or blonde something, will come home with me and turn up on my floor somewhere. There's something entitled about deliberately shedding your hair in public places. Groom before you get to class and stop pretending your ponytail needs redoing because you're tired and then extending your arm out past your mat to release the tangles in your hands. I walk through those urban tumbleweeds. Child's pose, rest in child's pose instead of molting all over the studio. I do not like seeing other people's hair in my apartment. I don't like it. At. All. That's my least favorite thing about teaching yoga. Story-topping the issue, seeing hair in a fridge violates something inside me that still thinks the world is a sacred, beautiful place.

On the spot, I decided to order myself a new refrigerator. It was one of those moments where my mind threw money at the problem. *I have a credit card, I'm an adult, and I'm buying a clean, new, working refrigerator.* There are things that, even cleaned, are never going to be clean. Of the three simulated wood kitchen cabinets, the one by the sink had water damage, the one above the sink had former food remnants solidified into circles and drips, and the other was just plain dirty.

There was one kitchen window with glass that was barely see-through, and like the rest of the windows, it had a similar metal brown frame. Only that brown frame turned out to be white. All the brown window frames turned out to be white after three and a half hours of scrubbing each one. Each one: three and a half hours of wearing rubber gloves and using lots of newspaper and water (which works fantastic). During the many, many, many hours I spent cleaning those windows, I hypothesized various scenarios that would explain how they went from white and clear glass to solid brown and sticky-goo blurry. The best idea I came up with is that the previous tenant murdered live poultry in the apartment. She killed them, defeathered them, gutted them, and then fried them over an open pit. Like the rest of the apartment, the kitchen window looked out on the air shaft and faced a brick wall. I didn't know which building came first, mine or the neighboring one, but to design an apartment where each and every window faces a brick wall is heartless.

Outside of the apartment, as my super and I were locking up and making small talk, I asked something about the building's security cameras. "Oh yes, the building is safe," he replied. Well, with all the brick walls surrounding the place, it was a little impenetrable. While it was in horrific condition, on paper the apartment had a great layout: a one bedroom with a living room, two closets, and an eat-in kitchen. The immediate problem was that the 48 hours I had before moving in wasn't enough to achieve the apartment's potential for cleanliness and livability. All the stress of finding the place was immediately replaced with the stress of the work ahead. Whatever condition an apartment needs to be in for a complete gut renovation, this one was close. Realistically, it needed weeks, months, to be live-in ready. The whole place was filthy and made me want to leave, to go home—except in two days, this would be my home.

It took money, a friend, one long New Year's Day of cleaning, a new refrigerator, two new floors, more money, the obligatory repeat trips to ikea, countless trips to hardware stores, tubs of spackle, three vats of paint, some more money, interminable afternoons trying to keep the dog on the sofa and his long tail away from wet paint, more cleaning... and then the place became home. The more I threw money at the project, the more I calculated that with every year I spent living in the apartment, the less the renovation cost on top of rent. Some funny math always helps. By mid-February the renovation was nearing an end. In that time I'd become friends with my super, a contractor, who I'd hired to do the big stuff, often acting as his handyman sidekick.

Now late winter, it was the perfect time to get bed bugs, because there really is no good time to get bed bugs. My building manager said I brought them in, and one friend was positive they came from the moving truck, while another theorized that they were there before me. Meanwhile, I thought I got them at the big-box hardware store in the Bronx. As a minimalist with barely any belongings, I owned two pieces of furniture where bed bugs could thrive: a bed and a sofa. Every time the exterminator came, we tore these pieces of furniture apart and never found bed bugs. We'd take flashlights and slowly pore over every inch of everything. We never figured out where they were coming from, where their nest was, where they lived. I even unscrewed electrical outlets, put double-sided tape around edges, and still could not find them.

But I had them. Or, as it was, I'd have one at a time. A lone bed bug out traveling during its gap year or on a reconnaissance mission in the middle of the night. It took until September, eight months, to be rid of the bugs and huge welts the bites left on my skin. Between the renovation and the sleep deprivation that accompanies having bed bugs, I was feeling unhinged by then. Was it worth it? A one-bedroom, rent-stabilized apartment in New York City, where I could take my dog for a hike in the woods across the street from me and be in midtown in 20 minutes on the subway? It was absolutely worth it.

Around the end of my bed-bug tenure, one of the tenants in the building and I had a disagreement about her renting out her apartment on Airbnb. Lease and law wise, it was illegal. My issue was the constant stream of people and their who-knows-from-where-previous suitcases coming in and out of the building. Were they bringing in the bugs? For the eight months I fought bed bugs, I never got a restful night's sleep. I slept with a light on and clear packing tape nearby. Every single bed bug I caught, I put it between pieces of clear packing tape and photographed it, documenting. As the bug squirmed inside the tape, I'd hold it up to the light and provide a ceremonial goodbye, "Fuck you and your fucking friends and your fucking night life. I hope you die, slowly. Namaste." The problem with catching a bed bug was that I only knew one was near after I was bitten, started scratching in my sleep, woke with a start, and then hunted through my bedding for the culprit. Often, I'd fry my eyes with the cell phone flashlight and disabuse my dog's trust with the sudden unmaking of the bed in the middle of the night.

Once I knew the bed bugs came at night, I'd jolt every time a dog hair brushed my skin, or the sheet fell to a new position after I had moved. Sometimes, I jolted over nothing at all. I tried pushing the bed into the middle of the room, putting double-stick tape around its legs, and never letting the bedding touch the ground. But one night, with the light on, staring at the ceiling, waiting for sleep, I noticed two bed bugs. They were crawling along the ceiling in order to drop into my bed with an aerial attack. That's when my bed bug issue turned me into a crazy person. That night was a turning point for me. Those bed bugs were cunning, played dirty, and didn't fight fair. The act of being asleep became a restless vulnerability. I'd lie in bed desperate for rest with the knowledge of the apple-seed-sized bugs' ability to crawl on my face without my knowing, and bite me multiple times, which happened twice. In my fried state, wondering and questioning where the bugs came from, I emailed management to complain about my Airbnb-ing neighbor, in essence ratting her out.

The bed bug issue was resolved after eight months of sleepless nights, three exterminating treatments that had to be spaced out, three expensive doggy day care afternoons, three afternoons at the Laundromat drying every fabric I owned on high heat for 20 minutes, two huge purges, and wearing a scarf and/or long-sleeve shirts, often in the summer heat, to teach yoga and hide the disgusting bites, when in the end I didn't so much defeat the bed bugs as fostered an armistice. They moved on to the apartment above mine. Under different circumstances, my neighbor renting her place probably wouldn't have crossed my radar the way it did during that time. Had I not had bed bugs I don't know if I would have said anything.

When the neighbor confronted me outside the building about our difference of Airbnb opinion, it got ugly. I antagonized her and she came right up into my face, threatening. I get it. Whatever her situation, she needed the money, and renting out her apartment was working for her. Except, giving keys to the building to so many strangers, most of them from out of the country, and none with accountability, did affect me. Aside from it not being safe, I found out from my super there was a history of bed bugs in other apartments, including hers. She told me stop complaining and I egged her on, "What are you going to do?" I didn't back down, or deescalate or do anything yogic. I matched her anger with a condescending tone. Embarrassingly, because I didn't have an outlet for my anger about the bed bugs, incensing her was a wonderful release of tension for me. After our confrontation I pursued finding her Airbnb listing. This was the issue that kept management from taking action; they couldn't find her ad. I couldn't find her ad either. So I emailed a friend in London to ask if she saw an ad for my building. I wondered if there was some blocking happening in the United States. My friend found her ad immediately, and I sent it along to management in equal time.

On September 19, 2015, 11:52 am, my building manager wrote:

Subject: Re: This is the listing...
Wow thank you for this I have spent days looking for some proof...I promise I won't mention your name and never have again thank you.

My decision to retaliate against my neighbor started everything; it was the butterfly flapping its wings. I don't think of karma as a bitch, or instant like oatmeal. I don't think of karma as a laundry list of deeds, a tally of two columns good and bad. I think of karma, the yoga of action, as energy. The energy you put out into the world is the energy you receive back, without the constraints of linear time. My neighbor was forced to stop renting out her apartment. She then stopped paying rent and was eventually evicted. Throughout, she was vocal to neighbors, openly blaming me.

In February 2016, new tenants moved into her place, across the air shaft and one flight up from me. They moved in loud and stayed loud. Not loud like a party loud, or loud like I've had a long day at work and need to hear this song loud. It was everything loud, all the time loud. They were noisy people. My first thought was that I was probably just as loud when I moved in and tackled the renovations. Doesn't everyone move in loud? Give them two weeks, I thought. They're just trying to settle in.

By the end of two weeks, it was still the same. The sounds of kids screaming. The sounds of two adults screaming. The sounds of kids and adults screaming. Phone calls on speakerphone with the volume turned up, and screaming. Dinnertime was the worst. Everyone, and it sounded like there were a lot of people up there, congregated in the kitchen. Everything they did was loud, whether it was putting a fork down on the table or turning on the faucet. After dinner, the sounds of cleaning were just as loud. Following dinner, there was a banging noise in the kitchen that went on for a couple of hours. They never spoke to one another without screaming. I wondered how this played out at work, school, the library. Since it looked like it wasn't going to get any better, I emailed management:

On February 15, 2016, 3:13 pm, Marcy Tropin wrote:

Hi My Building Manager, The new tenants in [Airbnb neighbor]'s old apartment yell at one another all day long. I have my windows closed, they have their windows closed, and I can hear them screaming. Both kids and adults. They also do something that requires a lot of slamming and banging things for hours on end in the evening. Their kitchen abuts the air shaft. Could you please let the new tenants know that unfortunately all sound carries through the shared shaft in their new building? We can hear every single thing they do through two sets of double-paned windows!!! If this is how loud they are with all windows closed, it's going to be worse as it warms up. Please help. -Marcy

By February 18, I hadn't heard back from my building manager. I was in my kitchen trying to write. The window was closed, but I could hear the neighbors screaming and couldn't get anything done. So I went upstairs and introduced myself. I was invited in by the mom, my neighbor. There were five kids running around, her husband, and her sister. There was also the delivery of a new 52 inch television. I found out they had just moved to New York from Florida, their belongings were coming, and until then they didn't have any furniture, except loans from the sister who lived nearby. I explained the air-shaft situation—how sound carried, unfortunately, easily throughout our side of the building. I explained it was worse when the kitchen window was open. She was empathetic. It all went well. I came back downstairs and emailed my building manager to say the issue was resolved.

But it wasn't. Nothing had changed. They kept being loud.

When I told my super what was going on, he said I wasn't the only person complaining about the new neighbors. The apartments below and above were getting the worst of it. In the apartment above the loud neighbors were two absolutely lovely gentlemen. Every morning, they received the New York Times, often wrapped in a long plastic bag that was perfect for dog cleanup. After a casual inquiry as to what they did with those bags, they started leaving them on my doorknob, tied in cute little knots. I loved that. It felt cozy and community like. They greeted my dog Buster like he was part of their book club, and they were just divine to run into. Even when I had the chance, I never asked them about the neighbors above. They worked regular hours, leaving early in the morning and returning in the early evening. I assumed that whatever intrusive noise hell the neighbors below were causing them, they didn't want to spend more time than necessary focusing on it. And I didn't want to contaminate our wonderful little relationship of cordial hellos in passing.

After the Airbnb neighbor moved out, I tried to maintain a low profile around the building. I was on good terms, as far as I knew, with everyone else. I'd been associated with a ton of negativity since the Airbnb neighbor was evicted and hoped it would eventually be forgotten. I didn't want the current tenants to think I was looking for an issue, seeking out rumors. In fact, I was conflicted about my role in my neighbor's eviction. I wasn't necessarily to blame, but I did walk into a grey area, turn on the light and point. With that in mind, I never brought up the new neighbors to the gentlemen who lived above them, even though it would have been impossible for them not to be affected.

As for the neighbor below the noise, Dewan (all people's names have been changed), he grew up in his apartment, left for some time, came back recently to take care of his mother, and stayed after she passed away. Dewan was the nicest guy you'd ever meet—endearingly loquacious and sweet sweet sweet. We'd already had conversations about everything, two chatty people living across the hall from one another. Even when he was talking about something terrible, he'd be jovial. Also, he liked my dog and my dog was smitten with him.

When I connected with Dewan about the neighbors above him, he was already in the thick of it with management. While I just heard screaming and banging, he and his equally sweet girlfriend endured all-night pounding. The kids jumped on the floors and played with bouncing balls at night. Dewan and his girlfriend would hear furniture being dragged across the floors at all hours. Since my bedroom was in the back, I could get a break from the neighbors' noise at night. I could hear them a little, but not as bad. As for the tenants who lived below their apartment, they endured noise day and night. It was wearing on them.

We wondered why they were so active indoors, and so loud. Why didn't they take the children outside to the many playgrounds nearby, to the park, for a walk? Why did they continue when there had been so many complaints? Dewan's girlfriend had to leave their apartment in the middle of the day and go to the library to study. Meanwhile, he had a record of phone call and email complaints to management and 311 (New York City's public-service hotline), and he documented conversations with our super. Having dealt with issues in the building before, he kept a running log of what transpired. We agreed to keep one another in the loop about the neighbors, and I agreed to start contacting 311 so it wasn't just him making the calls.

It was becoming hard to enjoy being in my apartment. After a renovation and bed bugs, this speaks to both my tolerance for riding through stress and how bad the noise was. The sounds of my neighbors screaming permeated my air. Their yelling followed me from the kitchen to the sofa, from the sofa to the bedroom. Pleasures like reading, phone calls, leaving a window open for air, or telling my dog out-loud how cute he was were invaded. The neighbors' noise was so bad I couldn't watch a movie on a laptop using earbuds with the windows shut. I couldn't hear the movie being piped into my eardrums over their screaming. In the beginning, I tried to put a spin on it. Nice! They have dinner together even though they yell the entire time. But as it got worse and I needed an outlet for my frustration, I started taking short cell-phone videos of the brick walls outside my windows, recording the neighbors' loudness. Documenting the issue felt like being proactive. I emailed my building manager with evidence:

On March 2, 2016, 12:47 pm, Marcy Tropin wrote:

Hi Building Manager, Sorry to trouble you with this again. The neighbors aren't any quieter. Here's a one-minute cell video from my kitchen windowsill. Both the husband and my neighbor are speaking to someone on speakerphone. You can hear every single word. And I'm across and one story down! Can you please help? Can you please convey to them the intrusiveness of their yelling loudly all day and night, with the sound carrying into their neighbors' apartments? -Marcy

Nothing changed.

Twice in March I went online to file a noise complaint with 311. Former New York City Mayor Mike Bloomberg launched 311 in 2003 as a phone service to register complaints

30

about environmental issues such as toxic chemical smells coming from New Jersey (ahhh, my home state), double-parked cars, bed bugs, barking dogs, loud music, noise complaints, noise complaints, and other various noise complaints. By 2009, the service was available online.

Registering a complaint with 311 felt exactly like hunting down my neighbor's listing on Airbnb. It didn't feel good. When people choose to live in cities, they're not necessarily choosing to endure endless injustices, though it seems implied that they should. After all, the catchphrase for New York City is "If you can make it here, you can make it anywhere." What does that mean, really? Personally, I think it's more about how hard it is to get around. So if you can make it from here, to here, to there, if you can figure that out, you can figure that out anywhere. You can make it to any place else from any other place else. Does it mean if you can tolerate living in an apartment in less than desirable conditions you can live anywhere else? It seems like the phrase implies rather low expectations of treatment.

The thing is, my lease had a "warrant of habitability" statute. While it can be a matter of pride in this city to tolerate a bad living situation as if the real world were a sitcom, the fact was that my lease granted me a tolerable quality of life just as equally as it required me to pay rent. As entitled as my neighbors were to interact in their home as they saw fit, I was equally entitled to a quiet environment. The less I was able to have what I felt entitled to, the more I wanted to inhibit what they felt entitled to.

Tuesday, March 15, 2016

The intercom buzzed, my dog ran to the door and started his weird whining noises. I calmed him and pressed "'talk" asking "Who is it?" Then took a half second to calm my dog before pressing "listen" and heard "Police." Took another half second to calm my dog before pressing "door." Was it really the police? For me? I'd just gotten back from teaching, hustling to therapy afterward, and then dragging myself to Mysore ashtanga yoga practice after that. By the time I got home to take Buster out, I was both emotionally and physically spent. I'd gone from the high-energy feeling of being a beloved yoga teacher to the completely different world of talking about your shit, to physically working through your shit.

I think of yoga as my health IRA. They both work best when done consistently, with cumulative results. You may not remember what you did for that hour last Wednesday afternoon or the $50 you spent last month, but if you use these for health and finance, both will pay off in the long run. After all, a body is a long time to spend your life in, and the parts are hard to replace. Even cars eventually get new tires. Don't expect to get 20 million miles out of your knees if you don't take care of them now. With the door opened I waited with Buster behind me, adhering to a sit-stay command in his own dachshund-stubborn way by moving a ton in one place. Buster loves rocking the meet and greet, but startling a person with a gun as they round the corner up the stairs isn't a good plan. Even though my mutt was smallish and as aggressive as a throw blanket, I kept him behind me, much to his chagrin.

Two policemen greeted me and explained they were there for the noise complaints I'd made to 311. The first order of business was to release the hound. "Are you okay with dogs?" I asked, and Buster came bouncing out from behind me. While he was wiggling for hellos, I left my apartment, giving the officers the one-minute sign, to knock on Dewan's door across the hall. Turning back around, I said that both my neighbor and I had contacted 311 and I'd like to include him in the conversation. Dewan opened his door and I introduced everyone as if we were all heading out for an evening stroll and cordials afterward. We decided to convene in my kitchen.

When I renovated my kitchen, I didn't do cabinets and countertops. The walls weren't flat. Over the hundred years the building had been standing, there had to have been a hundred years of different cabinets, repairs, water damage, replacement pipes, and spackling over all the above. No edge was straight. The walls were like puddles in heavy traffic. A friend of mine gave me the advice to design my kitchen the way I liked to cook. I don't like to cook, so that left a burden of figuring out how I managed to stay alive and what exactly I was doing in this particular room to make it happen. I ended up putting a big island in the middle of the kitchen, with storage on one side and a place for two stools on the other. Without so many wall cabinets, the small room felt roomy. The kitchen was designed to function like all of my previous art studios: large work space in the middle and lots of free wall space. It turned out I liked to make food the way I liked to make art: prepare and assemble.

We all stood around the kitchen island, me near the window and sink opposite the doorway, Dewan between the fridge and doorway, kind of to the opposite left of me, one officer near the stove and doorway, kind of to the opposite right of me, and the other officer standing in the vestibule, facing the living room, at the ready. It felt like I was hosting. Except, you can't engage police officers conversationally the way you do with unarmed guests. I wanted to offer beverages, even though I didn't have any, and snacks, even though I didn't have those either. Outwardly I was more giddy than appropriate for the context of the company I was having. I guess you shouldn't be jovial when cops are in your home. I should have been more solemn and low-key.

Dewan and I gave the officers a little synopsis on the issue with our neighbors. In my head, I was trying to tone down how inviting I felt, telling myself, "Dude, you're not entertaining these people." Buster had the same issue, wanting the officers' attention, wanting Dewan's attention, then circling back to the officers. While my dog wouldn't want me to get another dog and share affections, he would love another human around. He was beside himself about having extra company, making long vibrating noises no one understood. Then I'd have to act like his interpreter as if he was my foreign exchange student houseguest. "He wants you to pet him," I explained. I speak a little dog.

Dewan launched into a story about former tenants living above him. A woman named Delilah and her sons. They were loud as well, and when Dewan went upstairs to complain, they came after him with a baseball bat. Delilah got back at Dewan for complaining by flooding his family's apartment. She turned on the bathroom and kitchen faucet and let them run over. *Wow*. Looking down, he said he did not want to go through that again. After listening, the police offered that they couldn't really do anything. They said if it was noise from a boom box—and 1981—they could do something. Talking loudly wasn't under their jurisdiction.

Annoyingly, the neighbors were pin-drop quiet during this exchange. "I don't hear them now," an officer noted. Perhaps he didn't quite get the noise-carries-in-the-shaft-even-with-the-windows-closed issue. The neighbors knew the police were in my apartment. Everyone knew the police were in my apartment. They came into the lobby with their walkie-talkies on loud, the static of their background radio conversations announcing their arrival. And they stomped up the building stairs in thick black-soled shoes. Apparently reverse-stealth is how the academy trained officers. From a neighbor in the building who received frequent visits from the police, I knew they knocked on doors like they were tenderizing meat, which was why I had mine opened. The whole building was quiet while they were in my apartment. With the exception of my dog, everyone else was laying low.

We discussed options, all of which had been pursued to their ends already. The police offered to go upstairs and speak to the neighbors. I thanked them for offering and said maybe it would help. Maybe it would bring the issue some gravitas. I didn't use that word, though. In my head I was hoping it might shake the neighbors up a bit. We mean it, you guys are loud, crazy loud. The police went upstairs. Dewan and I hung out in my kitchen, chatting.

The officers came down and went over what they told the neighbors, that I had been complaining. Me. They didn't mention Dewan, the neighbor below. I could feel my eyebrows furrowing. The police made the decision to blame their presence entirely on me. They could have said multiple neighbors have been complaining. It would have been protective, and true. Instead, they might as well have gone to my neighbors window and pointed to my apartment, "It's her." Dewan reiterated that he had made multiple 311 complaints. *That's great, they don't know about those, they only know about me. They think it's just me. They think I called the police on them.* We thanked the officers for their time, and they asked us to stop contacting 311 about the issue. Then the officers left, Dewan left, I prepared food, and the neighbors continued being loud.

Nothing changed.

Saturday, April 2, 2016

Not being able to write in my kitchen, I purchased a table to put in my bedroom. It was a desk on Craigslist that was by a familiar company, and the owner offered to include delivery in the price. When the guy drove up to my building, he simply carried this steel-legged, real-wood-top, quite heavy thing in a rush from the back of his car, up the two flights of my apartment building and inside my place. It was a compelling feat of strength and will. Then he took my cash, got back in his car, and drove off to enjoy the rest of his Saturday. Having moved furniture my entire life, and I mean, my entire life, I put old thick wool socks under two corners, lifted the other side a bit, slid the desk to the back of the apartment. Then I used similar tricks to get the desk angled through the tiny area in the back and into my bedroom.

When I was a kid, my mother owned a consignment shop and thrift store in Keyport, New Jersey called "Fabulous Finds." This was where I learned how to move anything of any size or weight. Instead of having a babysitter, or perhaps some educational program, I was at the store all the time. On the weekends she'd take me to garage sales. This was in the late 1970s when people were remodeling their homes and switching from antiques to, feel their pain, Formica furniture. It was also a time before the internet, before the home computer. No one really knew what they had, and it was my mother's prerogative to take advantage of that.

Long before yoga and I fell in love, my mom taught me how to bargain, negotiate, play someone—whatever it took to relieve people of their goods and fill her shop. We had code words and signals. For example, if she held out a cup to me and gently shook it, I was to ask how much the cup was while making sure the seller didn't turn it over, where it was stamped with "Made in Occupied Japan." Imagine a four-year-old with a squeaky voice, shy like a rising soufflé, offering a quarter for your porcelain cup. It worked, every, single, time.

My mother's talent was to play good cop/bad cop as one person. She could talk crazy one moment, then softly and empathetically the next. She'd change subjects, confuse, and dominate the conversation. Among her more notorious deeds was the time she purchased a lamp for six dollars at a yard sale, took it to Bamberger's at the Monmouth Mall, and returned it for $84 because it still had its tag on. I remember being in the customer service waiting area during the whole thing. My role then was to stay put in the waiting room chairs, not get taken away by a stranger (in my day, the onus was on the child to prevent kidnapping) and not bother her while she was, more or less, screwing the store over.

In the early 1980s a drunk driver in a white van blew through a red light, hitting my mother's car head-on. The accident physically ended her career of hauling furniture for sale to her shop. I think that had she not been so devastatingly different after the accident, I'd have followed in her footsteps towards a life of using shakti (energy) to create meaningless scores that were good for stories but not for souls.

When she was out of the hospital, my father took my mother and me to where her car was being kept. She drove a blue Oldsmobile, the type with the long front, except the front was completely smashed into the driver's area. All of it, accordioned into the dashboard. Why the hell you bring your little kid along to see that, I don't know, but it stayed with me. Her accident took away the innocence I'd had in not knowing bad things can happen to your parents. Once that leaves, kids start becoming adult-like. After the accident, my mom was in constant pain, and for some reason, wanting me to bear witness. I'd watch her in the living room, lying on her belly, using a rope to reach back and try and bend her cartilage-free knee more than 90 degrees. She was screaming in pain and I was holding my Kermit the Frog stuffed animal for dear life, crying to myself. It was around this time I took to playing alone in my room more and more often.

Sometimes, over the course of 15-plus years of teaching yoga, I wondered if I was just trying to save my mother in extending myself with care and patience to students. Wanting to get back the woman who proudly brought me along everywhere and taught me everything she knew, which was about being a strong, independent woman who never, ever, took any crap from anybody. Even when people thought they had the better of her, she was in control. After the car accident, a bitterness towards life, and my perfect health, fomented our relationship. We were no longer a team. My mother withdrew herself maternally from me and my brothers. In what must have been such a terrible time for her, she took her manipulative negotiating skills and turned them on her family. Her children were never useful or caring enough to help quell whatever demons she was fighting. From the accident on, my mother fought the world.

With my desk in my bedroom, more and more I was sequestering myself in the back of the apartment, confining myself to one room.

Monday, April 11, 2016

Back in January, Exhale Spa, where I taught group yoga classes, had scheduled me to teach a workshop, though workshops are usually called "master classes" these days. So instead of a "Yin Yoga Workshop," I was teaching a "Yin Yoga Master Class." This implied a master was teaching it. Hardly. When I did my yoga teacher training in 2001, we were advised to find a niche. This made sense: there were close to 40 of us students in that training, never mind how many other trainings were going on in the city at the same time—or the trainings that were just finished, or the ones soon to start.

Yoga teaching back then replaced waiting tables as the job to have if you were trying to pursue something involving auditions. Except you can't repeatedly last-minute sub out your class for a casting call. It doesn't work for students to have a teacher they can't count on, and it doesn't work for a studio to have an unreliable teacher. It also gives students the impression you don't really want to be there, waiting for fame to release you from the "trenches." When in the early oughts performers started using yoga teaching as a side job, the sincerity of the "product" lessened as the availability of "certified" teachers increased. For the most part, students are drawn to classes with beautiful people who can do beautiful poses, never mind whether they can teach or really want to. This makes their classes about them and not about yoga. For me, whenever I got asked about how my writing or art was going, I'd change the subject back to the student. It should be about them.

I worked hard to outlast the posers. I subbed their classes and won over their students. I spent the first two years of my career not having a day off. If you're a studio owner and you have the choice between a blonde, bosomy woman with a chewing-gum-commercial personality and a short, wire-hired, sassy lady who wears a lot of black, you're going with the girl-next-door babe. Even though I get it, I still harbor resentment about how easy it was for those women to get classes. In surface appeal, yoga is no different than a lot of other professions.

My initial yoga training happened before studios realized they could charge a fortune and offer less. It was nine months long with 20-hour weekends every other weekend, 13 papers, two oral exams and a final three-hour written exam (that I wrote after becoming the studio's Gal Friday). It was a long, tough process made even more challenging when 9/11 happened halfway through it. On that Tuesday morning, I was on an express train going from the Upper East Side's 86th Street down to 14th Street. Except the train wasn't running express, it was taking forever. I was trying to get to one of the studio owner's 9:30 am classes, which was required as part of my teacher training, and it was looking like I was going to be late. Because of this, I exited the station bolting towards the northwest corner, heading away from downtown. I'm not that great of a runner and it was noticeably harder to run around all the people facing me, standing still, looking to the sky. I stopped and asked a guy, "What's going on?" He offered the easiest solution to my question by pointing behind me and saying, "Look up." I turned around and in 180 degrees everything changed.

I remember seeing one of the World Trade Center's twin towers with a huge hole in it. It was the craziest thing to witness. I didn't understand what caused the hole, and I immediately went into shock. I mean, I was less than a mile away, and it was a huge fucking hole. At first I thought of Godzilla, that it looked like the monster had taken a bite out of the tower. Then I thought about how it could be fixed; how the hell were they going to fix that thing? I've been through a lot of stressful, traumatic events, and my mind will disassociate and chat with me when trauma reoccurs.

Standing there, watching the towers burning, I told myself I was too sensitive to visual information to stay. I told myself to get to class. I'm so grateful I did. The towers went down while I was hidden away in a room practicing yoga. I don't think I could have handled seeing that in person. While I was affected by being in Manhattan that day, and all that happened after, I did get off relatively easy. I'm aware of that.

The teacher trainees with families and those living off the island retreated to their homes after 9/11. With the studio still wanting to stay open, they reached out to single-lady me, who was available to sub. From September 12, 2001 until the end of the month, I taught over 50 classes. Often I'd teach a power yoga class as a mindful, flowy retreat. Students were coming to the studio to be with people, to connect, to have a place to grieve that wasn't religious or dogmatic. This time period informed how I would approach classes for the rest of my career: meet students where they were at, teach to the energy of the room.

That September I taught and taught until one of my mentors pulled me aside and lovingly chastised me, "You're not dealing with this, you're not processing what happened, and it's affecting you." She was right. I was working nonstop and not sleeping well. When I got into bed at night, I'd close my eyes and see people jumping from buildings. Then I'd open my eyes. This went on and on throughout the night. I slept as a matter of passing out from exhaustion. After being confronted, though, I went home and cried the night through, for my city and all the people who were lost on that day, and all the people who would never be the same again, including myself. I mourned a way of being in New York that went down with the towers.

When my training covered restorative yoga I was completely hooked, smitten. This was a type of interaction with the body that wasn't aggressive, goal oriented, or adversarial. It was restful, healing, squishy. You did every single pose supine, with the support of props, often under a nice heavy woolen blanket, in a softly lit room, and…zzzzzzz. I'd found my niche. With most physical activities, we're taught to look for more. Even in yoga there's "more." Either through comparing yourself to the person who folds "more" next to you, or creating an internal dialog that involves the desire to fold forward "more." I loathe "more." "More" is not better, it's just more. If you keep practicing, you'll fold completely forward. It'll happen. Looking for more though, that fosters injury, desire, needless competition and the idea we have somewhere else to go that's better than where we are now. With restorative yoga you can try to look for more, but you'll probably fall asleep two seconds afterward. For the most part, there is no "more" in restorative yoga. Well, except when the class ends and you want "more." It's a way of healing and being in your body that is completely non-confrontational.

After that first teacher training, I went on to get certified in restorative yoga in 2004 and yin yoga in 2007. I eventually developed a style that was an amalgamation of the two. I told students to do less in the poses, that the poses didn't need their help, to get out of their own way, and let their bodies open feeling safe, and comfortable—the way you can relax on your sofa. From my own past, holding my body tightly in anticipation of arguing or violence, I found I opened "more" in restorative yoga than I did with an active practice. Feeling safe, learning to relax—that's what I needed. I then took that to my own active practice, becoming softer, with less fighting, less tension. The physical practice of yoga, hatha, is not intended to foster an adversarial relationship with your body, to make you push and twist and move harder, faster and deeper in each and every pose. Yoga is a practice that balances our energy. After all, "hatha" is union of "ha"/sun and "tha"/moon.

When my Yin Yoga Master Class was first put into the calendar, it was early in the year, and I had plenty of time to prepare. I went home and did all the grunt work. Researching, picking poses, testing them out, developing modifications, doing little stick-figure drawings, and then making notes for things to say. I also wrote notes on how long to hold a pose before things turned homicidal. Yin is not restorative yoga. It's right between an active practice and snuggling with a bolster. Yin poses are challenging and it's important to know exactly how long to keep students in them. Not too short or they don't give up the fight; not too long or they start fighting. For a workshop, I like to do all the planning ahead of time and then do nothing until a couple of days beforehand.

The master class was coming up on Sunday. I had a full week ahead and decided to spend Monday afternoon testing the poses out again and doing sequencing. The idea was to teach a more challenging version of my open-level "chill" class. In a group class I can have a student with a daily practice, a pregnant woman, and another lady who says she can't bend her knees (happened). Teaching to all levels lends itself to poses that can be modified for all levels. I call this being the Statue of Liberty of Yoga Teachers: "Give me your sick, your tired, your hip surgeries, your hamstrings, yearning to be free." Because my group classes attracted a broad range of students, this was an opportunity to teach people who were not infirm. I was looking forward to it.

Monday morning I went to Mysore practice, came home, ate, took Buster on the trail, chilled, and then got to work. I had an evening class on the Upper East Side from 7:35 - 8:35 pm and then a private client near Washington Square Park at 9:30 pm. This student was a woman I really wanted to work with, as she was suffering from neck issues, back issues, stress—all at too young of an age. As a result of the noise issue, I started working in my bedroom, re-reading some articles, going through my notes. When I was reading, I'd plug my ears with my fingers so as not to hear the neighbors screaming. Still, I could hear them through closed windows, the closed bedroom door, and my middle fingertips.

When the time came to sequence, I pulled out props in my living room. With a big desk in there now, there wasn't enough space in the bedroom to properly test out the poses. I needed the open living room to play around on the floor, with two blocks, blankets and a bolster nearby. The more I did the poses myself, the better I could talk people through what they might be feeling, or know if they were going to throw their backs out. I was my own crash-test yogini.

Lying on the floor in my living room, perpendicular to the sofa, I played with a supine triangle pose. Instead of doing the pose standing, I was recreating it using the sofa edge as "the floor." My left foot was flat and flexed against the sofa, while my right leg was out at an angle, with my right foot and ankle on a bolster, and a blanket for weight on the leg to keep it there. My arms were out like a "t," palms up. It was the same shape as triangle pose, only as if the person fell over sideways, perfectly to the ground. As I lay there wondering what someone could possibly find uncomfortable about this divine position, all I heard was the neighbors yelling. Over two months of nearly non-stop yelling. I couldn't take it anymore. Like Popeye, but with better grammar, I could stand all I could stand and then I couldn't stand it anymore.

I stood up, grabbed my keys and cell phone, shoved them into my sweatpants' pockets, left my apartment, and headed up one flight to my neighbors' place. I positioned myself outside their door where the security camera could see me, about two feet away, and knocked. The mother, my neighbor, answered the door and immediately started cursing. I thought, how naive of me, of course she's pissed and harboring resentment towards me, especially because she thinks I called the cops. Maybe she even thinks that I'm the only one complaining. She was yelling that my dog barked all day. There is a dog who barks a ton, but it's not mine, and I said so. She said it was mine. Okay I said, what times do you hear my dog barking, let's suss this out. I was proud of my exemplary openness to hearing out her concerns. This is how problems are resolved lady, we talk. She slammed the door shut. Standing there, staring at her door, I was pissed. I knocked on the door again, harder, and said, "Stop screaming."

Immediately, my neighbor swung her door open. She was screaming at me, she was telling me she was going to fucking kill me. Past her left shoulder I could see her husband sitting on the sofa, wearing only underwear, holding a baby, trying to keep it calm. Whereas before my neighbor had only cracked the door open to bitch me out, this time she was standing with the door opened to her right shoulder. A large woman, filling up the space horizontally, in a complete rage. It was an interesting juxtaposition: my neighbor screaming at me in the foreground, and the father doting on his baby, down a hallway, in the living room, in the background.

I stepped back and said, "If you're going to threaten me, then I'm going to film you," and took out my phone and started recording. She took out her phone and started recording too, and then said she was going to call the police. Fine I said, call the police. I had her threatening me; I had the 311 requests and the police's prior visit. There was a history of complaints in a short amount of time with this one tenant. Go ahead, call the police, you're an issue in the building and they are aware of this. I walked back down the stairs, into my apartment, grabbed my laptop from the bedroom and brought it into the kitchen. Typing away at the island, I began to compose an email to my building manager. I was going to attach the video of my neighbor threatening to kill me.

Halfway through the email I stopped to sync my phone so the video would be on my computer. Except looking at where the video should be, I only saw one photo, blurry, of my neighbors' doorway. Instead of capturing a moving image, I'd accidentally just taken a photo. Well that sucks, I thought. Then there was pounding on my door, the police. With Buster doing his whining schtick, too much going on, I opened the door while crouching on the ground, holding my dog and rubbing his belly.

There were two officers. They said they had spoken to my neighbor and wanted to know what happened. That was fast. I was confident in my version of the situation. I told them about the noise issues and how she had threatened me. They listened politely, nodding along. Then they asked for my ID, "Can we see your driver's license? Do you have a driver's license?" In my head I thought, this doesn't feel like the right next step, this doesn't feel right at all. I said sure and asked why as I stood and grabbed my wallet. "Because she says you hit her kid." Just like that, it's a completely different situation. "I didn't hit her kid, I just knocked on her door." They said they understood, nodding in agreement, took my ID, asked if I had any warrants, any priors, any arrests. No. No. No. They said everything was going to be fine, they were going to check and come back. I closed the door. When they said they were just going to check it made sense at the time, or I didn't question it. It was like they were saying: "We're going to check on the soup." I went back to the kitchen and finished sending the email to my building manager:

On April 11, 2016, 3:54 pm, Marcy Tropin wrote:

> Dear My Building Manager, I went upstairs to ask the neighbors to stop screaming, and the woman cursed and threatened me. In my lease agreement there is a warrant of habitability. If these tenants continue to disrupt the habitability of my apartment because I cannot hear anything but them screaming, I will put my rent in an escrow account and go to housing court. I've already had the police speak to them. This tenant is a problem. Especially physically threatening me. Please do not ignore this email. -Marcy

I had the idea to call my super, hoping he was around and in the building. Then I could take the police officers to where the security camera's footage was stored and showed proof of my just knocking on my neighbor's door. During the day my super is usually at a contracting gig, but he happened to be home. In a rush of words he probably only heard police and cameras and the sound of my voice. "Wait, I'll come up," he offered. In person, and slightly calmer, I explained to him what had happened. Could he check the cameras? The cameras are my proof. *Help!* Then he said the worst possible combination of words: "They aren't hooked up." I started to cry.

We'd spent weeks working together renovating my apartment. That's to say, I kept Buster on the sofa so he wouldn't stop my super from working with requests for long, love-fest belly rubs, and I occasionally came over to steady something or hand over a tool. The longer my renovation went on, the more my super understood I knew how to use tools and take directions and wasn't put off by getting my hands dirty. I learned a lot and saved some of his time. Throughout, he never saw me lose my humor or patience. Not when we ran out of paint (if the contractor miscalculated they'll say the walls were thirsty...whatever) and not when I snap rented a car, hauled it to a Bronx paint store, and then hauled back with gallons of paint. Not when we ran out of flooring underlay (that was on me). Not when Ikea forgot to mention that I didn't order a kitchen countertop with the sink when I thought that was what I was doing and we had to drive there, grab one, come back and install it all in the same afternoon. Not when my super accidentally blew out the electricity in half my apartment for a day and half. (To be fair, we were trying to re-install suspect antique wall lights.) And not when I came home from work to see Buster had found the dried-liver treat bag, and had eaten the whole thing while my super and his colleague worked in the kitchen. "Didn't you think that was a lot of treats?" I asked. "I thought you did that so he wouldn't bother us," he replied. It was a two-year supply. Two. Years. That little fucker. I didn't lose my humor or patience after the renovation, when the apartment was perfect, and the neighbors above me left their sink running, flooding my bathroom and causing bubbling and leaking to the newly painted living room ceiling. Not even when I had bed bugs and wasn't sleeping. For the most part, I kept my humor and kept moving forward.

"They're going to arrest me." My body felt numb. I had that feeling of being able to see everything around me clearly. My super stood just a couple of inches taller than me, but about two feet broader. He's a solidly built guy. He, too, was never rattled. Seeing me cry, he dropped his arms to his sides and tensed, his hands made fists. He exhaled out, almost like an air gauge relieving pressure. He said he would go upstairs and talk to the police, tell them about the lady, explain I was a good tenant. He said it would be okay. I closed the door.

It was not as though I thought his plan was going to work, but there wasn't anything else to do. I didn't know what to do. I hadn't showered in two days—don't judge—but thought that might be a little weird. What if the police came knocking and I didn't answer because I was in the shower? Would they break down the door? I hadn't eaten since the morning and decided to inhale a Clif bar. My dog was going to need to be fed and let out before I went to work. All of the things I wanted to do, things I normally do, felt wrong to do. The police having my driver's license didn't feel right either. It felt like they'd already made up their minds.

As I paced in my living room, the door pounded again and Buster did his thing. I opened the door, again crouching down, holding my little dog back from wanting to greet everyone. There were now two more police along with the original two, and a sergeant who did all the talking. The first thing he wanted was for me to come out into the hallway. I said sound carries and I didn't want to talk there. The sergeant said he didn't want to come in because he was scared of dogs. He asked if I could put my dog somewhere behind a closed door. Could I lock him in the bedroom? My spine straightened a bit; I never compromise

47

Buster's well-being. Behind a closed door, in his home, away from me, with all of you guys here? That would upset him greatly. All this dog wants in life is to be at my side, and in return I get unconditional love and loyalty. It didn't seem necessary to pacify the fears of an adult law-enforcement agent concerning an obviously non-aggressive small dog. While I didn't want to appear difficult or defiant, I made the decision to be protective of my dog's wellbeing. Also, the sergeant was unconvincingly sincere in his request. It felt like the he was trying to get me to leave my apartment and the whole dog fear thing was made up. I held onto my stance that my dog was not going to harm him and I wasn't locking him away. Besides, there wasn't a water bowl in the bedroom. Nope, my dog was staying by me.

There was a back and forth about this. I ended up putting Buster's harness and leash on, showing that he was restrained, and speaking to the officers at my doorway. I showed the sergeant the emails to management, the brick wall video recordings of screaming, and the 311 documentation. I retold the same stories showing a history of issues with this tenant. The sergeant nodded along. When I was finished with my powerpoint presentation, the sergeant had his decision at the ready, "So this is the situation," he paused to make sure the other officers were now paying attention, "she says you hit her kid, the kid has a bump on her head, and we're going to arrest you." I took a step back from the doorway, folded over a bit, holding my hand on my belly, "That never happened," I said. I began crying. Then the five officers walked into my apartment.

The police entered. Just like that. I walked backwards, towards my living room closet door, and stood there, perfectly still. People say that during life-changing events, time stands still or it feels like time slows down. Of course time is moving along as it always does. To me, it feels more like my ability to process speeds up: the environment, feelings, decisions, questions. It's like how they do slow motion in film. Normally it's 24 frames per second.

For slow motion it can be 120 frames per second. More frames. More information. The more you show, the slower it goes. I froze at the closet. With five officers surrounding me, with five men surrounding me, with five men carrying guns surrounding me, I stood and waited. Don't move, I thought. Don't give them an opportunity to be aggressive. Wait.

It seems natural to resist arrest when being falsely accused. My neighbor says I hit her kid, I didn't, but I'm about to be arrested and I'm not allowed to contest this. In any way, at all. That's a wide berth of authority. I mean, people haggle over iron-clad return policies. Toddlers negotiate. We're not really designed or reared for finality like this. The children's game spud is the closest you'll come to preparing for an arrest. One kid throws a ball in the air, all the other kids run, that one kid catches the ball and yells "SPUD," and everyone freezes. On a personal level, with my resistance to authority, even recipes, I would have guessed in a situation like this that I'd be a pain in the ass. Instead, my reaction was to be almost pathologically compliant and polite. I addressed officers with "sir" and at least outwardly appeared okay about going along with their plan. All the yoga I had in me, I was going to use every bit of it.

The officers asked me to put some shoes and socks on. I was barefoot. One asked me if I had shoes and socks to put on, "Do you have shoes and socks you can put on?" I didn't move unless directed or approved. We were going to play a version of Mother-May-I, "May I go to the bathroom?" I was wearing a well-worn cotton long-sleeve black top without a bra and black sweatpants without underpants. That's it. It was an in-the-apartment ensemble, not an out-of-the-apartment ensemble.

Then there was my hair. About a year before this, I had the fabulous idea to cut all of my hair peach-fuzz short, except the top and the little flat circle part near the back, letting those areas grow back to show my naturally curly hair. Almost a year later, the little farm on top of my head had blossomed into about five inches of ringlets, which stood out in all cardinal directions. It was a hairstyle similar to that of Johnny Galecki during his Roseanne years. The idea was to grow out the top so it was long enough to pull back. That way, it would be hard to tell the rest was short. This brilliant plan came about after I had grown bored of my short pixie cut, missing my curly hair, but not being able to commit to a full head of it. I thought I'd have the best of both worlds: part of my head wearing short hair and part of my head wearing long hair. In retrospect, this was an absolutely terrible idea.

I was allowed to go to my bathroom. An officer followed me. I was not allowed to be alone. When I got to my bathroom I told him I wanted to put a bra on. He stood at the doorway, two feet away. I wasn't allowed to close the door out of the police officers' fear that I might commit suicide or get a weapon. Thus, I had to take my top off, be topless, put a bra on, and then put my top back on, all in front of this man. Wearing a long-sleeve crew-neck shirt hid most of my tattoos from the police. I already had a weird haircut and was happy they didn't know how much ink was on me. It just didn't seem ideal to have them know at this particular moment. I had the choice of either flashing the officer or turning away and showing my back, which was in the process of being covered with a new tattoo. None of the choices felt ideal. They all felt like a violation. I didn't put up a fuss or question any of it. But I hated it.

My bathroom door had a clothing rack on the back that prevented it from opening completely. Using this, I took off my shirt while turning and tilting my torso behind the door. This gave me some privacy. I managed to stay awkwardly tilted while putting a bralette and my top back on. I chose to end the show and not put underwear on. In the mirror I caught a glimpse of myself and decided to glue my hair down a bit. Grabbing some aloe vera gel—the best hair gel in the world for having nothing to do with harming animals, and no chemicals—I dolled out a dollop and patted things down, then washed my hands and dried them off. The finished product: I looked and smelled pretty bad. Somewhere after I put my bra on and got out the hair gel the officer had disappeared from the doorway. I guess the real protocol was to humiliate me.

I exited the bathroom by first taking one big step out with my right foot like I was testing the safety of frozen pond water. There I stood, in the little vestibule area, facing my living room. There, in the middle, all five officers stood, facing one another, talking. A circle of white men, in dark navy blue, Matisse's dancers. I watched them. Their shoes on my rug. Their hanging out in my living room. Their casual body language. When they weren't gesticulating, their hands rested on belts filled with gadgets, and weapons. We switched places while I was standing there. It was something about how present and comfortable they were in my space that alienated me. It felt like I was interrupting. I wasn't sure what to do in my own home. How to move in my own home. I wasn't free to move in my own home. I couldn't walk into my bedroom or stroll across the living room to the kitchen. Once they noticed me, they would direct me, verbally marionette my movements. Standing there I was annoyed at their personal conversation, how they didn't notice I'd left the bathroom. I was annoyed by how they didn't notice the art on the walls, my art. I wanted them to turn to me and ask about the pieces, make compliments, question materials and process, explore ideas. I wanted them to ask what I was currently working on, but they were standing there waiting to arrest me.

I stepped into the living room, and the cops dispersed. They directed me to my front door. Buster was by my side throughout. At the front door was a pair of old sneakers and well-worn socks. Hanging on a coatrack was a pink puffer vest and a black fuzzy fleece scarf, the things I grabbed when taking the dog out. While I was crouching down to put my sneakers and socks on, the sergeant stood in the doorway with an officer to my left, while another officer was in the vestibule area with me, and the two other officers stood to my right at the entrance to the living room. Five officers there to arrest me, to watch me put sneakers and socks on.

I was asking the sergeant how long I would be detained because I had to go to work later. He replied repeating, "We just wanna get you in and outta there. We just wanna get you in and outta there." *Great!* I reached up and grabbed my fuzzy scarf. The sergeant asked, "What do you need that for?" It was a chilly day with rain in the forecast, but instead of pointing out the obvious, I said, "Because I'm feeling vulnerable and it'll be nice to have." Shoes on, scarf on, standing, I went into autopilot, putting my vest on, snapping up the middle buttons, grabbing my wallet and putting it in its usual place, the right pocket, grabbing my cell phone, putting it in its usual place, my left pocket. For a moment this familiar getting ready stuff felt normal. The keys were on the coatrack's first hook. I grabbed them and then made a gesture like, "Okay, you guys go out and I'll lock up," motioning my left arm towards the door. The sergeant shook his head. My body went cold. The officer in the vestibule with me held his handcuffs up to my face. They were black metal with scuffs on the edges showing silver underneath. I started to cry again. They were going to handcuff me in my apartment, not allowing me to lock up or properly say goodbye to my dog. Why?

Holding my keys in my hands, I found the one that locked my door. I held it up to the air, and the officer with the cuffs handed it to the officer behind him. My key chain was a round silver glop medallion that had "be here" on one side and "be now" on the other. It's a riff on the Ram Das book about being in the moment. The irony was not lost on me; the last thing I wanted was to be in this particular moment. It was time to put the handcuffs on me, but I asked (with incredible politeness and through tears), if I could please text my neighbor friend, Hope, asking her to let my dog out if I wasn't back by a certain time. I was allowed to do this, grabbed my phone out of my pocket, and texted two lines while shaking. Then I put my phone back in my pocket. Though I'd never been arrested before, I automatically put my arms behind my back and turned so the officer could apply the cuffs. He started with my left wrist and made them so tight it stopped me from crying. It hurt. The right wrist, he did a little looser. I assumed I wasn't allowed to give feedback on the comfort of being in handcuffs. Making the cuffs a punitive experience felt contradictory to the whole innocent-until-proven-guilty thing. It was also kind of childish and like a TV cop stereotype.

The handcuffing officer walked me through the apartment doorway with a hand on my back. I was now uncontrollably sobbing. Snot was pouring out of my nose, running down my lips, my chin. With my arms behind me, there was nothing I could do about it. My chest was convulsing. When I first started crying I remembered that my shrink had asked me if I cried recently. Except she used the word "emote," which cracked me up. Who uses the word emote anymore? It makes crying sound like an act of shedding tears in a circle. I hadn't emoted in quite awhile and happened to have spent the past weekend trying to do so: watching a sad movie, listening to sad music. Nothing came out; I was emotionally constipated. Or maybe just not sad. Or dead inside. One positive aspect of being falsely arrested for allegedly harming a child was that I got all of my crying done, for years, in one afternoon.

Outside my apartment everyone turned around to watch the door closing. At some point I'd taken Buster off his leash, but his harness was still on. Before the door closed he made a break for it, and I saw him, ears pinned back, head low, cutting and weaving around navy blue polyester pants legs and black shoes, trying to get to me. I can still see him doing this, desperately wanting to find his way through to my side. This crushed my heart. My chest hurt so much I couldn't stand up straight. I couldn't say goodbye to my dog. I couldn't reach down. I couldn't touch him. I couldn't make it better for him. He had nothing to do with any of this. My dog didn't know what was going on and I couldn't comfort him. Before this moment I never understood what choking back tears meant. That it wasn't just a phrase. I tried to sound completely normal while telling Buster, "Go lay down." To the officers' credit, they also started using that phrase softly, "Go lay down, go lay down."

In the kitchen was a dog bed for when I used to write at the island. I'd left it there because Buster really likes to be absolutely comfortable at all times. When I'm preparing meals or eating, he curls up, but in a position where he can keep abreast of what's happening food wise. The dog bed can be seen through the front door. Buster went over and then came back a couple of times, but he finally went to his bed. I started to sob again but kept saying, "Good boy, good boy," as the door closed on him, sitting on his bed, confused. Once the door was closed, I was turned around towards the stairs. Two officers would walk me down, which was helpful because I could barely steady myself and didn't have my arms for balance. Once my door was locked Buster started barking and whining. I winced, closing my eyes for a moment, my body tensing towards itself, feeling the sounds of his stress as much as I was hearing them.

Walking through the lobby, I realized that I was about to be put in public with handcuffs on and officers surrounding me. I hoped not to see anyone, for anyone to see me, even strangers. I just wanted to get inside the squad car. There were two patrol vehicles double parked outside the building, all for me. The yoga teacher who was practicing poses for a workshop but then decided to "shove a door open and hit a child." When we got to the door, I wondered about hitting my head on the frame as I got seated, or whether an officer might do that to me "by accident." With the handcuffs tight on my left wrist and with just being arrested in general, it felt like anything goes. I wasn't just being escorted to a police vehicle; I was being taken from one world to another. In this version, I was not in control of anything. Not where I would go. Not how long I would be there. My personal comfort. My boundaries. My time. Eating. Peeing. Sitting. Standing. I couldn't scratch my nose. I couldn't rub my eyes. I wouldn't get to say hurry up. I wouldn't get to know anything about what would happen to me next.

It was like the feeling of being made late for work by traffic. The feeling of wearing a plastic muumuu at the doctor's office. Of not finding your phone in your bag, waiting for your date to show up, trying to make a return without a receipt, going through airport security, running for a bus, double parking to "just run something inside," leaving your credit card at the last place, or so you hope, withdrawing cash, at night, at an outside ATM, or going to a new gym, but all of them, multiplied by waiting for test results that insurance doesn't cover. It's mistiming your jaywalking, turning around at a museum and not seeing your kid, and accidentally bumping the angriest person on the subway. It's every moment of vulnerability distilled into the finest, pure, fight-or-flight, sympathetic nervous system response. Uncut, clean, hopelessness. That's what it felt like to be handcuffed and put in the back of a police car. Except a moment like that has no clear end, it's happening in darkness because there is no other situation you've been in that's similar. Not darkness like a beach house at night, but pitch black where you can't see. There's no end and no beginning to objects without the presence of any light. It's just more darkness. Would I be released in time to teach class? Would I be held overnight? Would I be able to make a phone call? Would they let me have my cell phone so I could find a number? Would my dog be okay? How far was this going to go? How long? How much worse would it get? What were my rights? Should I even have considered what was right and wrong? To answer any of these questions I would have to reach out in the dark and feel around for something, to shape the space around me. But before I could reach for that object, before touching it, it felt like the moment was never going to end. I could be reaching out for a long time. I might be going to jail. Right then I could be on my way to jail. For knocking on a door twice. It was like there was nothing in front of me. My chest was tight, and I couldn't stop crying.

The car door closed. The officers turned to one another and began chatting again. They stood right outside the window of the car I was in. It was like they were picking up conversationally before arresting me. From the bits and pieces I heard it sounded as though they were retelling a story from the weekend. The sounds were humorous, jolly. Here I was thinking I was the priority. I looked around a bit. The back seat was clean. I was grateful for that. There was thick safety glass dividing the front and backs of the car. The car's windows were closed. It was hot in there.

I'd been in the back of a police car only one other time in my life, when I locked myself out of my mom's house as a latchkey kid. There happened to be police cars on my street for reasons I don't know. I went up to an officer, explained my dilemma and asked for a ride to where my mom worked, a real estate office some two towns over. Sure, the officer said, opening the back door and gesturing for me to hop inside. Then he closed the door and I was locked in there, on a warm spring day, for a long time. He forgot to mention he might be awhile. I sat there, now in the back of a police car on the street I lived, not happy about the whole thing. By the time the officer drove me to my mom's office, it was close to the end of her workday and I then got to wait there until she was ready to leave. Later I would hide a key somewhere in case I was ever locked out again.

For years my mother liked to tell the story of how I was escorted into her office by a police officer while she was speaking with clients. The whole office, desks in an open room, turned its focus towards me. Conversations were stopped in midair, phones just held up, mouths opened. People walking to the copier froze. My mom had a little smile on her face as we walked right to her, in the center of the room. She knew I didn't do anything wrong, I never did anything wrong. She also loved drama. When I said I was locked out, she repeated it loudly, "She's just locked out, locked out, forgot her keys!" Didn't think things through then; didn't seem to think them through now.

The back of a police car feels a lot like the back of a taxi. They both have that not-quite-black-but-not-navy pleather upholstery. The kind of material that can be hosed down. The seats are deep and at just the right angle, like an Eames chair, so that you can't lean forward at all. Your weight tips into the spot just above your ass, making it seem as though you want to be relaxing back there, when, in both the case of riding in a taxi and being arrested, you don't want to be there at all. For a person under arrest, that means being tilted back against your arms and hands, against the handcuffs. With my arms behind me, the cuffs tight, I couldn't find a position where I wasn't putting weight on my wrists and causing the metal to cut into my skin. There just wasn't anywhere to put my hands. They're not supposed to be behind you when you're sitting. Maybe in bridge pose lying on the floor, but definitely not in a car. I tried moving my arms left and right, but held together they weren't long enough to get out of the way unless I leaned in the opposite direction. I tried bending my elbows a little to see if I could get my hands in the small of my back, but that only pulled the cuffs taut between their two-link chain, causing more pain. After a short time, I realized the pain and discomfort I was in came along with the situation I was in. Maybe that's the point. The whole experience is meant to dehumanize, to shame.

Looking through the car window, watching the officers, seeing my street, my building, wanting air, water, comfort, my mind trying to process all these needs, the situation, everything, but at the same time being in shock, my thoughts split into two different dialogs: one that was losing it, and one that was trying to hold things together. As if the parasympathetic (calmer) and sympathetic (the sky is falling) nervous systems were having a symposium. Or an emergency meeting. The part of me that was losing it wanted immediate results; the calmer voice was thinking long view. They exchanged ideas about the handcuff situation:

> CRAZY: You know, I could easily slide my hands under my butt, around my legs and in front where they'd be more comfortable.
> CALM: Do. Not. Move.
> CRAZY: Wow they're chatting up a storm out there. I could easily get my cell phone out of my pocket and text people.
> CALM: Do. Not. Move.
> CRAZY: It's stuffy in here. Shouldn't I tap on the window to let them know I'm kind of suffering?
> CALM: Nope.
> CRAZY: So this is how a dog feels in the car.
> CALM: Shhhhhhh.

Eventually their conversation broke up and two officers got into the car, closed their doors and took off. As we began to drive I noticed no one, including myself, was wearing a seat belt. I wasn't able to put on a seat belt so it wasn't by personal choice on my end. This concerned me as we made a sweeping, illegal U-turn at a green light, with oncoming traffic, to head back to the precinct. Without a seat belt, or free hands, I didn't have the ability to stop myself from moving around. If we got into so much as a fender bender, nothing would prevent the movement of my upper body from being thrust forward except, eventually, my face smashing against the safety glass divider.

It's like when I was little, in the back of an Oldsmobile station wagon, my cousin and I would dramatize the car's slight movements by throwing ourselves around. Laughing, silly, innocent fun. After the U-turn, I slouched as far down in my seat as I could to protect myself, which also relieved the pressure on my wrists. Now I looked like a criminal in the back seat of a squad car. So this was why people slouched in the back of police cars. Not because they didn't want to be seen, but because it's unsafe and uncomfortable to sit up. They're not low in the seat sulking; they're concerned about a vehicular accident.

We drove into the police station parking lot. Two gas pumps in a middle island, a ramp to a door, and an overhang for inclement weather. The 33rd Precinct is shaped like a quarter slice of a pie. The parking lot is in the back, near the center of the pizza, at the point. The front is the round crusty part. I would have all the glory of entering through the back of the precinct. An officer opened my door, but in keeping with my "Mother May I" politeness, and not wanting to be roughly handled, I asked if I could come out of the car. Now, now I had foresight. With the "all clear," I swung my legs towards the door and out of the car, but I was still really deep in the seat. So deep, with my feet touching the pavement, my knees were practically at shoulder height. I was going to have to problem solve getting out of the car with my arms behind my back, my weight going backwards, and my feet and legs already out, but level to my torso. In one motion I threw my chest forward towards my thighs and pressed on my feet a bit. Then with the strength of my quads I caught the weight and torpedoed it forward, standing up right before I face planted. Had my arms not been bound behind my back I would have raised them in achievement: "Nailed it." The officer took my right arm—now he helps me—and led me to the back door. As we began walking, my scarf unraveled and started falling off. "Excuse me Sir, can you please help me with my scarf?" It felt kind of diva of me, like I was trying to make a big entrance and had asked the backup dancer to fix my feather boa. The officer did so politely.

We walked up the ramp and through the back door. Entering, we passed by two doors on the left, painted blue, with long rectangular glass and chicken-wire windows near the knobs. Then we passed a larger tan painted door with another glass window and a two-way mirrored wall after that. On the right, in the center of the space, was a large, round tall desk area. It was set up about two feet above floor level, in case of flooding, or to have everyone behind the desk look down on everyone not behind the desk or to give everyone on ground level the feeling of looking up to authority. I couldn't see over the thing.

We stopped in the middle of the room. I didn't have time to notice the atrium aspect of the architecture, and how you could look up two flights to the other floors, where people could look through glass walls down at the action. Just as we were stopping, the tan door opened. The sound of the heavy metal door dragging against its metal frame attracted my attention. I turned. Through the door came a woman about 5'2 tall and 5'2 across. She had long dark thin hair that was gelled flat and shiny to the top of her head and pulled facelift-tight into a ponytail. As she walked through the door, she was finishing putting on blue surgical gloves, letting them snap against her wrists. Had I not been handcuffed and at a police station, her entrance would have seemed comical. It was like a parody of a tough female officer putting on surgical gloves to imply something unpleasant was to come. Instead, it was reality, and she was walking towards us, towards me. My eyes widened. Was she going to strip search me? As the saying goes; "Shit just got real." My mind again split into two dialogues:

> CRAZY: If she's coming to strip search us, I don't think we can handle that emotionally, I mean, I don't think we can return from that to where we are now mentally.
> CALM: Totally agree.
> CRAZY: If that's what's about to happen, we're dropping to the ground, balling up in a fetal position, and releasing our bladder. We'll piss the floor if need be.
> CALM: Totally okay, we're all in agreement here.

Thus I made the executive decision to reverse course on being the polite wonderfully easygoing arrestee and move on to

Plan B, which was to act unstable, using body fluids. Having done performance art in college, I was positive I could tap into an unstable persona. This wasn't even a question. A past filled with endless personal space violations that I was still healing from as an adult inspired this stance. I couldn't have one more unwelcome physical contact. My fear was that being stripped searched would tip me over into another person, a person who may no longer function well in society, a version of myself I wouldn't recognize, in a place emotionally that might be unreachable. In the moment, I needed to protect myself from what would be an act of physical and sexual abuse, no matter how it was framed. As an adult I was trying to have less issues, blend more. Already, being arrested was traumatizing enough. But in the adult world, there is no calling "uncle." You can't tap out of unpleasant situations. Best-case scenario is your nervous system prepares itself.

As the female officer walked towards us, I felt a drain of life, as if whatever was holding me together all those years, like my ability to see humor in anything, was desiccating itself and leaving my body. Handcuffed, at a police station, encircled by men, and facing the possibility of an aggressive and unwanted sapphic interaction, I was preparing to either not be myself anymore or to fall to the ground and make a mess.

Before the female officer reached us, I turned to an arresting officer and asked, "Are those for me?" My voice, cracking with fear, sounding like that of a 12-year-old boy who'd just hit puberty. "She's just patting you down." I felt relieved. I mean, I was ecstatic. If you think someone's going to put their hands into your asshole and vagina, and nose, and ears, but hopefully not in that order and with multiple pairs of surgical gloves, and then you find out they're just going to touch above the clothes, it's Christmas, even for a Jew.

First, she emptied the pockets in my pink puffer vest and handed them to an officer behind the round desk, many feet above us. Then she crouched down at my feet. She started on the left side, at the ankle, one hand in front, the other in back. Before her hands could move up my body they had to touch me at the same time. While this could have been a nice bodywork moment for me, her hands made contact with my body like they were desperately wanting to touch one another. It was like she was trying to applaud an inspiring performance and I was in the way. This went on from bottom to top.

I remember going from casually annoyed to bracing for each next "pat." It felt like something between a self-exam and a vertical tackle. I counted the exchange as sufficing for part of my yearly annual doctor's checkup. Afterward, she wanted me to take off my socks and shoes, but an arresting officer chimed in that it wasn't necessary because he saw me put them on. Thank you officer. Then she tugged a couple of times at the string holding up my sweatpants and said "If those don't come off, we're going to have to cut them." I looked down to where the white strings came out of my black sweatpants, dangling harmlessly in the air. They were no longer tied into a casual bow. It occurred to me, seeing how things were going, that I wouldn't be led to a dressing room where I'd throw my pants over the curtain bar and wait for them to be altered. If the string did not pull out from my pants, I'd still be in the pants when the cutting happened.

My possessions had to be documented: one cell phone (goodbye world, goodbye free world, goodbye email, camera, contacts, friends, entertainment), keys, and wallet. The officer behind the desk was filling out the forms. They needed to know how much money was on me. Some bills in the bifold area and some change in the coin area were counted. However, I owed a friend $20 from dinner and had one folded up nicely, tucked in behind the little coin-purse area. That way I wouldn't spend it because I'd forget about it, but hopefully remember to give it to her.

I mentioned the $20. The pat-down officer, who now owed me dinner and a movie, went about finding the $20. I gave her a hint, telling her exactly where it was, behind the change part. Thus began the adult version of an object permanence test: she looked in the bifold area, then the change area, back to the bifold area, then the credit-card slats, back inside the change area. I tried to rephrase my directions like I do when teaching yoga, explaining "It's under the change area." She repeated the same exact search, but with more vigor this time. She kept taking two fingers and putting them into the change area to show me nothing was there. We all watched this woman fingering my wallet over and over again. "There's a pocket in back of where the change area is." She turned the wallet over. Had she been a toddler we would have all recommended classes to improve cognitive skills, wondering if as an adult she'd be able buy groceries or live alone unassisted. My goodness why was this befuddling her? "Can I just show you where the $20 is?" My arms were still behind my back. I just wanted to put this lady out of her misery. Didn't she own a wallet? Weren't there different places to put things? Or a coat? Anything with pockets, compartments, like her belt with the lethal weapon? Not that I don't sometimes have issues with everyday tasks, but this person should not have been authorized to carry a firearm.

While the pat-down officer was getting personal with my wallet, I recalled a piece of paper tucked into another "secret" area. It was a script from my shrink. However, instead of it being for drugs, it was a personalized note. Therapy was cold-showering my creativity. I couldn't write; I didn't even want to write. So I wouldn't feel badly, my shrink wrote an inspiring message for me, reminding me that I would write soon and that it was cool not to now. It was like a doctor's note excusing me from feeling obligated to be creative right now. Well, it was exactly that, a note from a doctor. The idea was to put the note on my fridge but then that seemed weird if someone came over. Without a good spot to place the note I just left it in my wallet for safekeeping. Only now, it wasn't so safe. If I thought the refrigerator in my home was too vulnerable of a place, having a gaggle of officers see it while I was handcuffed was going to feel worse. Boy, I really didn't want to have to explain that note. I didn't even know how to tackle an explanation and I also wasn't in a position to be private or vague. Should I go with nonchalant, like yeah, sometimes they write you notes? Or should I pretend it was all the shrink's idea, oh yeah, that thing, I'd forgotten about it? Looking at my wallet in the hands of someone else, I kept thinking, "Please, please, don't find that note." I also made a mental note to take it out of my wallet after the whole arrest thing.

She found the $20 in the pocket behind the coin area. Best time: six minutes, nine seconds. Possessions accounted for, I was led through the same tan metal door the pat-down officer came from and into an enclosed room. Entering via escort, I was facing the right wall. The first thing I saw was a small holding cell. In there was a young man, lying down on a long bench. Though he was the only occupant of the cell, I thought that kind of cavalier of him. That he decided to catch up on rest and snooze in there. Moving counterclockwise, to the left of his cell, along the same wall and divided by cinder blocks, was another holding cell. After that and along the same wall was the bathroom. Across from the entrance was another door leading out of the room. To the left of that door, in the corner of the room, was a smaller room with two walls. One had a glass and metal window and the other was solid cinder block. Through the window I could see a bunch of electronic equipment, and an officer sitting at a computer, doing officer things. Against the solid wall of that room was a bench, then some junk here and there. Once the door closed behind me I saw there was a desk in the corner that faced the wall. Around the area a couple of "wanted" printouts were taped to the wall. In the middle of the room was a large support pillar, and a tall floor fan on full blast. A 32-gallon trash can on wheels was near the pillar.

I was led to the bench and turned around. My handcuffs were removed. I did the thing where you reflexively rub your wrists after they're uncuffed. It does make them feel better. On my left wrist I could see where the cuffs had cut in. There were painful leftover red parallel curved lines. The pat-down officer instructed me to take off my pink vest, scarf, and the laces of my sneakers. I did the first two and put them in a nice little pile on the end of the bench. There wasn't a coat hook or any accommodation for treating your personal property respectfully. There should be, though…unless being arrested means your coat gets to go on the dirty floor?

To take off my laces, I sat on the bench and removed my shoes. Once the laces were off I noticed a pile under the bench of previous tenants' laces. Because I wanted the same pair back, I made sure to tie both of my laces together in a double knot. All the rest of them were just dropped into the pile. Assuming people like to keep their shoes on, I wondered about the pile of laces. They didn't go in the property registrar, and they didn't go along with their owners. Were people released from jail without shoelaces? Either that's a business opportunity wherever there are jails, or it's another crappy thing about being arrested, or it's both. The pat-down officer asked again about the white string holding up my sweatpants. I tried to pull it through from either end, but it seemed to be sewn into the fabric in the back somewhere. That was nice of whoever designed the sweatpants, to make sure the tie never came out or pulled all the way one way. It wasn't so great though for my situation.

Even though I demonstrated a clear inability to remove the tie, they were going to have to cut it. Suicide protocol. I assumed they had safety scissors for such an occasion. The pat-down officer grabbed one tie-end and held it out into the air. I watched, looking down, feeling sad for my sweatpants about to be ruined. Another officer pulled a decent-sized black metal knife out of a holder on his thigh, making a zing sound. No safety scissors. I held up my shirt a bit and he told me to stay still. This is the kind of advice used in action movies, and I find it annoying. Someone's hanging out of a helicopter, another person is trying to pull them in, but the helicopter starts doing evasive maneuvers to avoid the bad guys barrage of bullets. In order to assuage this transition, from pulling in to holding on, the person in the helicopter yells out, "Don't let go!" I think they get that. I think that's all the person dangling in the air is focusing on.

When the knife came close to me and my exposed flesh, I reflexively exhaled out, pulling my belly in as much as possible. There was never a moment, enough time, to express my concerns over this plan going wrong. I could feel my armpits start to emanate my nervous smell: something very sticky and stinky to keep people away. The knife was overkill for the situation and exactly the kind of decision-making people fault police officers for. It was also dangerous and scary having that blade so close to my body, the contrasting black metal and my office-paper white skin. Even though I wasn't wearing any underwear (and though I was grateful for the iffy elastic band in my sweatpants), had I known what they were going to do, I would have held my pants out, so only my thumbs and fingers would be in harm's way. The officer wanted to cut the tie as close as possible to the sweatpants, about an inch away from gutting me. If they were really worried about suicide, or if I was really inclined to kill myself in the holding cell, the sweatpants themselves would work for hanging. The stupidity of fetishizing weapons to the point of inappropriate use angered me. Okay buddy, you got to play with your toy today, good for you. Me, I wanted to curl up in a ball and rock for a couple of hours.

String removed, I was ready to be held, like a turkey after basting, covered in dried snot and sticky nervous sweat. The empty cell was opened and I stepped inside. The door closed behind me. The cell wasn't small but it felt small. There were vertical bars, and then horizontal bars, and then over that was some wire-mesh fencing. Aside from the grid of metal in front, all the other walls were cinder block. The cell was rectangular shaped. Near the back wall was a long bench that was about eight inches deep with a five-inch gap from the wall. The top was wood, well worn, and held up by two thick black metal poles bolted into the floor. The cinder block walls had a lot of graffiti. There seemed to be a contest as to who could put their name up higher and further away from the bench. Names and dates of prior residents were scrawled about. Of all the places, this is where you want to say, "I was here?" And how'd they get markers and pens in the holding cell? Each corner of floor had a mountain of black gunk. What the hell could that be a buildup of? The floor tiles, whatever original color they started as, were now dark brown. The place was filthy and smelled like cigarette smoke. I chose to sit opposite the exit. At first I didn't want to lean back. This was tricky because the bench wasn't designed for anyone's ass; it was too damn narrow. I sat straight up, with great posture, legs separated and at perfect angles, my hands on my thighs. It felt like I was waiting at a Soviet-era bus stop. I was bewildered.

I'd been given four squares of toilet paper to finish my crying with. Otherwise there was nothing to do. I thought about the removal of the string on my sweatpants and the logistics of trying to commit suicide. You'd have to be able to climb high on the metal mesh fencing stuff. It would kill your fingers before you could kill yourself. The challenge would be trying to tie something near the top while holding on. There wasn't really enough space to put a foothold unless you took off your shoes. I guessed that you'd have to tie whatever you had around your neck first and then climb up. You'd have to be really good at climbing, strong enough to hold your weight with one hand and possessed with the dexterity to push clothing through the tiny holes of the mesh wiring with the other hand to tie a knot, something that could hold your weight. Most articles of clothing would suffice: my long sleeve shirt, my sweatpants. You would also have to be sure the length of the thing around your neck wasn't so long that when you let go you just hit the ground. Thus, it also involved some measuring.

With nothing to do, this pondering helped me pass a couple of minutes. It was like negotiating how to deliver Ikea furniture into an apartment building without a doorman or street parking: rent a car, hoodwink a friend, double park the car, run stuff up to the apartment. But what if I needed the friend's help carrying the furniture? Okay: double park, unload together, have the friend wait with the stuff, return the rented car, get back to the building, carry the stuff up. How long was I going to be in the holding cell to think through hypothetical tasks?

I worried a ton about getting to my class at 7:35 pm. There was a clock in the electronics room, facing sideways. The glass window blurred its hands. Worst-case scenario, I'd teach dressed as I was: smelly, with no underwear, and no tie for my sweatpants. Hopefully, my neighbor Hope would have let my dog out. I just wanted to teach my class. I desired that more than anything. I had a three-plus-years record of never subbing a class out. That's not an easy record to maintain. I taught six days a week and went away never. I respected my career as a yoga teacher and the students who showed up. Surely it wouldn't take the police hours to do whatever they were going to do with me, would it? Was I going to be here for the night? No one told me what was happening. I was just sitting in a cell. No water. No food. No one phone call. No control. No freedom. Just me and my thoughts.

The end of Hitchcock's Psycho popped into my mind. Anthony Perkins as Norman Bates, wearing a blanket as a dress, hearing his mother's voice as his own in his head, "They'll see, why she wouldn't even harm a fly." It did feel like I was being watched, and I was aware of how my behavior would be viewed. Like Mr. Bates, I too wanted to prove how harmless and amenable I was. In reality, I really was being watched. There was a camera trained on the cell; there was the officer at the corner desk, playing on the computer, his back to me, but aware of my presence. He was scrolling through different pages of guns, occasionally looking over towards me, or coming over to talk. There was the officer behind the glass on the computer, technically facing me. Various officers who walked through the room. I was a zoo animal. Like Bates, I was getting cold. With the room air conditioned, the floor fan pointing toward both cells, my fear and vulnerability at record highs, my puffer vest across the room, and dehydrated from crying, I noticed that my teeth started chattering. I said nothing and sat there miserable.

The corner officer perusing guns got up to stretch his legs and asked if I was warm, did I want the fan on me more. "No thank you," I responded. "Actually I'm freezing, can I please have my vest please?" He looked back at my bubble-gum-pink sleeveless coat on the bench, and said "Hold on." He left, I guessed to ask permission, and came back with another officer to look my puffer vest over. They examined it, feeling around for any contraband and then decided it was okay. It was approved to be in the cell with me. The corner officer approached the door, unlocked it. I only got up after the door was unlocked and went over to get my coat. The door was closed and locked again. I put my vest on and zipped it up to my chin. I placed my hands in the pockets. I was so happy to have it on me. The corner officer moved the fan direction away from my cell. I got back to my sitting.

As time wore on, and I couldn't tell how much time, I couldn't stop playing with my hair. When I'm nervous I have a lot of tics. I have a lot of anxiety in general. In conversation, it'll manifest as sarcasm, and I'll say things I don't mean, without thinking. I used to bite my nails but keep them short now to do bodywork. I can sometimes go to town on a cuticle, though. When my hair is short, I'll scratch at my scalp. Now that my hair was long on top and there were curls, I worried those. I couldn't stop playing with them. I'd take all the curls on one side and spin them into one large curl while staring off into space. Then I'd snap back into the moment, realize what I'd done and how it probably looked from the outside, one big curl sticking out of my head. I would feel embarrassed, separate the big curl back into many curls and promise myself not to do it again. Then I'd try to be productive and practice some calming breathing techniques. After I wore myself out with focusing on breathing, I'd get up and stretch a teeny tiny bit. Stretching made me feel self-conscious, more self-conscious. I didn't want it to seem like I was having a good time in there, like I was on a retreat. After stretching I'd sit down again, zone out, and start twirling my hair unconsciously, repeating the scenario all over again. Twirl, breathe, stretch, sit, twirl, breathe, stretch, sit.

I was annoying myself with the circular neurosis of activities. I decided to cut my hair short again when I got the chance, because at the time I blamed my silly haircut and curly hair for making the situation worse on me. Surely I would sit perfectly still if I didn't have the opportunity to twirl my hair. The more I played with my hair, the less aloe gel was on my hair and the more my hair stuck out. It was growing into a big shrub with every nervous episode. Why didn't I grab a baseball cap like usual? Between thinking about the end of Psycho and watching myself being a nut, I came to the conclusion I wouldn't last a day in a real jail. At least not without the highest dosage of Haldol my body weight would allow.

The corner officer took another break from weapons perusing to ask me what happened. Story time. I love telling stories, but didn't he already know what had happened with me? It looked like a very slow day at the precinct, and as I was able to view firsthand, officers like to chitchat. He stood at the corner opposite me, sometimes playing with the wiring, sometimes leaning against the bars. A young white guy, gung-ho about his day job. This would be the first of many times I'd tell people what happened, but it felt like the millionth. I was drained as I explained to him, "I knocked on a neighbor's door to ask her to be quiet, and she told the police I shoved the door open and hit her child." The officer began a long lecture on how I need to learn how to tolerate city noise. He told me about an older guy in the neighborhood who called the police every day to complain about the traffic noise outside his apartment. They've been to his place a couple of times. Nothing they can do about traffic noise, but the guy keeps calling.

Personally, I agree that cars honk when they don't need to, but as close to an analogy as it was, it wasn't the same. The noise I was experiencing was making it hard to live in my apartment. Traffic sounds I learned to tune out decades ago. Nonetheless, I was literally a captive audience to whatever opinions and unsolicited advice this man had to offer. He didn't know I'd been living in cities my entire adult life since the age of 18, but sure, he could let me know what I was doing wrong, what I did wrong, how I was in the wrong. He was assuming a lot with the authority of someone on the right side of a jail cell. While I had his attention, I asked for some water and he grabbed me a bottle. I began to guzzle, but then decided to keep a little bit, pace it out.

The corner officer went back to his computer, to his official internet surfing, and turned on some music, loud. Yeah, I got his point. He was air drumming and thrashing to music that sounded like it was trying to be classic rock, but the lyrics didn't have the gravitas of that time period. I tuned him and his childish lesson out. Focusing back on my environment, I noticed the officer behind the computer kept leaving that area with a paper in his hand, walking through our area, out to where the front desk was, and then coming back not too long afterward and heading to the electronics room. It seemed curious, especially since nothing else was going on, and there was nothing else for me to do except muse about him and his paper.

Now that I'd had water, I needed to pee. Sometimes, it feels like my body's desire for liquids contradicts its ability to contain them. When there was a break in the music, I politely asked if I could use the bathroom. The corner officer left to get permission or a female officer to help me. I had very low expectations of how this was going to be resolved in regards to my privacy. Did a female officer need to supervise my peeing? The

71

corner officer came back and said he couldn't get a confirmation, but was going to allow me to go anyways. He grabbed the roll of toilet paper that was hanging around, the one from which I got a couple of squares to cry in, and came to unlock my cell. The door opened. I got up and walked towards him. He handed me the toilet paper, pointed to the bathroom that was next to my cell and said, "Just don't commit suicide in there."

After being told the jail version of "break a leg," I entered the bathroom and closed the door. It was nice to be alone. It was a small square room, completely tiled. In the middle of the room was a singular stainless steel unit: a toilet and washing station all in one. There weren't any knobs, only a lever on the floor to flush and another lever to turn on the faucet. Very few moving parts, or parts to remove. I went about my task as fast as possible so as not to attract any attention from the other side of the door. If I had the choice, though, I would have preferred to be held in the bathroom. It was the first time since knocking on my neighbor's door that I felt like I was safe. Look at me, I thought, I'm in a bathroom by myself, I do this, this happens in my life, this feels familiar, normal.

Finished, I opened the door and stood in the doorway. The corner officer was rocking out to his music, singing the chorus. The computer officer was sullen, busy at his screen in the electronics room. I froze for a second. Maybe if I walked out a little bit, someone would notice me? I stepped out and nothing happened. Not knowing what to do but fairly sure I shouldn't be "free," I left the toilet paper on top of the poop-and-wash station, held up my arms at right angles, and walked into my cell, pulling the door closed. It felt a little too casual and some part of me was disappointed, annoyed. If they were going to keep me locked in a cell, with guards, and no scarf or laces, then I was a threat, and I wanted them to please treat me like one. Once back inside the cell, I went back to my sitting.

The corner officer eventually came back to the cell, locked the door, and then chatted me up again. He was leaning against the bars, asking me what I did for a living. Great, this was going to be the definition of ironic: "I'm a yoga teacher." Oh really, he said, his girlfriend was a yoga teacher. I wanted to hear about his girlfriend teaching yoga like I wanted a sigmoidoscopy, "Where does she teach?" His girlfriend lived upstate. She taught classes there. He wished he lived upstate. "Why don't you?" I asked. "Because this is the greatest job in the world," he replied. I was listening to this guy, smiling, feigning interest, but internally, things were very different: *Yeah, keeping an innocent woman locked up under false pretenses, that's a good job to you? At the end of the day you're going to feel good about yourself? I help people get out of pain, relieve stress and feel better in their bodies, that's a great fucking job, buddy.* His cockiness was beginning to wear on me.

The corner officer said it's not so bad being arrested; he had been arrested. Hadn't I been arrested before? No, no I hadn't. He countered, "It's not so bad." It wasn't like I was a four-year-old being prepared for a flu shot. I was behind bars. I was in a holding cell. It was bad. He explained to me that they had two bosses: one out in the field and one in the station. "And the one here is tough," he said. "The guy walking in and out, he's a rookie, and he's writing up your arrest report. The one in charge here doesn't like the way the rookie is phrasing things and keeps making him rewrite it." They handwrote their reports?

Now, when I watched the rookie walk back and forth, slumping a little more each time, holding his test paper in hand, I felt sorry for him and even apologized at one point. The writer in me really wanted to help out with the essay portion of my arrest. I mean, I was there and everything. It took a lot of me breathing not to offer, a lot of just telling myself to keep quiet. There was also a good chance I was not going to like what was being written, and it would be better not to know.

This fell alongside some advice my mother gave me at a deli when I was little. We'd just ordered two sandwiches and were watching them being made, with the guy grabbing bread and slamming down meats. Then my mom turned to me, which in turn made me turn to her, and said, "Never watch your food being made." That's some sage advice, and it's true. We turned our attention to the glass storefront and to the goings-on outside. This same principle was also why I never go into the locker room after teaching. While I may catch some compliments, I may also hear some complaints. If you want to have your cake and to eat it too, don't watch it being made.

I asked the corner officer what time it was. Even if it was not getting close to the time I would have to leave to make it to my evening group class, it was probably getting close to the time I'd need to contact work and let them know there was an issue. If I couldn't make it to class, the studio would need all the time I could give them to find a sub. Until this point, I had been able to maintain some disillusionment about my situation. Surrendering to not getting to class was the responsible thing to do, and very difficult. I called the corner officer over. "Excuse me, sir." He came to the cell. I was at the bars. This was a delicate moment. This was where I wanted to cash in all my good behavior. All my amenability. All my nice listening skills. I didn't look him in the eyes, but made sure he could see my concern, "Sir, I understand the severity of my situation, but I'm supposed to teach a yoga class at 7:35 pm. If I don't show up, no one will be there to teach the class. Can I please let someone from work know I won't be able to make it?" He went to the front desk area, then came back. Then he went into the electronics room and brought out my phone. The cell door was cracked opened enough so that I could hold my phone. I was told to make it quick. The corner officer watched everything I entered, including my passcode. The first thing I saw was that the text I sent Hope asking her to check on Buster was still there after I composed it. In the stress of the moment, I didn't hit "send." She didn't know that I'd been arrested and that she needed to check on him. Argh. Crap. I sent it. Then I composed an email to three different supervisors at Exhale:

On April 11, 2016, 5:42 pm, Marcy Tropin wrote:

Hi, I have an emergency and can't teach this evening. I will not be able to send another email. Please find coverage for me!!! Marcy

With that, I made sure to hit send and hear the swish of an outgoing message. I handed my phone back to the officer and thanked him profusely. The email I sent was very far away from how I normally communicate, but it was the only thing I could think of to write in the moment that would accomplish getting a sub and not create an email dialogue in which I couldn't further participate. My cell door closed, I went back to my sitting. I couldn't even recall the last time I needed a sub, never mind a last-minute sub. This was just not my style. I've shown up to teach in various states of physical and emotional messes: with a stress fracture in my left foot, after re-tweaking an old neck injury, after saying goodbye to a friend's dog on speakerphone before she was put down, after my doctor told me some bad health news, after being dumped over the phone, after being dumped in person, after being tattooed, with laryngitis, with cramps, exhausted, feverish, stoned (that was by accident), with back spasms, and after I flipped over my bike and split open the skin on my elbow to the bone (as a matter of fact, I taught three classes in a row after that one). I have a strong work ethic, and I like teaching.

Sitting there, wondering who would be able to sub my class at the last minute, I was relieved to have been able to send the email. Then the pendulum swung back to how real my situation was. If I'd been able to get out with enough time to teach, I might have been able to stuff this experience down under the pile of denial, push it away a bit. Of course, I didn't know for certain if teaching class would have been a salve, but it wasn't an issue now. It was optimistic anyways to think that maintaining my schedule would afford me a boundary from the experience, as if it never happened. With the stress of getting to class somewhat out of my head and definitely out of my hands, I was suddenly really hungry.

The next time the corner officer came around to chat, I asked if there was anything I could eat or purchase through a vending machine. Even old crackers would do. He told me he'd check and left. When he came back some time later, he mentioned something about allergy issues, like peanuts, and said, "We're gonna get you outta here soon." With that, I sat down and finally leaned back against the wall. Maybe the kid in the other cell had the right idea, resting. Or maybe he was in there for so long without food that his body just gave up. Maybe he'd started off like me and then collapsed.

Another "criminal" was brought into the room. I couldn't see him, but I could hear the conversation. He sounded young. He didn't have any identification on him and officers were trying to get him to call someone to bring an ID in. He was not enchanted by this idea. One officer was saying, "You don't want us to put you in the system without a name, trust me." Another officer drove the point home, "You don't want us to bring you downtown without a name." The word "downtown" was used like a threat. The kid was being a little inconsistent with his knowledge of English, which was trying on the officers. "C'mon, give us a name, we just wanna get you out of here as soon as possible." They repeated the phrase. I remember the first time I heard that, when I was putting on my sneakers. Was I naive to believe them? To believe police officers?

The corner officer came over and said he was going to help with the fingerprinting and photographing in order to speed things along. The report was almost done. *Cool, thanks.* The cell opened and I was escorted into the back electronics room. I was thinking of all those 80s cop shows—Barney Miller, Cagney & Lacey, Hill Street Blues—where fingerprinting involved messy black ink. I didn't want black ink on my fingers. Wasn't that unhealthy? Also, I was positive I wouldn't be provided with proper cleaning supplies. Knowing how much I play with my hair and rub my eyes and face, I would be smudged all over for days. Inside, the room was heavily air conditioned to keep all the electronics happy. We stopped in the middle of the room. Against a wall there was a machine that would scan my fingerprints and palms. Oh right, modern technology.

As we began, my fingers were too oily for a good read. My body was still secreting nervous, get-away-from-me liquids. In the scheme of human evolution, I don't know what period, maybe Upper Paleolithic, made being stinky, sweaty, and sticky a natural form, a helpful form, of self-defense, but it was useless to me now. Each finger had to be sprayed with a pine-tree window cleaner and rubbed dry with a paper towel before being scanned. Soap and water might have done a better job, but I went along with the process. It seemed as though the scanner was being persnickety about getting an exact and clear image. Some fingers had to be done over and over again. Instead of worrying about ink and my skin, I was now worried about a chemical cleaning agent and my skin. Some fingers were rubbed red raw to get them dry while I stood there watching. When I noticed the officer becoming frustrated at the machine, nervous his energy was going to keep being transferred into my fingertips, I began to help out. I politely reached out my free hand for the cleaner and assisted with the spraying and placing my fingers on the scanner. Squirt, squirt, squirt, dry, place, hold steady, stop breathing, repeat. After awhile, the room began to smell of a Swedish mountainside.

To pass the time, the corner officer asked me who I was voting for in the presidential election. This was a tricky moment. Two young, white New York City police officers—and one Jewish, not-straight lady, who was also an alleged criminal. I didn't feel like this was an appropriate subject for small talk, lest our politics ruin what had already been a lovely early Monday evening. Personally, I just wanted to get outta there as soon as possible. So I didn't seem standoffish, I offered the usual response I gave people when I didn't want to discuss the election: "I think of the presidency just like any other job application. Just look at the resumes and pick the one with the most experience." "True," the rookie at the computer chimed in. Phew.

We moved on to my portrait. In the corner, amongst a lot of computers and yet very few monitors, was a blue screen that I was supposed to stand in front of. While I was not enthralled with memorializing the event, I did think I was in good company with all of the musicians, artists, and activists arrested before me. Even though my arrest was a lot less sexy than drug possession or advocating for those who don't have a voice: the environment, animals, the disenfranchised. Hopefully, I wasn't leaning towards any group of infamous awful people. Normally, I dodge a portrait. I started studying photography when I was 13 as a freshman in high school. By my junior year in 1990, I'd exhausted my teacher's knowledge and did a Summer pre-college program at the Parsons School of Design in New York City. Then I did a year of college before I burnt-out and moved on to different mediums.

The second someone holds a camera up to me, I'm critiquing their technique or lack thereof. I know they're going to put my head in the center of the frame and most photographs of me are with my lips moving, saying not to. The other issue that bothers me is when people will watch through a camera. You're supposed to capture the moment, not be a voyeur. While they're standing there doing nothing, and I'm supposed to be standing still, my eyes begin to water and my mood grows dark. I'm really good behind a camera and really grumpy in front of one.

There have also been some tense moments where people wanted me to look pretty. When you photograph a mountainside, a goldfish, a teddybear, a plate of food, a flower, a guy, you never tell these subjects to look beautiful; you take them as they stand. Women are instructed to look pretty, to smile, to present themselves in an appealing manner, an obligation that eludes my interest. I grew up hanging around my brothers. I must have been playing catch with them when all the other little girls were being brainwashed into wanting to be objectified. I don't understand the cult-like focus on wanting to look beautiful. When I was little, I thought models were supposed to look beautiful because that's their job and the rest of us could have our own pursuits. The only time I pose for a photo is at the DMV, for their "proof of life" style ID cards.

I stood with great posture and my awful haircut. In one little afternoon, I'd surrendered to a lot of things. Each hour brought a new milestone. Instead of the photo being like a DMV portrait and affording me the freedom of driving and drinking, but not at the same time, this photograph was documenting when my freedom was taken away. We did front, left, right. Then we were done. I was sad not to hold my arrest number in front of me and for the photo not to be in black and white. It would have been great if there were period costumes to put on, but as the day revealed, the police are very literal in their world perceptions.

From where my photo was being taken, I could see my cell phone and Ziploc bag of personal effects on the table, next to where the rookie was working on the police report. I could also see it was now nearing 7 pm. I'd been held for about two and half hours, mostly so one guy could write four sentences. Class trip over, I was now being led back to the holding cell. If I did get out soon, I could still make it to my evening client at 9:30 pm. Wanting to work gave me something to focus on. I mentally prepared what needed to be done: letting my dog out if Hope hadn't, eating something, showering, re-gluing my hair down, and re-hydrating.

A short while later, I was released from the holding cell. Freed. I found my laces and stuffed them in a pocket. I threw out my sweatpants' strings, grabbed my scarf, and wrapped it around my neck. The corner officer came over while I was grabbing my things from the bench and presented me with a DAT—a desk appearance ticket. Instead of being held overnight and being arraigned in the morning, I was allowed to leave. There was a date and time on the ticket. I was not really absorbing this information, figuring I could look it up later. I just wanted to get the heck out of the police precinct.

The corner officer escorted me back through the door I had entered while handcuffed and up to the officer at the front desk. There, my items were poured out of the Ziploc bag. I put my cell phone back in my left pocket, keys in my right pocket. Before I could grab my wallet they wanted me to count my money and sign to confirm that it was all there. I tucked the $20 back in its secret hiding spot. It was all there. I signed for my possessions.

Then the officer behind the desk started telling me something about where I could go, I think, for legal services. But by then, I was woozy from not eating. I was fried emotionally. I wasn't processing anything, so I cut him off and said, "Okay, thanks," without really thinking. He raised his voice and leaned forward, saying, "You know, you're lucky, we could have taken you downtown." What was this downtown place? I didn't even know what he was talking about in order to understand the threat. "I'm sorry sir, did I say something wrong?" The corner officer mediated, and I was free to go. I guessed that was the tough sergeant I was warned about earlier. Tucking my scarf into my pink puffer vest extra tight for warmth, I walked towards the front of the building, through a short black metal fence and turnstile, to the front doors and then outside. It was dark now and raining. The walk home was about 20 minutes, with the park on my left side. It was an incredible relief to be walking away from the police station.

As I headed home, I saw texts from Hope but decided to call my friend Nancy first. She's a dear friend, and a shrink. We met over a decade ago when she was a student of mine and became friends when, for a very brief no-doc mortgage minute in 2006, I owned a house in a nearby town next to her and her husband's place in Connecticut. Even though there was about a 30-year age difference between us, we still formed a great friendship and close bond. She answered the phone and was being funny about something when I said, "I've been arrested." "What?" she yelled into the phone. I started to cry and told her the story. Nancy spends a lot of time, her entire professional life, hearing unpleasant things. She's not easily rattled, but hearing my story made her raging angry.

When I was finished she told me a story about almost being arrested many years ago. Her then new office had an enticing (yet off-limits) balcony. Seconds after she was on it, her landlord came knocking. The woman was screaming in Nancy's face while holding a baby, and Nancy just wanted to slap her. Of course she didn't slap the woman, but her desire to felt dangerously close to committing a crime. She ended the story with, "That's not exactly the same, is it?" I didn't answer. It was the first in a long line of such stories I was going to hear that began with, "I was almost arrested once." There's a side to empathy where people want to explain they get what you're feeling by saying a similar thing happened to them. It's not necessarily story topping, but if it's not the same, it can come off that way. Almost being arrested is like kissing some one. Being arrested is actually fucking. Until you've been arrested, you're still at first base and don't get it. What happened to me was that my neighbor had me arrested and fucked me over. We got off the phone, and I looked at Hope's texts. What I originally sent her, right before being handcuffed, wasn't as clear as I'd thought.

ME: (sent at 5:41 pm, when I was in the holding cell)
I'm being arrested. If you don't hear back from me by 6.

That's it. That's all I wrote. I thought I had in there something about Buster. Nope. In my head it said, "I'm being arrested, if you don't hear back from me by 6pm, please let Buster out." Or please take care of Buster. Or Buster. Buster!! Buster!!! Hope had written back immediately, "What??" And then a little while later she typed, "I am just now getting back from the grocery store and will be putting dinner together. If I have not heard from you after that, I will go check on and walk Buster if you're not around. Hope you are OK!"

I called Hope and told her what had happened. It was hard to read her reaction. On the one hand, she has four grown children and has probably received a couple of crazy phone calls in her day. On the other hand, it sounded like I had interrupted dinner. After we got off the phone, she called right back to ask if she could come over, and I told her I was going to head out to teach. This probably sounded a little ill-advised, but I wasn't cancelling the appointment.

I was almost home, checking email as I walked. A sub was found for my class. That was a relief. They were concerned about me. *Me, too!* As I approached my building, I became frightened. I slowed down. There was a change, a difference. I was hesitant to walk into the building. I was scared to go home. Apprehensive, fearful, nervous, to go home. The place was stained now, emotionally. Having lived on the same small island for nearly two decades, I sometimes pass street corners where I think, oh, that's where I made out with so-and-so. That's where I rode my bike off the curb and didn't know there was about a two-foot drop, where the front wheel got stuck and I flipped over, but landed on my feet, facing my friends, who were frozen in their own Edvard Munch screams. That's where I found 15 bucks, that's where I was spit on when someone didn't time things right, that's where I used to buy and sell used books. Places hold memories just like photographs. That's where I had a huge teenage hissy fit when my mom and I came into the city for a show and a meal, and I still can't forgive myself. That's where a small publishing house used to be, where I made bank and did a terrible job. That's where I had dinner with a friend who'd eventually commit suicide. That's where I taught that famous guy. That's where a short friend fell into a curb puddle that went up to her knees and then fell again trying to get out, like she was diving for a penny, and I almost died on the spot laughing so hard. That's where my bike dumped me onto my elbow and then I decided never to ride a bicycle again. That's where I adopted Buster, when he rescued me. That's where they have a good deal on frozen blueberries. And, of course, that's where such and such a restaurant, a bar, used to be that I loved.

There's a concept of time to which I was introduced during my yoga training; an idea that it's happening all at once, but to understand it on this plane of existence, we need it to be linear. When I see those places and recall those memories, I wonder if they are happening at the same time I'm passing by. It's not quite a solid theory in my head. If that were true, wouldn't part of me have known something bad was going to happen in the building before I moved in? I don't know if that would have stopped me. I didn't have any other option.

I entered my building like I was sneaking in. The arrest got put aside as I climbed the stairs and couldn't wait to see my dog. When I opened the door, Buster greeted me and I cried seeing him. Usually he waits on the sofa, watching until I've taken outdoor stuff off and crouched down, then he jumps off the couch, stretches a bit, and does a happy, bouncy walk toward me. This time he was right there and I sat down, in the same area where I was handcuffed hours earlier, telling him what a good boy he was, rubbing his belly, smothering him with love.

From the floor, I was looking around at the apartment as if it wasn't mine anymore. It felt cold to me; or maybe I was cold to it, like it was supposed to protect me and it didn't and I felt betrayed. I checked the time and had to go into work mode: let Buster out, feed him, shower, dress, grab another Clif bar, and leave. I also spoke on the phone with my shrink, whose voice dropped very low when she asked, "What did you do?" I made an appointment for the next day and headed out to the subway. Since I had run out of time for a proper meal, I was wondering when I would get to eat real food again. I was probably in shock, but maybe that made it easier to focus on what was in front of me, what needed to be done, what responsibilities needed my attention. I'm used to this reaction. After violent and extreme nights at home as a child, I would go off to school the next morning like nothing had happened. I needed to do an awesome job working with this woman. Then I could come home and be a mess.

The private went well. It was a vacation to focus on my client, to be a yoga teacher, to do something I know how to do, to be in familiar skin. After the appointment, nearing midnight, New York City felt charming and quiet. I was heading toward the A train, walking by Washington Square Park, to a side entrance more frequented by locals as it can be easy to miss. There was one of those large-slice places next door and I grabbed a slice. It had been a very long day and the pizza tasted Michelin-star good. As I was standing on the subway platform, chewing the last bites, I could feel the shock wearing off, I could feel my body again. I didn't have to keep up appearances, pretending I was cool with being arrested and in a holding cell. Hope and I had made a plan to walk our dogs on the trail in the morning. I was looking forward to some human contact that didn't require so much work. Every move I made and everything I said at the police station had to be carefully thought through. I could feel how fried my nerves were, but I was wide awake. I had spent most of the day worrying about trying to get to work and being prevented from doing so. Now I wanted to get home and curl up with my dog. I also wanted to go online and read about what a DAT ticket entails. What was going to happen? How bad would it get?

Tuesday, April 12, 2016

In the morning, I reached out to someone who I used to practice Mysore yoga with, and who worked as a public defender. Not long after I sent my email, she called me. Apatia worked for a nonprofit legal aid group that I'll call the League of Lawyers. It had been about four years since we had seen one another and my first concern was to reassure her I hadn't gone down a dark path. Then I wanted to know whatever she could tell me about what was about to happen, but our phone conversation was brief. She asked when my DAT was and said she would try to be there. It sounded like she couldn't be my lawyer, but since I didn't understand the process, I didn't know why. She didn't explain. I was remembering television shows where lawyers came into rooms and introduced themselves with, "Hi, I'm so-and-so lawyer and I've been assigned to your case." Wasn't that the case if you didn't have a preference? I was still too fried mentally to muster the cognitive energy to ask better questions. It seemed like I should get a lawyer. It'd help me not worry, for one thing. I wanted a lawyer right then because I wanted to not worry. I wanted someone to relieve me of my stress with their knowledge and confidence. Since I didn't find the conversation all that helpful, I laid down on my bed and stared at the ceiling, trying to think of who I knew who was a criminal lawyer. I had taught a lot a people. Surely someone was a lawyer.

On Wednesday, I had a private in the evening with an old student of mine who was an immigration lawyer. I didn't want to mention the arrest during our session because that was not why she was hiring me, but I would figure out a way to ask her later. I'd been teaching yoga since 2001, and this would be the first time I'd reach out to students for something personal. It was always important to me to never break the boundary I fostered with students, so they could have at least one hour in their day to take a break from their roles as professionals, parents, and partners. Giving people that respite was my job, and very rewarding.

Bad things happen and you still have to get groceries, go to work, do the laundry, walk the dog. I kind of knew I wasn't doing great, but I switched my focus to teaching my Tuesday afternoon class. All I had to do was keep it together for one hour. Then therapy afterward was where I could unpack it. As I got ready for work, I could hear my neighbors yelling. Did they watch me leave the building in handcuffs? Did they feel satisfied with lying? Did they think they had won something? Did anyone else in the building notice my being arrested? It was the kind of news that I'd personally find interesting. The idea that being arrested had legs made me feel like an open wound.

My apartment felt like a hotel room, just a place I was staying in. I showered, ate, and got dressed, all from a distance. The weeks' events went by fuzzy. I'd gotten into a heated discussion with my shrink that Tuesday when she'd interrupted me to say I needed to move. I should move. Lots of people should move out of lots of difficult and hellish living situations. But I wasn't able to pick up and move. I wasn't even thinking about moving. I was thinking more about having an arrest record, a criminal record. Of course I wanted to move. That would have been great, preferably to a two-bedroom dog friendly condo near the Flatiron area of midtown, with views to the south and the second bedroom as my art and writing studio. I wanted a doorman building with a low maintenance fee. Maybe a cozy place at Walker Tower in Chelsea, formerly the New York Telephone Company building, with its 14-foot ceilings and 18-foot-thick walls. There, my dog could bark and bark and bark when we were playing, and no one would hear, and I would hear no one. I think more people want to move from where they are than don't. Especially in cities where you live where you can afford to, not necessarily where you want to.

My shrink and I also argued over my knocking on the door. All of sudden knocking on a neighbor's door was insane. "Who does that in New York City?" she asked. I'd always knocked on neighbors' doors without issue. Was she implying it was my fault? I mean, it was my fault, I did knock on the door. I thought I had security cameras filming me. Surely if you're thinking about robbing a bank, it occurs to you the outcome might be arrest, but knocking on a door, maybe it doesn't go well, but you don't have your neighbor arrested because they knocked on your door. Who does that?

In the evening, Apatia sent me an email checking in:

On April 12, 2016, 5:40 pm, Apatia wrote:

Been thinking of you today. Hope you got some rest and are feeling calmer about the whole situation...

And I responded:

On April 12, 2016, 8:57 pm, Marcy Tropin wrote:

Hi Apatia, thanks so much for checking in. I really appreciate it. I think I'm less numb. Wish I had something prophetic or yogic to add... Wish I didn't feel so naive about the situation, but then that's probably a good thing! -Marcy

Wednesday, April 13, 2016

Went to Mysore to practice in the morning. If I was putting off feeling something, it would come out on the mat. Everything comes out on the mat. All the emotions I'd been giving the one-minute sign to from my arrest manifested themselves into weight, and my body's relationship to gravity increased tenfold. The first movement in the practice is to raise your arms in the air with an inhale. Lifting my arms that first time felt as though I were pushing my hands through drying cement.

As I moved and progressed through the series, I got to the place where you have to step a foot forward from downward-facing dog, then inhale up into warrior one. From the outside, it might have appeared as though my limbs and I were no longer communicating through motor neurons. Instead, I had to reach back with a hand and grab my leg to bring it forward. Then I'd climb each hand up on a thigh and lift from there into warrior one. My right hip flexors ached, as they do when I'm upset. Fear, anger and sadness were rendezvousing at my heart, and my chest took on a heaviness. After about ten minutes, I dropped to my shins and rested my torso onto my thighs for child's pose. In addition to being a great break in the action, child's pose is a white flag. I was done. Sometimes, I can rally back after a little time out, but this time, I went into the finishing room to do some closing poses. Then I lay on the mat for savasana. Instead of closing my eyes, putting my practice to sleep, and transitioning into the rest of the day, I stared at the ceiling.

Afterwards, I waited in the doorway between the two practice rooms to catch my teacher's eye. When she came over, I gave her a two-sentence synopsis of what had happened. She didn't know what to say and was completely shocked. She offered to reach out to her mother, who was a judge in Brooklyn. I was compiling in my head a list of all the law-related allies I could gather. One more to the list.

Wednesday evening, I taught my immigration lawyer client, Esther. She told me she signed up for my workshop on Sunday. Oh yeah, that workshop. Maybe afterward, there would be a moment to tell her what had happened and ask for her advice. Timing my question was important to me. Also on my list of people to reach out to was Frankie, a former student of mine who'd just moved to Cleveland with her husband. Prior, she lived ten blocks down from me in Washington Heights. She used to come to my Tuesday afternoon class. Walking out one particularly hot and sunny day, both of us heading uptown, I hoodwinked her into getting fish tacos and hard cider at a neighborhood pub. We bonded over bad haircuts, messy childhoods and low alcohol tolerances.

The problem with hard cider is that it tastes apple juice yummy with a sneaky high alcohol content. It also has a way of letting you know about the high alcohol content after consumption. I stood up from lunch and needed to grab hold of the table. The drink hit me hard, as its name intends. I walked home in a stammer, laughing at myself. When I opened my apartment door, Buster came bounding over to play, "Oh not right now honey, take one for the team buddy, take one for the team." I woke up hours later, sprawled on my bed, feeling as though I'd fallen off the Empire State Building and kind of lived. It wasn't even 5 pm yet, too early to be hung over. Alcohol intolerance, one of the many benefits of a dedicated yoga practice! Though Frankie no longer worked as a lawyer, I was sure she did some criminal work previously. I texted her:

> ME: Hey. It's Marcy from NYC. How's Cleveland? Question: were you a criminal attorney here??!!
> FRANKIE: Hey! How are you? Cleveland is good, finally some signs that it might start warming up soon. Yes, I was a public defender in the Bronx!
> ME: Short story: was arrested. I'd love to pick your brain and understand what happens next. Can we please set up a time for a phone chat this week?
> FRANKIE: Sure. How's tomorrow for you? I'm pretty wide open. Did you already see a judge or did you get a desk appearance ticket (DAT) to go to court at a later date? Were you in Manhattan? Do you know what the charge is?
> ME: I have a DAT. I don't know the charges. Arrested in Manhattan. How's around 3pm tomorrow. East coast.
> FRANKIE: Sure that sounds good

ME: Cool. Thanks. You're not going to believe what happened...
FRANKIE: Oh, you're going to leave me wondering huh?
ME: Mmmmhmmm.

Thursday, April 14, 2016

I didn't feel great about texting Frankie to ask for help. Especially since she was in her second trimester. There was a huge milestone happening in her and her husband's lives, along with transitioning after a big move. I didn't want to bring negativity into her space. However, when we spoke on the phone, all apprehensions left. She was super excited to talk about anything other than the impending baby. We spoke for over an hour, her patiently explaining and answering my questions. I mentioned the lack of info from Apatia. She said that her colleagues were so used to the process, day in and day out, that they often forgot people outside of their world had no idea what was going on.

The first thing she recommended was that I get contact information from my super and Dewan. Then she explained how I would go to the courthouse and place my DAT paper ticket in a basket with other DAT tickets. Then I'd sit and wait. Whoever picked up my DAT ticket was the lawyer assigned to me. This sounded fantastically simple, even quaint. Nothing scanned, no bar code. Like putting your name in a hat. She added that I might need to bring along, or have handy in my phone, the 311 calls, management emails, and my tax return. She explained that my neighbor would be reached by the DA's office to get an official statement. If she was uncooperative, the case would be dismissed. Bring someone along to post bail, Frankie suggested. "Can't I do it myself?" "You can, but it's tricky." Wait, bail? Like bail bail? Money to make sure I would show up in court instead of them holding me in jail until the next court date, or simply trusting I'll show? I think of bail as a formula calculating charges times flight risk, plus network, notoriety, dual citizenship, and previous record. In my case, bail should be zero. Zero.

Next she gave me a heads-up about an order of protection. It was common in these situations for the DA to request one, but because I lived in the same building as the defendant, I had to make sure the order of protection was subject to incidental contact. That way, I would not be arrested walking in the hallways or leaving my building if I passed my neighbor. It was hard to breathe through all this. A lot of the words she was using were familiar. I've heard or read them in fictional contexts. Applied to real life, my life, their definitions escaped me. I know the word bail. I know the word protection. But I felt like an idiot when using them in sentences. It's like when a company says their jacket color is lupine and I can't tell from my phone exactly what that looks like, so I have to do a search for the word to see that they mean purple.

Frankie went on to say she saw these kinds of cases all the time as a public defender in the Bronx. Neighbors wanting to get back at neighbors would make up stories and have the person arrested. Then they never followed through with the complaint and the case was dropped. That sounded like a terrible way to use and abuse the system. It also meant your neighbor would be missing work or needing childcare. Couldn't they do the passive aggressive anonymous note thing? Frankie also explained that if police are dispatched for a violent offense of any kind, they have to bring someone back to the station. That's their job. Then they pass it along in the system. It didn't matter if what my neighbor was saying was true: that she accused me of harming her child was enough. They had to arrest someone. Considering how much yelling went on in that apartment and that I never shoved the door open, it's my neighbor who should have been arrested. Perhaps someone did cause that bump on the child's head.

While my call with Apatia felt like I was hungry and given rice, one single grain of rice, with Frankie it felt like I'd been invited over for dinner. Information is power, and being informed is being empowered. I wanted as much knowledge about what was about to happen as possible. I needed it for life decisions. I needed it to focus and try to be calm.

After our phone call, I grabbed my clippers and kitchen garbage can and headed into the bathroom naked. There was a need to do something, to feel proactive. If I was going to have to appear in court I wanted to look as boring as possible. I needed a simpler hairstyle. Prior to my arrest, I'd been thinking of fully committing to letting my hair grow out, allowing the short parts to catch up to the top. The DAT was three months away, it wouldn't be enough time. I was still numb from Monday. Holding scissors, I grabbed a long curl and cut it off, emotionlessly throwing it in the trash. Then the next one, then the next one. There was a mechanical machine-like feel to my actions. I could sense, from far away, that I was not happy about what I was doing. But I didn't stop myself. Clippers plugged in, I shaved everything to the same length.

Finished, my hairs were about a quarter of an inch long everywhere. I looked in the mirror and rubbed my head. Then I noticed the patch. I'd been slowly going grey since my early 20s. It never bothered me. I thought it was fascinating that one day my hair would no longer be brown. With the top shaved, there was a new large silver circle in the middle of my head. It looked like either a cult thing or a wannabe monk thing—or terrible. With the curls long on top, it all blended. It took a year for those curls to grow out, and in that time, the center of my head had gentrified. Looking into the mirror I said, "Well, that sucks." Then I showered and cleaned up.

On my way to a client's place that evening, I kept telling myself, "Don't say anything, do not say anything." This client and I had a more casual gig. Instead of teaching him an active practice, I do healing bodywork. Most of my clients preferred this, though not the tactics. I have pointy elbows and man-sized hands and usually work with clients on a yoga mat on the floor. If you didn't know what I was doing and passed by, it would look as though I was pro wrestling with my clients and they were losing, terribly.

Since I was little, I'd been able to use my hands to help remove pain from people's bodies. When I was around seven and at sleepaway camp, I was sitting on the top of a picnic table with a bunch of other kids. A counselor came over and sat down in front of me on the bench. With no candy to eat, in a rare moment of unscheduled activity time, I instinctively began rubbing my hands into the knots around her neck and shoulders. She quickly turned around and said, "Where the hell did you learn how to do that?" No one taught me how to heal with my hands. As hokey as it sounds, it's simply a gift.

Usually before I began stabbing my client in the back with my pointy elbows, we would eat dinner, small talk, turn on some sports, procrastinate, and procrastinate some more. My client and his wife were the nicest people you'd ever meet. I knew I was upset about the arrest, but I wouldn't acknowledge it. Also, because I was arrested for child endangerment, I didn't know how to talk about it. It was a serious charge. Privately, I just tried to keep doing normal things. However, when I found myself around people, it was really hard not to talk about it after all the internal bottling up.

It was Thursday, just three days after my arrest. I hadn't been sleeping well. I could barely practice. My home felt unwelcoming and cold to me. Normally, I don't invite private clients into my own crap. I'm there to flush away their crap. Who wants to pay someone a lot of money so they can complain about themselves for an hour? My rule of thumb is the advice I once gave my mother when she called asking if it was okay to wear white to a third cousin's wedding, "No, don't wear white. You're the smallest balloon in the parade. You're not Kermit. You're not SpongeBob. You're like a candy cane. Lay low. Fly under the radar."

In any given situation it's good to ask oneself, "Which balloon am I in the parade?" At someone's home, as their private yoga teacher, I was like one of those little star balloons. For the most part, I was doing great keeping it together during the session. Halfway through, my client's wife came around with one of their adorable dogs and hung out with us. When she asked, "So what's going on with you?" it was as if the safe had never been locked. I busted out, "I was arrested on Monday." She let out a nervous laugh and asked, "What?" I liked this response, the hoping a funny story was going to follow. "I was arrested" isn't exactly what you'd expect to hear from your husband's yoga teacher. When I finished the story, she added, "On Marcy, that's horrible." Later, I berated myself for blurting out the whole thing.

Friday, April 15, 2016

I texted Frankie to thank her for her time:

> ME: Frankie!! Thanks again for yesterday. It really helped and calmed me down. You have a lot of patience for explaining; that's a gift. Not a lot of people spend an hour on the phone going over the ins and outs of things
> FRANKIE: Oh I'm so glad it was helpful! I'm always happy to explain this stuff because I know how opaque the system can be if you're not an "insider" (and even when you work in the system, it can honestly be a bit befuddling)

Saturday, April 16, 2016

By Saturday, I still saw the black metal handcuffs being held to my face before I was handcuffed, with the scratches in the black, along the edges, showing the silver underneath. I still saw my front door in the background and the sergeant standing there. I

94

could see myself being cuffed. Wearing the pink puffer vest. Crying. I could still feel my heart sink when my dog dodged around the officers' legs to follow me. I could still see Buster's snout, his ears tucked along his sides, his quick weaving, his moving toward me. I still felt the sadness and frustration that I couldn't, with my arms behind my back, reach down and touch him. I could still hear my cracked voice trying to calmly tell him to go lay down. I could still hear the officers repeating the phrasing after me. Each time I relived this flashback, my heart went through the same crushing, over and over again. For this act of love and loyalty, my dog was rewarded with being sent to his bed, having the door closed, and being left alone. He didn't do anything wrong, but I couldn't let him know that, and this was terrible for me to live with. I didn't feel badly about knocking on the door given my naivety about the outcome. I felt badly that my dog didn't know what the fuck was going on. That I disappeared on him.

I did keep thinking about knocking on the door. I couldn't stop replaying what happened, going over our exchange. My neighbor is at least three inches taller than I am, with about 60 pounds on me. She's a sturdily built woman. Her weight is distributed in a linebacker-like way: mostly upper body. When she was telling me she was going to fucking kill me, it was intense. Had she backed up those words with actions, I'd have been pummeled. It's hard to understand how the police believed her. Did she put on an act? Did the family participate? Still, how did they think I shoved a door past this woman? It would have been as though I were pushing a refrigerator against a concrete wall. The physics of it, the logistics, the logic—none of it worked. That door was open to her right shoulder, meaning her right shoulder, right arm, and a portion of her right side were behind it. The doorframe is 32 inches wide; she's almost 32 inches wide. The door was not being shoved open, at least not by me. If I had pushed on the door while she was standing there, it would have begun and ended with her right side stopping me. Even if I caught her off guard and got the door open, there wasn't enough space between her and the wall for a child to be behind there.

This would bother me for months. I started replaying how I'd knocked on her door in a loop in my head. It wouldn't leave my thoughts. Finally it occurred to me that I never heard a kid crying. Wouldn't I have heard a child crying over her yelling? Even if I didn't hear her child crying, my neighbor never looked down. If her child was hit by the door, even by her opening the door, wouldn't she have looked down? Wouldn't the child have reached towards her for comfort? Wanting to be held, to be picked up? Maybe there was an adult I couldn't see who took care of the child. Wouldn't she have looked, though, to see? She never stopped screaming at me. She never took her eyes off me. It didn't make sense for her not to instinctually turn her head even for a moment.

Say I managed to shove open the door and it hit her kid who was somehow behind it. How did she not have a maternal reaction to the incident? It was inconceivable to me that she wouldn't have. Even I have involuntary maternal reactions when other people's kids take a spill. Once, I was walking down a sidewalk under scaffolding that was being held up by rows of metal poles, and a kid was flying towards me on a push scooter. The kid was weaving around the poles, with no helmet, no kneepads, no gloves, no adult nearby, and I yelled, "Careful!" It just fell out of me. After, I wondered when I had gone from being the child who would have been doing the same thing to becoming the adult whose nerves were instantly rocked by the laws of inertia.

Was my neighbor able to override her reaction to her own child being harmed to yell at me? Nope, because it never happened. I never hit her kid with the door. Even if she hit her kid with the door when she swung it open the second time, why hadn't she looked down? It would take a lot of anger to override that reaction. I understood she made up a story for the police that worked, that probably didn't take much from what happened. I didn't understand how it was believable.

Hope and I took the dogs on our usual Saturday morning hike through Highbridge Park. I updated her on what was going on. In the afternoon, Nancy and her husband were driving up from the Upper East Side to see my apartment for the first time and grab a bite at the little cafe next door. Mostly, they were coming to see how I was doing. After lunch I had a group class and then a private client at the studio. I was just inhaling and exhaling for the next thing, then the next thing, then the next. Checking off responsibilities, social engagements.

I didn't enjoy lunch very much. I wasn't in the mood to show off my apartment, where I'd just been arrested, and Nancy let me know she thought my hair was too short. *Thanks.* Then I headed to teach. At work I felt like I was impersonating the person who used to be me. And the person who was me was waiting after class, where we could meet-up, and go back to being confused and in shock together. Tasked with helping people feel better, I had to leave behind how I really felt, which was like the hallowed tread under a shoe that's stepped in horse shit. It isn't lucky to step in crap, that's just something someone told their kid, long ago, so they'd stop crying.

As my class was starting, and I stood in the doorway greeting students like a stewardess, I grabbed my friend Goldie as she was saying, "I'm really looking forward to this," and made her wait by the door with me. I began to conspiratorially whisper the arrest story to her, pausing to usher students in. There was a little multiple personality whiplash in the retell, between my venting to Goldie and the happy-to-see-you welcoming to everyone else. It was like I had to tell someone every 24 hours to keep sane. Goldie was enraged, which isn't nice to do to your friend before they take your yoga class. She told me a story about returning books late in college and almost being arrested. Then, just like Nancy, she realized it was not the same thing, and I agreed, just like with Nancy, it was not the same thing.

After my private, I walked through Central Park's southwest corner. It was the fastest route to the subway entrance on Central Park West and tourists rarely use it. Entering, it's two flights down then a bunch of full-floor turnstiles. Once through, I cut left to the uptown trains. The location of the subway entrance was perfect for where I needed to be at the front of the train. Since it was also the least-used entrance, it was quieter and less crowded at that end too.

When I turned left, though, I was facing two officers standing by the stairs. There were often police standing around the station, but this sighting after my arrest surprised me. I became terrified, wanting to run away. I told myself to focus on getting to the subway platform. Keep walking, look down, go to the stairs, hold the banister, take one step at a time, focus on the movement, not your thoughts. Once on the platform, I was trying to understand what was happening. I couldn't breathe, I was shaking and I couldn't stop pacing. I was having a panic attack. At the same time, I felt ridiculous to be scared of the police. But I was. In my pounding chest, it felt like they could arrest me and take me away. They had arrested me. It was possible. I was having a hard time talking myself down. I didn't feel like I had control over being taken away by the police.

Sunday, April 17, 2016

In the morning, I headed to practice. I was still not able to do ashtanga yoga's full primary series. I was just practicing until I needed to stop, and then honoring that. I had the workshop at 4pm and then a class right afterward. The workshop was poorly attended, but that was okay, at least for me, though maybe not so much for my employer. Coming in early to set up, I saw Esther in the back of the lobby, chilling on the sofas, knitting, and decided to tell her then. I walked over and sat down, trying to think of a casual opening. When I was finished, she berated me for not telling her on Wednesday. When I said that would have been inappropriate she responded, "You could have called me."

When the workshop ended, Esther got up and said, "I'm going to check on something. Something's not right." Then she left and I added her to my list of people who were able to help.

Monday, April 18, 2016

After my evening class, I was walking out with a student. He was in his twenties, smart, raised in Hong Kong. He asked me where I was last week and I told him about being arrested and asked him to please not mention it while I was at work. He had been coming to my class for a couple of years now and was funny tight. When you're young, inflexibility is entertaining, or so I've witnessed. He often waited for me after class so we could chitchat while walking up Madison Avenue until our directions diverged. He didn't understand why I couldn't speak about it to anyone at work. I told him I had to curate the audience because I wasn't arrested for demonstrating, protesting, or even a little weed possession. I was arrested for "hitting a child." Not every single person was going to believe me. There was always the chance that the narrative would get distorted and develop out of my control. Also, you can't spin harming a child. There's no joke in there. It doesn't make for a good "You'll never believe what happened to me" story. It doesn't give me "cred." I didn't feel badass about being arrested. My student and I hugged, and I headed to the crosstown bus.

Having a dog means you wake up, and leave. Having a dog means you come home, and leave. After teaching, tired from being processed through the gauntlet of public transit in New York City, I climbed the two flights to my apartment, opened the door, and grabbed Buster to head out again. As we were leaving the building, my neighbor's husband was coming in with their daughter. This was the small child who I had allegedly hit. The first thing I noticed was that her head didn't have a bump. She had sustained no scarring, no discoloration. Could this "bump" have healed perfectly in a week? Reflexively, I held the door open for them and said, "Hi." I wasn't even sure he knew who I was. *Hey! I'm the lady your wife called the police on.*

Sunday, April 19, 2016

I had dinner at my friend Sunny's place. She was recently engaged and moving upstate. We hadn't seen one another for some time, and there was a lot of catching up to do. It was really nice to hear about someone else's life, especially since hers was going fairly awesome. When it came time for my update, I used some fillers: where I was living, how work was going. Then I said, "Oh, yeah, I was arrested last week." This was a friend, not a client nor a student. The storyteller in me wanted to own what had happened by making it an anecdote, my reward for being arrested. The best-case scenario a horrible experience can harvest: the story and its details.

I'm the youngest in my family, with two older brothers. Both my mother and my brothers are very funny. Impossibly in their own ways funny. My mother has perfect comedic timing. Her delivery is killer. Like when I dragged her to the movie The Blair Witch Project. It was a popular movie in its time and the theater was packed. We sat just off center in the thick of the crowd. Throughout the tale of a camping and exploration trip gone very wrong, she was bored to tears. The woman never got scared. Me, I was holding my legs to my chest as if bracing for a collision, curled up in a ball.

When the ending was near (spoiler alert), there was a kid running towards a ramshackle house in the middle of the nowhere woods. Could it be the Blair witch's house? The theater was silent, except for my Mom. She saw the house, and was cracking herself up. From the corner of my eye, I could see her shoulders starting to shake, so I leaned over to her, my eyes still on the screen, and she leaned into me whispering, "Handy Man Special." Now she was beside herself. We got shushed by the people in front. She leaned back into me; I leaned back into her. "The value's in the land," she cracked. That I understood her real estate humor made it even sweeter. Unfortunately, because I got her humor, we ended up leaning over hysterically laughing, trying to contain ourselves, while the rest of the theater was watching the end of a scary movie. Three hundred some odd people frightened to the core, and two ladies who could not stop giggling. I will say, she saved me from seeing what happens to the kid once he enters that house, and from probably not sleeping for a week without the lights on.

My eldest brother is whip smart and can do accents. He's a couple of seconds ahead of you, and you can tell by his grin he's up to something. If you don't laugh at his first joke, he'll come at you with another. If you don't laugh at that one, he'll come at you with another. He'll keep going until you're laughing. We used to have these frozen burritos that were essentially dried tortillas wrapped around a half pound of frozen, refried beans. We wouldn't reach for one of those unless we were out of the Benihana frozen dinners. There was always a burrito of suspect age, freezer burned in its one-ply plastic packaging, available in desperate times.

In order to eat the burrito, you had to heat it in the microwave just long enough so that you could cut through the frozen center without overcooking the edges. If you burnt the edges, not only would the beans become molten hot, the tortilla shell would dry into something probably best suited as a scroll if you wanted to, say, send a note back in time to warn the Jews about Egypt. Frozen, the burrito was impossible to cut in half, even if you were pounding at it with a steak knife, a mallet, and a lot of teenage angst. Once the middle was warm enough to split in half, it went back in the microwave so the center could warm to at least room temperature. Then it could be served. My strategy was to microwave it somewhat, eat the warm edges until I hit Antarctica, then warm it again, eat the edges towards the middle, and repeat. The burritos were disgusting, but my mother didn't like to food shop. One morning, as I gnawed at the edges of my burrito, my older brother sat down at the table beside me.

At the time there was an 80s TV commercial called "The Switch," where patrons of a fine restaurant were served Folgers coffee. The idea was that they didn't think such good coffee could be an inexpensive, store-bought brand. Even though they were charged good-coffee prices, guests were pleasantly surprised at the reveal. The famous voice-over line goes, "We are here at [insert name of four-star restaurant], where we've secretly replaced the fine coffee they usually serve with Folgers crystals. Let's see if anyone can tell the difference!"

As my brother watched me eat, miserable as I could be, he was inspired to redo the commercial. Instead of replacing fine dining coffee with Folgers, he was replacing it with my breakfast. He started doing the voice-over, "We're here at Old Manor Restaurant, where diners don't know their coffee has been replaced with a burrito." He thought it was very funny. I found it annoying. In a home where people really liked to be funny, an annoyed family member was like a superfood. Being annoyed fueled our humor. For some reason we believed that on the other side, just over the hill of annoyed, was laughter. My brother went on all day with this joke. I wanted him gagged and locked away. Then he went on for years. Decades later, we were driving through the beautiful scenic landscape of Provence in France, and he remarked, "Remember when I made that burrito joke, and you got really angry? I thought it was hysterical." Smirking, he'd retell the whole thing over again right there, still trying to sell me on the concept. You gotta love the dedication. He never, ever, gave up on that joke.

Then there's my middle brother, the physical comedian. Absolutely physically fearless. Never gauche, though. The front door to my mother's house opened to a small entranceway and stairs. She ran a no-shoe household so the bottom steps were where we usually sat for lacing up to go outside. One day while I was putting on my sneakers, my middle brother came in and immediately put his hand on my head, looked up to the sky and said, "Heal my child, heal the..." He motioned about the room, praising the lord and asking for help so that I might be able to walk again. He bent at his knees to the sky, waved his arms to an invisible audience, pantomimed my rising up, and touched my head again. I was cracking up the whole time. He went at this one hundred percent, which is key. Whatever your funny is, you gotta commit whole to it. Eventually both laces were tied and I stood up. "She is healed, it is a miracle..." He raised both arms to the heavens and I was barely breathing laughing. Then I went outside and he went about his business. For all the hell going on in my childhood home, these were the funniest people, somewhat competitively, in their own very funny way. Except me.

I had nothing going comedically and this became a huge concern for me around age nine. I tried doing jokes and there wasn't a family member, friend, or neighbor from that time who didn't hear me ask, "What did the Pink Panther say when he stepped on the ant? ...Dead Ant, Dead Ant, Dead Ant." It was the theme song to The Pink Panther as a bug joke. After people heard the joke dozens of times, the only thing left that was funny was how much I giggled when delivering the punch line. Once that wore thin, if people saw me coming, they'd say, "I've heard it." This was the 70s and 80s, when children didn't get a trophy just for showing up and parents didn't know you were alive until you were hungry. It was a tough crowd for a nine-year-old. One joke was not going to give me cache in this family. Then came the 1983 Bill Cosby (I know) special Himself. My dad had cable TV at his place, and we watched it over the weekend with my brothers. I didn't get most of the jokes, but what I did marvel at was: a) Cosby didn't curse, which my mother abhorred and thought was cheap for laughs; and b) He was just telling stories. He retold stories, probably true events, not so much with embellishment as with killer description.

There was a whole other world beyond one-liners, accents and silly movements. There was describing. You could describe something for funny. Describing was an art form. I've watched Cosby's Himself many times over the years, and I'm still in awe of his use of silence and pauses. How much he had the audience at his pace. Pulling them into a scene, like getting kids ready for bath time, speeding up, slowing down, and then using a simple analogy to describe his wife hitting a tolerance wall. It's definitely less fun to watch now knowing who he is as a person, but comedically, it's brilliant. After that first viewing, I practiced describing anything with the slightest potential for funny. I'd do this over and over again in my head, each time trying to do it better. Being an engaging recounter gave me the two things I wanted most in my life at that time: more family attention and a place in the family comedically. It would also be a useful tool because later in life, my mother never, ever, wanted to listen to me unless I was entertaining.

At Sunny's apartment, when it came time to tell my arrest story, though, it was too soon for me to find the humor. As an adult, talking to a friend, I didn't need to be entertaining. I told the story of my arrest as it happened emotionally to me. Sunny listened. After telling my arrest story I got asked arrest questions. Was I read my Miranda rights? Nope. We both thought that was what was supposed to happen. Sunny asked if police could enter your home without a warrant. I guessed my proximity to the experience implied a sort authority about the experience in its entirety. I didn't know when the police were allowed to come into your home.

People didn't like what happened to me, so then they didn't think the police were allowed to come into your home and arrest you. I appreciated this version of empathy, friends expressing a distrust in the system, which isn't the same as knowing what your rights are. Saying, "They can't just come into your home like that and arrest you" is sweet, but not necessarily true. Can they enter your apartment without a warrant? Well, they did mine. Can they arrest you without reading your Miranda rights? Well, they did. Can they hold you in a cell for hours? Can they make you miss work? Can they deprive you of a phone call? Can they watch you get dressed? Appears that way. Most of the time during my arrest, I was crying and falling apart. This didn't give me great insight into my rights or proper procedures. Flashbacks to dried snot and the door closing on my beloved dog didn't leave me with a lot to go on. In the end, Sunny said I'd given her two weeks' worth of storytelling herself. "You'll never believe what happened to a friend of mine..."

Thursday, April 21, 2016

Esther emailed me on the 18 and said she had found a lawyer and wanted me to call him. His secretary made an appointment to speak at 4 pm on the 21. When I called, I was transferred to his office and heard him either ending a conversation with someone in person or on another phone. It kind of felt like part of a shtick. Why transfer me over if he was still on another call or had someone in the office? Right off the bat, I was told I needed a lawyer for these things and not to proceed without one. He said he'd just charge a flat fee for the whole thing. Easy. I asked him what the fee was, and he wondered why I cared. Unbeknownst to me, Esther had offered to pay it, all $7,500. The lawyer wanted to keep the conversation moving, and asked me what happened. But when I started with, "Well, I'm a yoga teacher and I was preparing..." he cut me off mid-sentence. Okay, I get that might be too "happened" for the "what," but ya asked. I stopped politely, and let him ask me questions that I gave brief answers to. When I had the chance, I emailed Esther an update:

On April 22, 2016, 9:45 am, Marcy Tropin wrote:

Hi Esther,

I now have to run out for a couple of hours and don't want to be rude in not calling so let me send a quick note…I don't think Gary is the best route. Prior to my speaking with him I'd had a long and thorough conversation with a friend who was a public defender in the Bronx. She was able to walk me through each step of the process and a lot of the variables. I had my notes out from that conversation when I spoke with Gary, and whenever I seemed to lessen an aspect of the process that he was using, in my opinion, to create fear, he ignored me. My impression was that he was happy to have you pay the $7,500 fee, but not prepared for my knowing a little bit about what happens. Not to say I'm a criminal lawyer, of course. I felt like he wanted to play on the emotional reaction to my arrest and when he wasn't able to win me over in that regard, he referred me to someone else.

He also doesn't think it's a wrongful arrest and doesn't want to sue the police because he represents too many of them.

I feel like this a very different impression than what you experienced, and I'm touched and appreciative that you would offer to cover my legal expenses, but I didn't end the conversation feeling like having him represent me would be helpful.

Another bit of research revealed to me that in wrongful arrest lawsuits, plaintiffs are awarded between $2,500 and $5,000 for every hour they are detained. In my case it was about three hours. You can then add emotional damages but it's not an amount that would be worth extending this experience for. What happened was wrong,

but as is often the case, I won't find resolution from pursuing legal action. The thing I have realized is that I have an incredible support system. I mean, everyone wants to do something to make this better and I love that! It's nice to know people feel that way.

-Marcy

And Esther replied:

On April 22, 2016, 10:22 am, Esther wrote:

Hi. Go with your gut and if he is not for you and you don't feel he would help, stay away. No matter my impression, you need to have full faith in your lawyer. I really mean that. I think it was still good that you spoke with him just to get a perspective! You'll be fine and know I will help in any way I can! See u next week. Esther

When I next saw Esther, she was pissed that the lawyer told me he didn't sue police officers. He had told her differently. She said you can't take on a client for false arrest with a bias that you don't sue the police. I thanked her profusely for having offered to pay the fee. It would have been easy to accept the offer, use Gary, and not worry about what was going to happen. Throw money at the problem, throw someone else's money at the problem. I had a bad feeling about him and went with that. It's the sixth chakra in yoga, intuition, and it's never wrong. Sometimes it annoys other people when it seems like I'm not taking the "smarter" more "logical" route because of a feeling, though I don't know where the hell my intuition was when I made the decision to knock on my neighbor's door in the first place.

Sunday, April 22, 2016

I ran into my neighbor across the hall, Dewan, while letting Buster out. We exchanged warm hellos and then I asked, "What have you heard?" "It doesn't matter until I hear it from you," he replied. This guy was a goober. We caught up on all things crazy neighbor. He told me the same week I was arrested, he had the police come to speak to them. I panicked a little, and asked, "Um, did they know it was you, or did they think it was me?" He said he'd overheard them speak, and when she asked which neighbor was complaining, the police said, "The one below you." Oh, relief! Dewan said our neighbor then added, "I'm complying." I didn't know what that meant, because they had never stopped yelling. Dewan said it sounded like they bought a treadmill. Over his head, on and off all night, he heard running. He looked worn. I probably looked worn, too. Dewan added that he also spoke to our super, who said management was trying to relocate the neighbors to a ground-floor apartment. That would be ideal for everyone.

Monday, April 23, 2016

One of my long-term private clients, a Chaplain, had just moved back home to Louisville, Kentucky. I'd been working with her for over a decade and then helped her move by selling everything she didn't want anymore in her apartment. She'd sent me an email on the 21 asking how everything was going. We'd grown very close over the years, and probably no subject was left unpacked between us. I did, though, make sure to put things plainly enough for the old lady not to worry:

On April 22, 2016, 5:50 pm, Marcy Tropin:

McClure!! Sorry for not responding to your first email!!! I thought after you left I'd have a nice quiet month but it's been very busy. The most interesting thing is that I was arrested. The short version is the building is having trouble with a new tenant, and when I knocked on her door and asked her to keep it down, there had been a buildup of animosity. The woman decided to call the police and contrive a story that I shoved her door open, and hit her child, or it hit her child. It's not clear, but I got arrested. Holding cell, fingerprinted, photographed …They gave me a desk appearance ticket for May 18 …Other than that… well there really isn't anything else I'm focusing on. Just trying to digest what happened and get grounded. How's that for news?!? xo -m

And McClure responded:

On April 23, 2016, 3:43 pm, McClure wrote:

Marcy...what a terrible nightmare!!! How could they do that to you? A perfect example of the overreacting by police in NYC that there has been all the talk about!! Are you totally traumatized? I hate this for you...feel terrible I'm not there to help you! Please keep me posted... do you have a lawyer friend to go with you...or someone? If you want to talk, please call anytime! I am outraged! Love you, me

When people expressed negativity about the police, I found myself defending them. The officers arriving had no idea what to expect. I may have shoved that door open. Except I didn't. That pisses me off, and it pisses my friends off, but it doesn't necessarily make the officers' reaction wrong. I guess I didn't want to fuel any anti-police rhetoric. I could be upset with how the situation was handled, as I lived it. But people needed to have their own crappy experiences with law enforcement to be upset by, instead of co-opting mine. I preferred to be the sole owner of the anger, the proprietor of the anger, for my experience. I wanted it for myself. Also, being angry at the police didn't help me. It was really my neighbor who deserved lots and lots of anger.

So far, listeners were falling into two emotional categories: upset for me or angry at the system. When they were angry at the system they went off on rants, complaining about the militarization of the police or overreaching. When they were upset for me, they were having their own personal reactions that felt overwhelming, and rarely helpful. I was finding it a chore to tell people. Here's this bad thing that happened to me, now I have to navigate your own reaction to it, along with the one I'm not processing, my own.

Tuesday, April 26, 2016

Nancy sent me an email to say that she was coming to the desk appearance and bringing all forms of currency, including bitcoin, so there was no chance I would end up in jail. Still, every night I couldn't fall asleep because I thought there was a chance I could end up in jail. I imagine jail as a much, much harsher version of the public school playground, with higher stakes, where you're surrounded by grownups whose moral compass presumably points down, and not children, who can be cruel but have yet to reach their cruel potential as fully formed cynical adults broken down by life. Like most people, I have a visual encyclopedia of prisons that comes from movies and television more than from personal experience.

There's the Charlie's Angels episode "Agnes in Chains," where they go undercover in a prison and find out the sheriff is forcing inmates into prostitution. I watched that around the age of nine. Or the episode "Caged Angel," where Kris goes undercover in a women's prison to identify a crime ring. While out on the activity courts, she's introduced to two nuns, who are the other Charlie's Angels in disguise. They hand her scriptures in the form of a pamphlet and advise, "But it is said the tears of true inspiration come from reading in between the lines" Later in the episode, Kris is taking a shower, in a private bathroom, and soaks the pamphlet to reveal a hidden map between the pages. I guess she couldn't have wet the paper under any other possible context but while she was naked in the shower. In the episode all the women are attractive, even the bully and the lady jock. There are massages with sapphic undertones, and sports and leisure activities. The women have a choice between khaki smock dresses or tight sweatshirts with the sleeves cut off and 70s short shorts. I was six when that one aired, and prison looked fun. For a while afterward, I was really taken with the secret map thing and tried to do one myself. But the reality is, if you wet paper, the ink smudges and the whole thing turns back into pulp.

Then there are the darker versions of prison. The one that sticks out the most and scares me the very most is from the movie Lady Vengeance, a film about an elaborately planned revenge by a woman, who is not a lady, but does have vengeance on her mind. The head bully in prison has other female prisoners doing her bidding, such as fanning her, making sure mosquitoes don't land on her, and performing cunnilingus. An ex-girlfriend gave this film to me. I don't know which was more disturbing, the movie as a gift or the movie itself. When I think of being in that scenario, a daymare, I imagine winning over the bully with my ability to do bodywork. Surely, she has a lot of tension and knots in her muscles, being in jail, being the meanest, and all. The scenario always turns to me hitting a tough area, causing her some pain, and then she breaks my thumbs. Afterward, I try to convince her I can still do bodywork with my elbows, but it's all downhill from there.

More recently, there has been Orange is the New Black. But whenever I think of that, I imagine being processed through a New York jail like Rikers before heading upstate. Rikers is a real fucking jail. Since the arrest, I'd been lying in bed most nights with Buster squished into me, staring through the dark, having circular conversations about how it was unlikely I'd go to jail and then questioning my naivety until I eventually fell asleep.

Tuesday, May 3, 2016

Getting home after 6 pm, hungry, I was pacing around the kitchen, eating anything that could be consumed without prep: a pile of raw almonds, some watermelon, a leftover smoothie. As my belly started to ease, I noticed arguing in the hallway. The apartment diagonal to mine had been leased by a long-time female tenant. There was a man's voice in the arguing, so it must have been one of her rotating roommates. For awhile she would have a guest from the south come live with her for brief periods. About every three months, a new and different young man would stay. Then for weeks afterward, her doorbell would ring all day and night. It would ring either repeatedly, or the buzzer would be held down for one long ring. It was nearly impossible for whoever wanted to gain entrance to gain this woman's attention. Adding to the issue was that she didn't give out keys to her apartment to anyone. Her guests also had to buzz in every time. Those that came day and night would head in for a couple of minutes and then leave. Unfortunately, from my apartment, I could unwillingly hear the hallway conversations and her door opening and closing. She also ordered in for every meal. Thus, her doorbell was always ringing. While I didn't have any issue with or interest in what she did, I would have really liked it if she were more responsive to her guests' buzzing.

The doorbell ringing was annoying, but I'd gotten used to it. Sometimes, they'd ring my apartment by accident and that would get Buster going, but I still didn't care. Such is life in New York City. This trip around, the man staying with the neighbor across the hall had a lady friend with him. It was definitely them arguing in the hallway. The walls surrounding their fighting were the same walls that surrounded my kitchen and entrance vestibule.

From where I was standing, I felt involuntarily involved, frozen by the violent exchanges, standing in my kitchen, not knowing what to do. Things got louder: stuff smashing on walls, things hitting the ground, cursing, and then a woman sounding like she was being pummeled. I stood very still, not wanting to make any noise of my own.

Now the woman was screaming for help, repeatedly. I paced near the door. My first inclination was to open the door, but anyone who's watched a horror movie knows that when people check out noises, something bad happens. I questioned why this was my first "good" idea. It's not safe. Don't check shit out. Then there's the Kitty Genovese reaction, which is no action, bad things continue happening, and the woman dies. It's harder to make these decisions in real life as opposed to telling the movie screen what to do when, as a viewer, you know what's on the other side of the door. That being said, I will never, ever, find it reasonable to enter a basement in a negligee, especially during a storm, after hearing a noise, and without even an aerial spray for a weapon. I mean, c'mon, nothing good happens in an unfinished country house basement in the middle of the night.

Listening to the fight in the hallway, I settled on calling 911 and made a quick decision not to have the conversation near the door. I was hustling back to the bedroom, speaking in hushed tones (are there other tones?). The operator asked me to describe the attacker. Um, didn't I mention it was happening outside my apartment? I scurried back and looked through the peephole, then ran back to the bedroom to describe the man. I didn't know why the specifics were so necessary. In the hallway were two people. One was pummeling the other. The pummeler was a guy. Go on that! The call was taking forever.

The police had my apartment number, so I could buzz them in. Once I gave them my apartment number, I might as well just have opened the door. They would know it was me who called the police because they would hear my buzzer and then my dog.

This system wasn't working for me. Suddenly, the couple retreated back into their apartment. My doorbell rang, my dog barked, and I buzzed the law in. Many officers were heading up the stairs. I could see through the peephole that they were going to overshoot my floor because they were looking for a couple fighting. With reckless idiocy, I cracked open my door, pointed to the neighbors' door twice, and then closed my door. I was like a parody of what not to do when calling the police on your neighbors.

Now there were five officers in the hallway. The same number sent to my apartment, so maybe it was protocol. But because I didn't harm anyone and am not a large man, it felt like too many at the time. Buster was whining, so I took him to the back of the apartment, saying, "It's okay, they're not here for me." While I thought Buster's noise was meant to alert me that danger was coming, he seemed more concerned about himself. A long time ago, I asked a friend what he thought my dog was trying to tell me when he made that weird noise. At the time Buster was sprawled across his lap, demanding belly rubs. My friend looked up to me, down to my mushy dog, and then looked up again to offer, "Hide me?" It's like instead of air going out for barking, it's being pulled in. It's a very strange sound.

The doorbell kept ringing, and I kept buzzing whomever it was in. I was expecting a package. A box of dog food, dog cookies, dried liver treats (also for the dog) and maybe some hemp powder for me. This would be a crazy inopportune time for a delivery. By now, there was a gaggle of officers in the hallway. Some were staggered halfway up the stairs, some halfway down the stairs. Now there were too many officers for the occasion. Except the whole incident was suddenly over. I felt badly because it seemed like an entire precinct was surrounding my floor, and they had nothing to show for coming.

Then there was a knock on my door, and it turned out to be one of the arresting officers from that Monday. The man who stood in my bathroom doorway. When I first opened the door to him, I became cold and motionless and said, "Hi, sorry to see you again in the same month." I meant to imply sorry we're such a busy and problematic building. I thought he got my point. It felt strange to see him, the guy who followed me to the bathroom and watched me change, and then handcuffed me. Of all the officers in the 33rd precinct. It was like ending up in an elevator with the drunk guy who kept hitting on you the night before. You're not supposed to run into those people again. At least you hope not to. I was trying to confirm what I heard and saw, at the same time not wanting my neighbors to hear me confirming it. I was going to be the one left behind when the officers dispersed. Didn't anyone else call? A woman screams help me, help me, help me, and no one calls? I was not the only one home in the building.

All the officers left. The man who pummeled the woman opened the door, answered two police questions, and then closed the door. Then there was nothing. He refused to come out and he refused to speak to them. I didn't know that was an option. It was quiet now in the hallway. It was the third time I'd called the police for an issue in the building, though technically I'd called 311 and not 911 for my neighbor. The other time was when the college kids on the ground floor had a raging party and allowed their drunk guests to go running up and down the fire escapes. I was woken up at three in the morning, having to teach in four hours, with kids outside my bedroom window, some three feet from where I was sleeping. When I went downstairs to request shutting the fire-escape ride down, they thought that was a terrible idea. I called the police because I needed to sleep and to keep those idiots from falling to their deaths. It was a milestone: I'd done the same thing in my twenties, and now I was the annoyed slash concerned "adult."

Friday May 6, 2016

I was entering my building. In one hand, I was carrying a large clean-looking box that I needed for shipping. In the other hand, I was carrying a handheld Dyson vacuum cleaner and all its attachments someone left outside for grabs. My dog was attached to my pants with a carabiner. His job was to be fearful of the vacuum as it hung and swung above him while we walked back home. I approached my apartment just as Dewan was leaving his and we immediately began talking. Since I was used to being a sherpa in this city, carrying too much at one time, we had the entire conversation without it occurring to me that I could open my door, put everything down and let Buster off his leash. It was completely normal: I was just going to hold all this stuff in the air while we caught up.

We got into my arrest experience, and I mentioned that an officer followed me to the bathroom and watched me change. Dewan was upset and told me, "I know for a fact they need a female officer for that." I didn't know anything for a fact. Or, I preferred to defer claims of proprietary knowledge. I like a little wiggle room in my thinking. A fact is a thing that is indisputable, so says a search-engine definition. How did Dewan know that for a fact? How'd that come up in his life? Everyone seemed to have an opinion on whether or not aspects of my arrest were okay. While I'd only canvassed non-police officers, the majority seemed to think the whole thing was not okay.

And I was not okay. My mind was still repeating scenes of black handcuffs with scratches, my dog trying to get to me, the woman snapping her blue surgical gloves, the worrying about getting to work manifesting in nervous tics, and my fear hitting a level ten. Would these memories of being arrested ever stop singeing along my nervous system?

Tuesday, May 10, 2016

It was time for quarterly teachers' meetings at Exhale. Every three months, we were supposed to meet with our managers to go over class numbers, the amount of classes subbed for other teachers, the amount of classes a teacher needed subbing—just that one for me, when I got arrested—and goals. These were goals in terms of increasing the class size, retention, and repeat rates. Not personal or professional goals. There are often lots of numbers and percentages printed on a white piece of paper. I like to see where my class size averages are because I understand the business aspect of running a yoga studio. You could have the Buddha teach a class, but if he doesn't build, he's out. The other number that's important to me is the repeat percentage, or how many first-time students to my class return. That number is on me. But the other numbers are kind of out of my control. Pulling people into Exhale, offering packages and memberships that make it worth it to become regulars, that's on the marketing department. My manager was going over acceptable reasons to sub out a class. She had to do this with me every three months, and I would try to make it as easy on her as possible. The little mom-and-pop studio I became endeared to back in 2004 had grown into a national presence. There was a board. There were checks and balances. Along the way, I'd had to learn how to work for a corporation.

Yoga teachers, good yoga teachers, rarely sub out their classes. Often, when you sub out even one class, it can break your regular loyal students' routine. Some will come and try the sub, but most don't. Once you break a student's routine, it can be weeks before they return. Or they don't return at all. Sometimes they return and remind you that you were gone, saying, "I came three weeks ago, and you weren't teaching." Fair enough. They're keeping you employed in a kick-ass job, and want to make sure you're valuing their commitment and time. I loathe subbing. If you want a long yoga-teaching career, don't go away often. My manager ticked off the acceptable reasons to sub: illness, death (both yours and that of a loved one). Then came the unacceptable reasons to sub: got Hamilton tickets, got an opportunity to work privately, it was a nice day out. As she was going over these reasons, I thought about being arrested. She should have added "arrested" to the list of reasons a teacher would need to sub out their class. Being retained by the police in a holding cell—all of those were good reasons.

Thursday, May 12, 2016

I was up at 6:30 am to teach a private client. Buster and I were heading back into the building after his business meeting, and I saw my neighbor's oldest daughter heading down the stairs towards me. I held the front door open a little, and then walked past her. When she walked by me, my mind started a daymare scenario of answering police questions about something she accused me of during this exchange. Like shoving her. My brain tipped over into "the sky is falling" thoughts that I couldn't stop. They could say anything. I began to hypothesize about getting Buster out of state, if she accused him of aggressive behavior. Buster looks like a baby seal and occasionally acts like an entitled former child star, but he's all mush. Before leaving, I gave him a lot of mush love. Then I rushed out to teach, fearful the police were on their way to arrest me again, and again prevent me from getting to work.

While the people who knew about my arrest brushed off the idea of jail, it was not as easy for me. Maybe it was highly implausible, but since I had already been arrested, I was past implausibility. People have extreme life-course changes all the time. I was arrested for hitting a child. It's a horrible charge. It should be taken seriously. I assumed a judge was going to take it seriously. There were other factors, like quotas. Just like I have my class size to worry about, there are analytics in every job. Then there's the whole "being made an example of" scenario that could play itself out.

118

Friday, May 13, 2016

My desk appearance was in less than a week. The last exchange I had with Apatia, she said to send her a reminder on Monday about the date. It was Friday, my one day off a week, and I needed something to do with my anxiety. I decided to email her. I was hoping, so close to the date, that I could get into a dialog with Apatia and ask her more questions. I was not in a good place in my head about everything, or about making decisions.

On May 13, 2016, 1:31 pm, Marcy Tropin wrote:

Hi Apatia, Just letting you know my desk appearance is this coming Wednesday, May 18. DAT Serial No... I think I was only supposed to give you three days' heads-up, but then I started thinking... what if she's going away on vacation? Hope you're well. -Marcy

And Apatia responded:

On May 13, 2016, 4:11 pm, Apatia wrote:

You should be fine. The scheduled judge is very reasonable. I'll try to come check on the case Wednesday morning if I can.

Should be fine has a different feel than will be fine. It's just a word, but if a student asked me, "Will this pose destroy my shoulder?" and I said, "Should be fine," I think they'd feel the same way I did. Should is a probability. Will is an inevitability. If "should" and "will" say they're going out, I'm guessing "should" never leaves the couch. Should imbues opinion without accountability. Maybe there simply isn't a combination of words

119

that would quell my anxiety. It's a nice email, but it also feels like the lawyerly version of "Have a nice summer."

Then I had a little meltdown. It wasn't like I was trying to make plans with Apatia to have a drink and I wasn't getting the message. This was serious. I had been arrested, and I was heading to court. I circled back to the thought that maybe I should have just gotten a lawyer. Then I wondered if I should have emailed her back an honest and vulnerable query, saying, "You know, I thought I heard, though it has been stressful and there's a lot of new information coming at me, that I could get help from your office. Or did I hear incorrectly? Am I going to jail? Is the court-appointed person going to chat with me? Is this not a big deal yet? That would be good to know. Do you not want to help me? Are you just really busy? Did we have a falling out that I've forgotten about? (That's happened.) Are you premenstrual? Is your life going okay? And well…please help."

I decided to decide on Monday about whether or not to reach out again, realizing that could change. I structured the rest of my day around obsessing privately. It was nearing 5 pm. It had been a shitty day off. The questions I had for Apatia were fairly direct. Could I get the case dismissed on Wednesday or would that not happen yet? Could she offer any helpful strategy on how not to have a criminal record? Was it legal for the police to enter my apartment? Was it legal for them to watch me get dressed? Instead of the opinions I'd received, I wanted answers, empirical and definitive from a professional in the field. I wished she'd even offered to get there early, or given me the room number, or reminded me to dress nicely. Anything.

I went online and looked up DAT. Online queries are great if you're leaning towards feeling hopeless about any subject and want to be pushed over the edge into hysteria. Somewhere in search-engine algorithms is coding to have the worst, most unhelpful outdated results come first. Search engines, like the news, can foster fear, foster panic, foster stress. I often find it hard to navigate the World Wide Web away from negativity. It's helpful if you want to know how to repair something with step-by-step instructions and videos, watch old-timey news broadcasts (the infamous Kennedy versus sweaty Nixon debate, for one), or look up the nutritional value for golden beets (yummy when baked and then sliced with goat cheese). Mostly though, the internet is where people are using avatars to post personal questions on forums so a stranger can respond. "I don't know about it being weight-neutral, but I know a guy who died on that drug."

The first hits for DAT were, surprise, lawyer sites that emphatically told you not to go to court without a lawyer. It took some time, pages upon pages, to finally find an informative article: National Lawyers Guild, New York City Chapter (NLGNYC): IF YOU GOT A DESK APPEARANCE TICKET (DAT): WHAT TO EXPECT AT YOUR FIRST COURT APPEARANCE (http://nlgnyc.org/wp-content/uploads/2011/10/NLGNYC_WhattoExpectDAT.pdf). The all caps was overkill, but the article was concise. One sentence read, "If you plan to plead not guilty, you should decide whether you will hire a private attorney or acquire a National Lawyers Guild appointed attorney as soon as possible; some important strategic decisions must be made at your arraignment and you want to be prepared." Later on, there was helpful advice about shutting up:

"A Warning: Exercising Your Right to Remain Silent. It sounds clichéd, but you should take full advantage of your right to remain silent until your criminal case is resolved…This is also true of any videos posted on [social media]. Police are notoriously good at using [those] sites against criminal defendants. You may be well intentioned, but you may not realize that you are implicating yourself in the crime charged. You also should exercise caution in dealing with the Civilian Complaint Review Board (CCRB)—New York City's civilian police oversight. While it is common for those unjustly arrested to want discipline for the officers involved, it is best to wait until the conclusion of your criminal proceedings before you file a complaint. A complaint filed with the CCRB may be used against you in your criminal case and may encourage the officers involved in the complaint to be extra diligent in their attempt to secure your conviction...

Conclusion: Your first court appearance is a critical phase of the criminal process. You should be prepared to make some difficult decisions on what is best for you and your future. Carefully weigh all of your options, work with your attorney and make a choice that you will be happy with individually. While some people want to resolve their criminal case with as minimal impact on their life as possible...Others simply want to be declared innocent of any wrongdoing. No matter your choice, make sure it is the appropriate one for you."

I took a break from the search results and decided to poke around the League of Lawyers website, where Apatia worked. There were income guidelines. Oh, was this why I was supposed to bring my tax return? I had forgotten about that. It seemed like I should have visited that site a month ago. Why hadn't Apatia advised me to start there? The guidelines for LOL stated clients' incomes couldn't exceed $13,000. That disqualified me from being able to use them. Wasn't this an important detail that I should have been told during my initial phone call with Apatia, the day after my arrest? Maybe there was something I wasn't reading correctly. Having never been through this process and not in a great place mentally, I kept fuddling information. Now I was confused about using a public defender at all. Did the income requirement apply to every case? With the income guideline information, I thought I could contrive another email to Apatia. I was relentlessly hopeful that I could inspire her to help me, to peek from behind the curtain of her profession.

On May 13, 2016, 5:04 pm, Marcy Tropin wrote:

Hi, I didn't realize that the income requirement for the League of Lawyers was one person, about 13k. Would you have a recommendation for a criminal lawyer? Sorry if you had explained this to me. There's been a lot of information to understand. -Marcy

Apatia got back to me to let me know she was not allowed to recommend a lawyer but could give her opinion of a lawyer if I sent her the name of one. She also said she was sorry she couldn't be more helpful. Okay, no more reaching out to Apatia. It was frustrating. This person had a very dedicated asana practice, but was kind of cold off the mat. This is the kind of practitioner I have issues with: all poses, nothing else. Who cares if you can put your foot in your butt? It doesn't mean you're enlightened. In Patanjali's Yoga Sutras, the definitive guide on how to practice yoga, asana (the physical practice) is barely mentioned. What I find important to practice are the guidelines for behavior in how you treat others (Yamas), and how you treat yourself (Niyamas).

The five Yamas:

Ahimsa: nonviolence, causing no harm
Satya: truthfulness
Asteya: non-stealing
Brahmacharya: non-excess (e.g. chastity)
Aparigraha: taking only what you need, without greed

The five Niyamas:

Saucha: purity of mind and body, cleanliness
Santosha: contentment

Tapas: self-discipline, training your senses
Svadhyaya: self-study, inner exploration
Ishvara Pranidhana: surrender (to God) or a higher being

I started thinking of the endless times I'd stayed after class when someone asked, "Do you know any hip openers?" It's not that hard to be helpful. I was pissed off at Apatia. It was a nice safe place to direct my anger. I get that life is more complicated than "yes" and "no." In trying to figure out what was between those finalities, some insight into what the hell was going to happen on Wednesday, I wasn't getting anywhere. All out of ideas, I sat, staring at the computer screen. I was frustrated and defeated by not being able to prepare myself mentally and emotionally for the DAT.

I was also exhausted. Everything was about my being arrested. Every moment was about being arrested. Every thought was about being arrested. I was wearing it every day, going to sleep in it, showering in it. I started rubbing my head, like warming up an engine, moving my hands forward and backward, feeling the short hairs. The repetitive movement and tactile feel was soothing. I pulled my knees to my chest, bringing my feet onto the chair. I just wanted to talk to someone who didn't need me to take care of their feelings about the arrest. It wasn't the time for feelings. There wasn't time for feelings.

While still sitting in an upright fetal position, I decided to scan through those search-engine results more. It felt like I was doing something. The waiting and wondering made it hard to focus on anything other than what I was waiting and wondering about. For the umpteenth time, I jogged my brain for lawyers I might know. I felt like I knew a lot of lawyers. It seemed like in New York City, I would know a lot of lawyers, but I couldn't remember any of them, if I did know them.

I felt screwed. Like I was going on a camping trip without any gear. Or the tag was sticking out of my collar, or I buttoned up

my shirt and skipped one, or there was food on my sleeve, food in my teeth. I felt like my skirt was tucked into my tights, or I was caught singing out loud, off key. I felt like I had a credit card they wouldn't accept, my laces were untied, my shoes were dragging toilet paper, my bags were left open, and I had shown up early, but on the wrong day. If there was an income limit, wouldn't she, shouldn't she, have told me to seek out representation during our first conversation? What the heck.

Finally, I remembered a student I'd known since she was in law school, for well over a decade. But I only had her wife's email from when I was helping her with back pain. Goodness, how many people were going to know about my "hitting a child" problem? I sent an email to my student's wife, chastising her for not coming to class during her birthday weekend—we all need an opener—and then asking what kind of lawyer her wife was. That was subtle. That worked. Jan got back to me immediately, sending along her wife Carrie's email.

On May 13, 2016, 6:58 pm, Marcy Tropin wrote:

Hi Carrie, I got your email from Jan, hope that's okay!! I'm poking around to find a criminal lawyer and was wondering what type of law you practice and/or if you have any recommendations. -Marcy

Lawyer. Lawyer. Lawyer. The more you say it, the more it sounds like a sheepherder's call: Laaawwww-yerrrrrr. While all this pondering was going on, I had bicoastal clients in town. A couple from Los Angeles. Sometimes, like this morning, they'd book me for 6:30 am. This meant my alarm went off at 4:30 am, leaving an hour for morning stuff and an hour to get to them. Depending on whose schedule was the craziest that day, I'd see the husband or wife first, back-to-back sessions. Afterwards, I'd usually nap to catch up on sleep. Still, cognitively, I would be off for the rest of the day. It's strange to wake again around 11 am knowing I've already been out and about in the city, but am now back in bed. The strangeness is hard to shake off.

Yoga teachers have enviable schedules where they might teach very early in the morning and then not again until the late afternoon through the evening. It's technically the same number of work hours as a regular job, cut in half. On paper, it seems like there's all this free time, but it's deceptive. In the middle of the day, during those odd blocks of free time, you're catching up on sleep, laundry, bills, grocery shopping, and all the things people do after work. It's hard to make use of that time knowing that in a couple of hours, you're going to be back in front of bunches of people, talking and guiding.

Being ready to teach means being ready to hold the energy for students, extending it beyond yourself. I use my energy to pull students out of theirs, out of the places where their energy is stuck mentally, emotionally, physically. If I can do that with my energy, then I can create space for students to see themselves, their lives, their bodies differently, to feel differently. It's rewarding, but it also exhausts me. Wanting to write or make art or do any creative pursuit, requires being squirreled away with your own energy, like lovers. I never found an easy switch between the two, often feeling shameful about my free time, with nothing creative finished to show for it.

My brain was still groggy after the early morning appointment. I was blinking a lot. It was cold and rainy. My dog had circled himself into a bed pillow divot and was sound asleep. I ate a sandwich I didn't remember eating. There was a pile of white paper stuff on my desk that I was ignoring to my right, and a pile to my left that could not be ignored. I was still wearing the well-intentioned yoga outfit I'd planned on practicing in after those early morning clients. But instead of going to yoga, I went food shopping. I was running out of Clif bars and that's dangerous in my line of work. With constant movement comes the need for constant fuel. Something that can tide you over but not cause flatulence while you're demonstrating a twist or inversion.

On occasion, I've needed to release some vata (the energy located in the colon, which in excess builds up as air) as I walked to a corner of the room and then quickly walked away like a kid who has just peed in a pool. Gas happens. Especially in my profession, where there's a lot of focus on diet and nutrition. A lot of trying out healthy fads, cleansing, and rebuilding. Sometimes it felt as though I was fermenting on the inside. Like the time I tried eating only raw foods or the time an Ayurvedic doctor gave me some powder to take every morning and didn't let me know it was an herbal laxative. To this day, I'm still grateful to the woman at a sports club on 59th Street and Lexington Avenue—where I'm not a member—who let me use their bathroom early one Sunday morning before I shat myself. As a matter of fact, I say a little blessing every time I pass the place.

I didn't know if going food shopping over practicing was the best decision. I was stressed. It was now nearing 7 pm. Did I need a lawyer? I was also cold. It was spring, when buildings turn the heat off but when there are days that can still dip below 55 degrees. With the heat off and the sun not on, the walls were cold, the floor was cold. Nothing was keeping the building warm. I didn't appreciate being cold in my apartment. It seemed like that was one of the reasons why I went through the trouble of working and paying rent: shelter. I got up and grabbed one of those Clif bars.

Now that I was fueled for outdoor adventure, I headed to the sofa with Buster, who draped himself over my torso like a throw rug. His head was on my chest, and I was warming up. The neighbors were being loud in their living room, which is still loud, but better than their kitchen. I took the opportunity to tune into the Yankees radio broadcast on my phone. I was still trying to think of lawyers I might know. My jaw was killing me from clenching and grinding in my sleep. Years ago, during a particularly stressful move, Buster destroyed my $400 night guard, and I hadn't gotten around to replacing it.

My thoughts repeated the same questions. Was I just hearing the charges against me during the DAT? Was that all that would transpire? Then would I plead? What if my neighbor didn't show up? Did that mean the case would be dismissed? It was too late to really hire a lawyer for Wednesday, if I needed a lawyer. The biggest question was did I need a lawyer, or not? A lawyer would say yes. Maybe it was personal preference. Some people prefer mistreating their bodies, then they go to the doctor and fret about something being wrong. Those people feel comfortable having other people handle their business. But I'm not one of those people. I have my mother's disdain for unbridled trust and not my father's naivety for the spoken word of a man in a suit. It's a negative attitude, to feel like people want to gain my trust because they have bills to pay. Nonetheless, it is a motivating factor when I'm doling out advice. When I help students with injuries, it's often contradictory to the advice of a "professional." Without pause, I let them know why my opinion differs: "I don't have their overhead, I don't need an angle to generate repeat business. I prefer to heal you and then you refer me."

During this morning's private, the wife wanted to book me for early Wednesday, and I blabbed the whole arrest story. I'm not good at lying and I usually make myself completely available when these lovely and loyal students are in-town. Let them know it wasn't my choice not to teach. Well, I could have taught since she was requesting crack-of-dawn, but my energy would have stunk, and it wouldn't have been fair to them.

After the retell my client repeated out-loud "five cops" jokingly to herself, then added, "for all 82 pounds of you." I happened to be sitting on her at the time. With one exception, clients love it when I do this. In a group class, students will release their backs by pulling their knees to their chests while lying down. In a private, I have them bring their knees to their chests and relax their arms out like a "t." Then I separate their legs just a little bit. I have to do this whole thing with authority. Otherwise, if I step outside myself and lose the moment, it's kind of awkward, with me standing over them, opening their legs. Then I sit on their shins. My butt's pretty much in the middle of their legs, and it's my thighs that are making contact. I'm holding back my own weight by distributing it to my feet and using my quads for dear life. You can't just sit on someone and drop a 100 plus pounds (since technically I'm not 82 pounds). You need to make sure the student isn't clenching their glutes (ass) or hip flexors. You need to make sure they're not clenching anywhere. If they are, it tilts the pelvis up, away from the ground, putting pressure on the lower back. What I'm trying to do is get them to relax everything around their pelvis: those hip flexors, glutes, and abs, any tension and holding.

Once I've got my position steady, I gently lean from foot to foot, and a little backward. After a while, the repetitive rocking motion has gotten them a little mushy, and I can add just a pinch more weight. The whole thing releases the lower back into nirvana with style. I'm not just plopping on someone. I'm a professional. It's also a nice challenge on my legs. While I was doing this, my client was cracking herself up, saying, "You're a yoga teacher." She's worked with me for a long time, and the idea of my being arrested is, if you're not me and not the one who was actually arrested, kind of hysterical. I'm happily boring externally, as I live more internally. When you add the whole yoga teacher thing, it is funny it's me who's gotten arrested. Hardy-ha.

Back on the sofa, enjoying the rainy afternoon after my private, I felt Buster's weight on me and it was pure love. His energy calmed me, comforted me, got me out of my obsessive thinking. He was making squish noises as I scratched the area of his head that dips in, saying, "You've got a dent here, did you know that?"

The Yankees were batting against the other team's ace and shellacking him. Though people complain that baseball is slow and boring, I love it. If you know the game you understand all the chess matches going on, how it changes from pitch to pitch and batter to batter. It looks like a waste of time when a batter steps out of the box, but often he's doing it just as the pitcher looks like he's ready to start pitching, when he's "set." The batter is trying to throw the pitcher off his rhythm, get in his head. There's a lot of strategic antagonizing in baseball. You have to play until all outs are recorded, and you can't hurt another team's player to win. I prefer this over all other timed sports where you're watching teams go back and forth, back and forth, back and forth, until the last minutes when the time-outs and fouls and delays become interminable. I don't find it interesting for a team to win with clock strategy. That comes from the people on the sidelines, not the athletes. I want to see athletes play sports. I spend enough time on time.

These moments alone with my dog, feeling safe, were healing for me. I needed these moments. I needed this dog by my side. Since my arrest, I worried about wasting even one more hour being in a jail—losing my simple life of simple pleasures, just for knocking on a door. Stressed and hungry for information, I reached out again to Frankie in Cleveland with a long text:

> ME: Hey…I know the biggest day of your life is about to happen. But I just found out that the League of Lawyers can't help me bc I make too much, and the person who told me about them didn't tell me this. So I need a criminal lawyer, and if you happen to know of anyone…and aren't in labor, or feeding, or sleep deprived, let me know
> FRANKIE: Hey! That's silly. Who told you that? When it's a DAT, no one ever does an income check! I've never seen that…Or did you already have the court date?
> ME: Dude. The person I know has been really…weird. She said she would try to stop by on Wed. That's all. And then I looked at the income thing and asked her about it

and she said she can't refer me to anyone bc of rules. I don't understand, but for whatever reasons, she doesn't want to help me...

FRANKIE: Honestly I don't really have any rec for criminal lawyers because everyone I know is a public defender...So you haven't had the court date yet?

ME: DAT is this Wed. If it was you, would you have said something else to me, something more affirmative?

FRANKIE: Unless a judge tells you that you have to hire someone, just stick with the LOL

FRANKIE: Is your desk appearance this coming Wed?

ME: This coming Wed. And I don't think the LOL will help me. I think I'll be assigned a public defender

FRANKIE: Yeah, but if the LOL is covering that part that day, they are the public defender

ME: Oh

Should I have known that? Do you people know that?

FRANKIE: It's either the LOL or the City Redeemers, depending on the day...NYC doesn't have a public defenders' office per se. They contract out to those orgs

ME: Why are you giving me more information than her, from Cleveland and about to have a kid...Weird

ME: This is what she wrote: "You should be fine. The scheduled judge is very reasonable. I'll try to come check on the case Wednesday morning if I can."

FRANKIE: She doesn't sound very helpful

ME: I've been more helpful to strangers at bus stops with back pain

FRANKIE: But don't hire someone before Wed

ME: Got it. See that's f'n helpful!!

FRANKIE: Someone will represent you that day, and I doubt you'll be told to hire someone. But if you cross that bridge, then it would only be for court dates going forward

ME: Okay. Again, that's helpful

FRANKIE: If you do have to hire someone, I'm happy to reach out to former colleagues to see if they have recs

ME: Groovy. I've been reaching out to all the lawyers I know bc it wasn't clear to me how I should be prepared for Wed regarding counsel. This woman didn't even explain how there isn't a PD office, etc. Frankie, I want you to know how appreciative I am of your help!!

FRANKIE: No worries at all! I know how stressful this shit is!

FRANKIE: All I ask in return is that you send this baby some vibes telling her to get out!

I took Buster out for an evening walk, came back home, and realized my belly was distended, stressed, bloated, as though I was the one expecting a baby. Guess those good-feeling texts had an emotional shelf life. I was tense as hell. I could see why people sue for emotional damages. It was stressful enough being arrested, and my stress kept on growing while I didn't have control over my fate after the arrest. The vulnerability of not knowing, not being able to get a clear picture of the legal process, was killing my nerves. I practiced, I breathed, but I still didn't know what was on the other side of this. Lawyers wanted a fee, public defenders were a little busy, and online search results yielded advertisements and worst-case scenarios. Even if I was overreacting, I had been arrested. For the rest of my life, if I was ever asked that question, I would have to say "yes." And when I was asked what for, it would be for "hitting a child." My fingerprints were in "the system," as was my arrest photo with that lovely haircut. It was in my time line. It was not going anywhere. It was canon.

I scheduled therapy the day before my DAT because it seemed like a good idea. Maybe I should have scheduled it for afterward? It's hard to project into the future when one might be falling apart.

Sunday, May 15, 2016

I'd been waking up at the crack of dawn to teach the bicoastal clients for a couple of days now, and I'm loopy from it. This morning, I headed to Mysore afterward, went home for food, and crashed before teaching again. The scenario worked: all responsibilities were checked off. I was impressed with myself at keeping things going, especially with this fuzzy feeling, like I was wearing my brain sideways.

Today's schedule was like a teaching conveyer belt. In the afternoon, between classes, I got a migraine and lay on the sofa moaning to myself. Nancy called. She was checking in on me after my Friday loony-bin trip. I was not in the mood to talk about the DAT, though. I just wanted to lie on the sofa and whine before heading out to teach again. Nancy wasn't getting the message, and I regretted answering the phone. She was in the car, driving, had me on speakerphone, and was also talking with her husband, who's a lawyer and doctor. She was talking to both of us at the same time. She was asking him questions, I heard his replies as mumbles, then she was telling me his answers about whether I might need a lawyer and what might happen during the DAT. I thought she thought she was asking him questions on my behalf, but she hadn't gone through the process of asking if I wanted her to ask in the first place. It was as though I had called her. She just assumed I'd want to know what her husband's opinion was, even though he had never practiced law. It wasn't helpful, and I wanted to find a way to get off the phone quickly, but I couldn't get her attention.

Speakerphone is my Room 101. As is the case with mattresses for sleeper sofas, there isn't a speakerphone product that does a great job at both ends. There isn't one that cancels out background noise. To a speakerphone, it's all the same noise. It's technically a microphone with a better outfit. It doesn't work to direct your voice into the air as though your friend is in the same space with you, with the part of the phone that picks up sound somewhere nearby. Every time I've ever asked someone, "Am I on speakerphone?" they've replied, "Yes, but I can hear you." Of course you can hear me, I'm holding the device that transfers sound close to my mouth. It's me who can't hear you, but I can hear every single background noise, equally. My migraine was hating this conversation. If you love someone, don't put them on speakerphone.

I ended the conversation as swiftly as possible and changed subjects over to anything else, like asking Nancy how her laptop purchase was going. I'm her IT person. Mostly it's the age difference. For most of my friends over a certain age, I'm the go-to person for computer-related issues. It starts with a simple question, like how to log into your email account on a mobile device. Then the next thing I know, I'm setting up their wireless internet at home and writing down passwords on a piece of paper that's as good as lost before the ink dries. Nancy is a highly intelligent woman with a talent for fostering conflict with electronics. She's also got that shrink thing for sniffing-out deflection. Thus, she circled back to my arrest and to whether or not bail would be set on Wednesday. "I will hear my charges, and then maybe the judge will decide bail," I explained. These questions had answers that would take place in the future, so I was just making up answers now. I really wanted to get off the phone.

"Hear charges and decide bail" were phrases I never thought I'd say. I never thought I would refer to bail as anything other than a stack of hay, certainly not in the personal proper. We went back and forth about this detail a couple of rounds. It was really about her not wanting to head down to 100 Centre Street on Wednesday morning if she didn't have to and my desire to have her there for support regardless of the bail issue. I was using bail as a way around asking for help, because I'm not good at asking for help. I wasn't prepared for her to backtrack on offering to come. I pushed the envelope and jokingly said that without bail, I could end up at Rikers. This was to show I was scared. There was a pause in all the conversations happening at once. I could hear the sound of a car driving along a highway. Then Nancy said she was coming. She didn't know for sure what happens during a DAT. No one knows. It's a well-kept secret.

Monday, May 16, 2016

I had run out to the bodega for plain M&M's to ease belly anxiety. Normally, candy and I don't hang out, but when my belly's in knots, those little chocolate drops work really well. As Wednesday neared, my physical body was catching up to my mental stress. There didn't seem to be anything I could do to calm myself. It didn't help that I was living in the apartment where I got arrested, in the building where the tenant who called the police and got me arrested also lived. It was like a trigger party. And the neighbors were still loud, of course.

Walking to get M&M's, Buster smelling and trotting along beside me, I see my neighbor's husband. He was carrying one of the bodega bags in his hand. We had that two-second moment of "oh yeah, you," and then passed one another. The crazy thing was that he had good energy. With the exception of not having an inside voice, he didn't seem to have the anger that his wife did. When she was screaming at me, the image of him in the living room, cradling his youngest, bare-chested, big-bellied, was tender. It was hard to reconcile that this was the same guy who was always yelling. Heading into the store, I was relieved we weren't shopping at the same time. Good energy didn't stop him from letting his wife lie to the police and going along with it. I didn't want to be anywhere near these people.

Scenes from my arrest were still replaying in my head, especially the part when my neighbor opened the door the second time. Was that where the little girl got hit in the head? I was still trying to apply logic to it all. And I arrived at the same answer: it wasn't possible, the mother never looked down, there was no noise. But that didn't mean it didn't happen. Okay, so the kid got hit in the head, she didn't look down, it did happen. She did it, but she lied, and the kid lied, and the family lied, and the police believed it.

I was obsessing about facts the way my dad would. Beguiled by the spoken word, he gave too much of his trust to what other people said and got crushed for it a million times. Words are just sounds in the air. They don't have any weight unless you back them with action. Until the action, they should just float there. You shouldn't put them in your pocket for safekeeping. My dad would refer back in confusion to an opinion I had years ago, reminding me, "But you said you hated winters." As particular as he was about what other people said, he often spoke as though he was ready to fight and defend, even in moments requiring introspection or tenderness. "Is that because you can't get a man?" was how he responded when I said I was dating a woman. Instead of it being a reaction to attraction, a choice, desire, curiosity, the nineties, to him it was a matter of desperation. Logic. In order to understand a decision, you did the math and made a deduction. He was an accountant, understanding the world in columns of red and black. He believed you came to a conclusion, and then it was fact. There were grey areas he never considered, where information might be missing: I had dated men.

But because I'm my father's progeny, my mind gets stuck in the same ways that his did. My neighbor lied, told a story I didn't know about. Unable to account for the missing information, my thoughts fought in the empty spaces created by the lapses of knowledge, circling from the beginning to the end, start to finish, passing blindly around the unknown middle. They could not land. What if I liked winters now and hated them again later? It was about fluidity. The same applied to sexuality. We don't owe anyone a commitment to our opinions. I needed to stop thinking about the arrest, and I couldn't. I reenacted and reenacted without applying the lie, and then it didn't compute. She lied. I should get over it. People lie. Okay, so she said I shoved the door past her, a large woman, and the door hit her child, who was squished in there behind it, and I did not do that, and I couldn't get over it. She had me arrested.

I was putting away dishes from the day before, the mindless act let my mind wander, and it immediately played out a scenario where bail was set at $2,000, and I was led away, handcuffed. I didn't want to be handcuffed again. This reminded me of a student of mine who had something very tiny removed from her shoulder. She was distraught over it. It took me awhile to figure out that she wasn't distraught because of what test results might reveal. She was upset because it was her first scar when she was over the age of 30. I had trouble mustering any empathy, "You don't have any scars?" She had none.

The first decade of my life had been one scar in the making after the other. There was the one in the center of my forehead from a playground slide. I was an unattended kid at our temple's men's club picnic. I recall heading off alone to the playground, where there were two slides. I opted to go down the largest of the two, on my belly, feet first, seeing how far I could stretch before letting go of the ladder's side safety bars. Once I let go, I was tossed left and right as the slide swayed left and right. It wasn't bolted down. At the end, I slid out into the dirt and my head dribbled a couple of times on the end of the slide, which wasn't curved down and smooth, but worn to a sharp edge. Then I passed out.

When I came to, I just got up and started walking back to the festivities. Then I saw a woman running towards me screaming, "Oh my god, where's this child's parents!!" There were about eight of her in my vision. I had no idea what her problem was. I noticed I was walking as much laterally as I was forward. Then I remember touching my forehead with my right hand, and blood pouring into my eyes. After that, I felt my body fall backwards, and I passed out again.

The next time I woke up, what first came into focus was a small circle of beautiful blue sky. I couldn't understand why I didn't see more of it until a crowd, a circle of heads above me, all looking concerned, came into focus around that little circle. It was then I thought, "I must be really hurt" because in those days you had to be genuinely injured to attract that kind of turnout. My mom and I had to wait at the park entrance for a ride to the hospital. It was hot out, and I was parched. I remember being annoyed about the waiting. Climbing up on a fence and jumping off to pass the time, all with my head injury and possible concussion.

In the emergency room, I received six stitches to my forehead and zero painkillers for the procedure. I can still see the doctor's needle moving towards me, feel the pain, then see the needle move up and away, with the thread attached to me, then back down again, and pain, until the doctor was finished. The results were brutal: lumpy skin pinched haphazardly closed and thick black stitches. It looked as though I had done them myself, or Dr. Frankenstein, or Rambo. In lieu of being numbed, my mom cheer-leaded my bravery. As if complimenting the way one is handling torture assuages the victim. Compliments are nice. However, they do nothing for pain management. Instead of drugs, kids my age were promised ice cream after any trauma, and that actually worked. The promise of ice cream does indeed assuage the victim while she's being tortured. Decades later, the scar is just another age line on my forehead and now looks less like a third eye that was removed at birth.

There was the time I tried riding a yellow banana-boat skateboard down a steep suburban asphalt hill. My previous skateboarding experience was to take the thing up and down my flat driveway. I'd brought along the skateboard to a weekend overnight visit at a friend's place. I love that I thought I could go down a hill on the thing. I loved this time period of endless youthful courage, or ignorance.

Not very far down, the board started to vibrate violently under my feet. As it picked up speed, the vibrations were too much, and I decided to bail by jumping off. In order to jump off something, you inadvertently have to press against that thing. In the act of what I believed at the time to be a casual maneuver, my weight went into the board, the board flew out from under me, and for a very brief moment I was horizontal in the air. Then for a longer moment I slid down the rest of the hill on my right side, in short shorts and a T-shirt. By the time I stood up I'd burned a hole in my right ass cheek and elbow. It was some nasty road rash.

My friend and I walked back to her house to clean me up. There, her mother was pissed we'd be late to the swim club, so my friend patched me up with about thirty Band-Aids and zero adult help. That was a lot of pain, but I went to the swim club and probably had a great afternoon otherwise. Tattoos have long since covered those scars.

There's the scar from when my mother's father's second wife was trying to teach me to walk down the stairs. I was very, very short for a very, very long time and took stairs by stepping up with my right foot, then bringing my left foot up to my right, kind of like an aging butler. It annoyed adults. Maybe they thought I was going to stick with that moving forward, you know, for life, instead of thinking, she's a little tyke, her legs can't go one step each. At the time, it probably would have had me at full splits to do so. Nonetheless, my step-grandma took it upon herself to break me of this habit. She had the patience of Brie. The cheese. She didn't have any patience.

The stairs in question were covered in thick, burnt-red carpeting. That carpet was so plush my brothers and I would take sleeping bags, with a smooth nylon outside and deep quilted inside, and ride down the stairs toboggan style. Unfortunately, there was never enough room on the landing for us to stop properly and avoid hitting a wall. After a couple of crashes, we decided to wear winter hats to protect our heads and lined sofa pillows on the wall as our version of hay stoppers. My generation, pain didn't stop us from fun. Pain wasn't necessarily a negative experience, just an annoyance, like having to pee with a lot of cold-weather gear on.

Along the right side of the stairs was a black iron banister to keep people from falling off and onto the marble-tiled foyer floor. From the foyer, you walked up about five steps to the landing, which split off into a high-ceilinged living room that was used variously for furniture storage or as a place where three kids could do indoor sports and not get into trouble. If you turned left on the landing, there were 12 more steps to the upstairs. Going downstairs, that turn was challenging for me because of a gap in the banister at the landing that left nothing to hold onto. Heading down, I would stop at the last step before the landing and either not make the turn without an adult, or squat and butt ride it around the bend.

With my step-grandmother cheering on my three-year-old self by telling me I was, to paraphrase it, a wussy pain in the ass for hesitating at the turn, I cried and tried to do it. The banister gap wasn't finished with a nice flourish such as a curl or knob. It was just cut metal, and that's what it did: it sliced open my right pinky finger. I remember being in the bathroom with my step-grandmother washing out my cut and feeling quite happy about having been injured under her care. My concerns over tackling that corner alone had been vindicated. I still have that scar. It reminds me not to let other people rush me. Actually, it doesn't have any significance and I rarely ever think about it. But that incident did help foment a distrust towards authority, especially when my gut says otherwise.

My legs are a topographic history of a tomboy childhood, a life lived through the body by a mind that best understands things experientially. But I get it now. I don't want to wear handcuffs again as much as I don't want to ride a skateboard, as much as my student doesn't want a scar on her shoulder. It does seem like once something bad happens, it can happen again. My student who'd just gotten her first scar ever was upset at not having control over whether or not it happened the first time, and whether or not it would happen again. Not wanting what's already happened, equally upset about not having control over what's happened, and not wanting it to happen again. That was the story of my arrest, with its own emotional hangover, and then the fear of being arrested again. A fear can be like a scar, something you have forever. I absolutely feared being arrested again.

One of the first things I learned after graduating from college was to be leery of plain white envelopes with clear plastic windows. Crisp white envelopes sealed completely from corner to corner were always from student-loan offices. No matter how many times I moved, they were the first letters greeting me at my new place. Before cell phones and personal GPS, I had this theory that if I went missing, my family should just ask Sallie Mae or William D. Ford where I was because the people there knew how to find me.

With court just days away, I opened my mailbox to find a lone envelope, in the same white and windowed style, from the New York City Criminal Justice Agency. It was a reminder about my desk appearance. It also let me know that if I did not go to court, a warrant would be issued for my arrest. That was a good motivator. The letter was divided into two columns, with English on the left side and Spanish on the right. Just those two languages. The court appearance time on the letter was 9:30 am. The one I received from the police said 10:30 am. I'd already planned on being at the courthouse Black Friday sale early. I was hoping the DAT basket drop-off that Frankie had told me about meant this would be a first come, first served situation, like a deli counter, but for alleged criminals. If I got there early, could I get out of there early? Could I get out of there, period? I just wanted to get there and then get out of there. I didn't even want to be there. The letter wasn't as bad as those bright orange tickets under your car's windshield wiper, but it had the same effect: somber humiliation. I'd prefer not to be in correspondence with the criminal justice system. As I walked up the building stairs, I started scratching at my scalp before catching myself and breathing. It was just a piece of paper.

On Wednesdays, I usually had nothing in the morning, then clients in the evening. My schedule was clear enough that I could be in court until I needed to get back to let Buster out. I wasn't sure if that was an allowed reason to leave court, but I didn't have a dog walker. I liked walking my dog. Aside from scheduling issues, I was hoping (the secular version of praying) for bad weather because I can only dress nicely if it's chilly. And by nicely, I mean looking slightly not like a yoga teacher. Because I'm usually either going to practice yoga, have just practiced yoga, am heading to teach, or have just finished teaching, I have a bit of a lazy-Sunday look going on. This kind of snuck up on me, and it's harder to undo than it appears. After being seduced by comfortable clothes for the better part of two decades, my body now rejected constricting, form-fitted fabrics.

The last time I dressed professionally I had a landline and used a telephone book called the Yellow Pages, which had yellow pages, to look up business addresses and phone numbers. I'm past casual attire: I'm glorified laundry day. That's my fashion wheelhouse. Also, it's easier to cover my arm tattoos in chilly weather. Though I don't regret having had great artists draw on my skin with needles, I am often the recipient of strangers' unwarranted biases and unsolicited judgment about tattoos. While it's okay to spend five figures on a piece of animal skin that's been color dyed with a polluting runoff, sewn by slave labor, shipped to the States at a high carbon footprint, and is a nonessential item used maybe three times a year, having a pink lotus on my elbow that I'll wear every day for the rest of my life, so long as my arm is attached, is considered weird. My tattoos are references to art, books, spirituality, and beloved pets. There isn't anything on me about hate or death. Still, if you're tattooed at all, it's common to be grouped with all the people who are tattooed: gangs and criminals and devotees of ethnic cleansing. I thought it might be best to show up in court covered, looking like the nice Jewish girl from the Jersey suburbs that I am, under my skin.

Carrie, Jan's wife, got back to me:

On May 16, 2016, 11:22 am, Carrie wrote:

Hi Marcy! Sorry for the delayed response. I'm not a criminal lawyer (have only done civil stuff, and now focus on education law) and I don't have any personal recommendations here in the city for a criminal lawyer. One of my friends, who used to work for the district attorney's office, recommended this group... as having good defense lawyers. Hope this helps! Best, Carrie

And I responded:

On May 19, 2016, 2:25 pm, Marcy Tropin wrote:

Hi Carrie, Thanks! Hopefully that wasn't too... what is the yoga teacher doing asking about a criminal lawyer?? I promise it's nothing!! See you in class. -Marcy

If "What's the opposite of a criminal lawyer?" was a trivia question, I would never have guessed that the answer was "civil."

It seems like there's a lot of obvious information I don't carry around, don't know, or confuse, like fiction and nonfiction, wet and dry measurements, or how to spell words with "c" and "s" near one another. Here's what I do know: that a fathom is only six feet (so when people say "I can't fathom that," they have a limited imagination); that it's best to cough or sneeze into my elbow like the World Health Organization recommends (even though it's a odd gesture); the lyrics for Whitney Houston's "The Greatest Love of All" (but not one song from a band I listen to often); and the contraindications, modifications and counter-poses for a couple of hundred asanas. Normal, handy information doesn't stick. Sometimes, it feels like while I've been holed up in a room calling out poses for years and years, everyone else became an adult.

Tuesday, May 17, 2016

I had a panic attack on the way to my private client last night. It felt embarrassing to be a yoga teacher and have this issue. To feel as though I wasn't present in my body. To have a hard time being in my body. Since being arrested I'd felt more like I was in a constant state of fight or flight. The arrest plugged into my life and pulled a ton of wattage out, even on idle, while it was sitting in the back of my thoughts. I was an overburdened power cord. After my client I taught a group class. By the time I got home from work, it was after 10 pm, then I got up at 5 am to teach again.

My schedule wasn't helping. I couldn't process much beyond basic needs or let my nervous system get some real rest. I taught in the morning, then an afternoon class, had therapy, and headed home. It was a good decision not have scheduled an early morning private Wednesday, even though I pride myself on saying "yes" to my clients. Even though I like to earn a living. Regardless of how I was doing personally, I did need to pay my bills. So far, it looked like I would miss teaching one group class and a private. Court appearances could keep me from future work. If I worked less and let my arrest get ahead of me emotionally, I wouldn't be able to work much, shifting me towards becoming a lesser member of society, like an actual criminal. Thus, the justice system, by cornering a person's time and well-being, was a villainous enabler. I didn't feel inspired by due process. I didn't feel like it had my back. I felt like it was an affront.

It's like when I was applying for that no-doc mortgage back in 2006. I had the 20 percent down and excellent credit. But the bank quoted me a rate two percent higher than the national average, increasing the monthly payment by hundreds. When I asked why, the man in the suit said it was because I was a greater risk. So I suggested, "If I'm a greater risk then wouldn't it make more sense to have the payments easier on me?" The guy in the suit shrugged, and I took my business elsewhere. A higher rate, a bigger monthly payment, wouldn't have safeguarded against my defaulting on the loan. It increased the chances that I would. I ended up liking the idea of a rural country house more than the reality and sold it two seconds after buying. There is a theme here though, something along the lines of "we don't give a shit."

By the afternoon, I was anxious—anxious like 14 Chihuahuas in Michael Flatley's living room. It turned out it was a good idea to schedule therapy the day before my desk appearance. I'd been texting my shrink a lot since being arrested. I was needing a lifeline, to tell someone I wasn't doing well, so I could go to work and do my job. There's not a lot of room for falling apart when you're a yoga teacher, even though we have the same crap going on as our students. Well, hopefully none of my students had endured being arrested.

In therapy, my shrink asked me what would happen tomorrow. "Do you know what will happen at the DAT?" was competing against "Do you know any hip openers?" as the question I got asked most often. I couldn't wait until tomorrow actually happened, and I would have an answer to that question. Why were people asking me if I knew what would happen tomorrow? I'd never been arrested; they'd never been arrested. So if they didn't know, why would I know? I didn't know. I wanted to know. I wanted to know how it all worked and then do my own thing. I wanted it to be like using a microwave, where we have all these options—reheat, defrost, pizza, low, high, liquids—and most of us just push one one one "start." My shrink advised me not to say anything, especially if I was pulled aside by a detective. I'd already heard this suggestion, to shut up, which is funny advice from a person who professionally nudges people to talk.

After therapy, I trucked along to Mysore practice. The second I stepped on the mat, I was extremely tired. So I did what anyone would do after they'd gone through the trouble of getting to their workout and was confusing a long day with actual physical-well-being activity. I lied to myself. I told myself we only had to get through the 5A and 5B (Surya Namaskara) series in the beginning. Once that was done, I lied again to myself, "Well, you're warm now, just do the standing poses." After the standing sequence comes the fun stuff where you're twisting and binding and getting your stretch on. "Why miss dessert?" I thought, and kept on going. The primary series is long, and most weeks, you're supposed to practice everyday but Saturday. Sometimes, I break it up into small goals, like cleaning my apartment: do the vacuuming, check social media, put up a laundry, lie on the floor in a twist, take the garbage out, eat some dark chocolate. There's a difference between being mentally tired, emotionally drained, and physically spent. With the first two, you just practice.

Near the end of the primary series is a sequence of backbends: three wheels, standing up from the third wheel, then dropping back from standing into wheel, and coming back up to stand three times. Most practitioners, including myself, have had to really earn this transition. It's terrifying. Pushing off your hands from wheel and hoping the rest of your body works in unison to lift you into an upright standing position requires a lot of breaking through fears, not just physical strength. Because I have a healthy sense of self-preservation, in the beginning the whole thing seemed to be an ill-advised, illogical pursuit. Once you stand, though, it is a sincere "woohoo" achievement.

After the three drop backs, you stand with your hands on your shoulders, arms crossed on your chest, like a corpse, and wait for the teacher. The teacher comes over, you make eye contact, and then she holds your hips lightly and dips you backwards as far back as you can go, arms still across your chest, then brings you up. There are three of these: halfway back, up, halfway back, up, halfway back, up. It's the yoga equivalent of the trust fall. After that, you drop back one more time into full wheel while the teacher counts five breaths in Sanskrit (you can't really hear this), while in English she's saying, "Walk your hands in, walk your hands in, walk your hands in." This inspires you to go deeper into the backbend. Speaking for myself, I never want to walk my hands in. I feel like whatever I'm doing is worthy enough, but since she's asking nicely I'll move my hands a teeny tiny bit closer. After the fifth count, you get pulled back up to standing, feeling grateful to be alive.

Because ashtanga is the yoga version of Ginsu knives, after that last wheel, wait, there's more. Backbending finished, you sit down for paschimottanasana, a seated forward bend with legs straight out in-front, touching. The teacher walks behind you, kneels down, and lies on your back, slowly squishing you, all the way forward, chest to thighs. The first time I experienced this, it was a guy resting his weight on me, and I wondered if I was being cognizant of the moment before becoming a quadriplegic. Lying there, smushed into myself, I imagined a future where I'd be telling people who are wiping drool from my chin and draining my piss bag that I had a feeling right before it happened, which is right now.

In the mindset of going to court tomorrow, with all my fears and anxieties in tow, I attempted my first wheel and felt like someone had stabbed me in the belly. The second, it was like my belly was being torn open, shredded. I took a break after the two, lying on the mat, staring at the cracks in the plaster, rubbing my poor belly. The third wheel was fine, but I didn't stand up. I went for a forth and stood up.

The belly is where the third chakra is located: manipura, your power center. Whenever people have stress, it's usually stored there. Tension accumulates around the base of the neck. But if your boss is making your work life miserable and you feel powerless, your belly is going to kill you. Except you might not feel it until you have lower back pain. Because we're three-dimensional objects, anything going on in your belly affects your lower back. The belly is the front of the lumbar spine.

When I work with people who have bulging or herniated disks, I dig into their bellies first. If those muscles are tight, they are shorter, pulling the spine's lordotic curve flat. Once the lumbar spine starts being pulled straight, you risk having bulging disks followed by herniation. I can cure back pain by slowly working through the belly. It's challenging, though. Not just the pain, but the frustration and anger it brings up. People love having their shoulders mushed. Pain there can be superficial. Emotionally, back pain is deeper, stuffed down emotions. While it might seem harmful to keep moving myself through wheel pose, I know the importance of releasing those muscles and the relief I'll feel afterward. Desiring to be free of the tightness in my body more than I wanted to do a fancy pose, I practiced the wheels slowly, never pushing or being aggressive with my body, breathing into the space.

Afterwards, I wanted to connect with my teacher, so I leaned on the doorway of the practice room again, giving the universal sign for "Please come talk to me!" She came over, and we crouched down to speak quietly, her facing the students, keeping an eye on everything. The etiquette for these exchanges is to speak like Hemingway wrote: in short, tight, quick, to-the-point sentences. This is not my forte. Anytime I have to get to the point fast, I start sounding like Kate Winslet accepting an award, all out of breath and bemused.

I told my teacher I was going to court the next morning to hear the charges against me, but hopefully wouldn't be going to jail because I was bringing a friend along for bail. I said that I planned on coming to the afternoon practice and namaste. There was a pause. Yoga teachers hear lots and lots of personal stuff. Students feel comfortable and safe sharing with us. This, though, was probably the first time a student had said to her, "If I'm not in jail, I'll see you in the afternoon." She laughed and said, "At least you ended on a good note. You're just making a circle from here to there to here. It's an auspicious day tomorrow: the anniversary of our teacher Guriji's death." I asked if "auspicious" meant it was a good thing I was going to court on the day he died, or a bad thing. Maybe I'd confused "auspicious" with "suspicious." We stared into the room, watching students practice, my teacher thinking of a synonym for auspicious, and me wondering if we had, indeed, ended on a good note.

On the way home from practice, I strategized about my court outfit. Working from the base layer out, I thought I should probably wear a real bra, not one of the stretchy bralettes I prefer. There's a special place in my heart for the disdain I feel towards contemporary corsets. A proper bra, going back to the time of the greeks, simply wraps around breasts. These modern things are terrible. They remind me of how long ago men in advertising made women's underarm hair "objectionable" in order to sell powders and eventually razors.

Since a shirt over a women's bare-breasted chest is not acceptable in our patriarchal society, which has sexualized every part of a woman's body it can get its hands on and governed the rest, women are obliged to wear a bra. No matter that there are quantities of men who have larger breasts than I do, it's only women's boobs that aren't allowed to move freely under fabric. Sure, bras can be supportive for heavy chests, but for most women, they don't need to wear one. What if humans had to keep everything that moved freely under clothing locked-down, like testicles? It's as logical to make women wear bras as it would be to have a man wear a mini holster for his balls. Judging by how much time in public guys reorganize themselves, maybe they should wear something that keeps the boys in place. If it seems ridiculous to suggest men wear a device that contains their anatomy and causes discomfort, why isn't it the same for women?

How do bras work? With a constrictive band strapped around the rib cage, equally constrictive loops over each shoulder, and fastening in the back with itty-bitty hooks—hooks so small that four of them can fit in a row on a piece of one-inch fabric. But the breasts themselves, they're not completely covered. The cups usually start mid-mammary gland, because while it's not okay that they be seen moving freely, it's most welcome that they be seen. Breasts are ideally presented by being pushed up, forward, and held there via wires and padding. Never mind the childish obsession with cleavage, where the girls are framed against one another to attain a shadowy line between them. Breasts don't naturally move towards one another. In reality, boobs hang, sway, and just peter out in place, each side with its own mood and bearing.

It makes you wonder what the real purpose of a modern bra is. Is it to keep breasts contained, or to present them like hors d'oeuvres at a (pun intended) cocktail party? Presentation aside, the design of the bra restricts arm movement, causes shoulders to round forward, and inhibits breathing. Breathing is the act of bringing oxygen into the lungs to stay alive. If you place your hands around your rib cage and take a breath, there's a natural expansion as air enters the lungs. The ribs need to open to let air in. Imagine trying to blow up a balloon while holding it tightly in your hands. It won't expand. It won't inflate. Same goes with the ribs and your lungs. For me, the difference in rib circumference when I inhale and exhale is about two inches. However, bras don't expand two inches. You purchase them at 32 inches, or whatever, and that's it. You can wear the band loose around your ribs, but then your boobs annoyingly slip under the cups.

Women shouldn't have to wear a bra unless they want to wear a bra. Want to look sexy, awesome! There should be a very appreciative select individual—or individuals—in a woman's life who she chooses to show off her chest to. Not a boss, and not someone who happens to be standing over her on the subway. This constant, never-ending, marketing, and monetizing of the male gaze, fetishizes and objectifies women's bodies. It also takes the fun out of dressing up.

The other thing that takes the fun out of dressing up for me is unpleasant memories. People seem to like dressing up to be seen. I loathe being seen. After being tricked many times as a child into dressing rooms, where boundaries were crossed, and the lure of new clothing was an excuse to have me undress, I'm resistant to repeat anything close to that process as an adult. When in the early 80s clothing was worn loose, I adopted the trend with great fervor, wearing bagging jeans that dangled on my waist and were held up by thick black leather belts, oversized T-shirts I could tuck all the way into my socks, and men's extra large college sweatshirts on top. My association with being gazed upon was shameful and negative. I hid in clothing. I hid my body in clothing.

This changed when I became a yoga teacher. The first private I taught was in July of 2001. I was broke and couldn't afford any real yoga clothing, so one of my mentors gave me her hand-me-downs. Since I couldn't afford the subway, I rode my bicycle from 89th Street on the Upper East Side all the way down to the Lower East Side, below Houston Street, to what was then a very quiet and not-yet-developed part of the city. My student was a banker who raced boats. He had a whole room to work out in, with a mirror of walls. It was the first of many fancy exclusive homes I'd enter as a private yoga teacher.

For my client's first down dog, I went to spot him by standing at the front of the mat and resting the palms of my hands below his lower back. Then I leaned into him a bit to take the weight off his shoulders. In the mirrored wall to my left, my attention was distracted by a colorful, moving object. I looked over and realized it was me. I was wearing a fitted, red-capped, short-sleeved shirt, and tight purple bell-bottom yoga pants. I needed to blink for a second to reconcile my reality with that of the woman dressed as her favorite Care Bear character, Hopeful Heart Bear, with her hands pressing professionally close to a guy's butt. Then with a squint and a sigh, I surrendered to the whole thing and went back to teaching. Thus started my career in form-fitting comfort clothing.

Teaching yoga often requires demonstrating the proper alignment to students. Alignment in yoga poses fosters safety. It's also a way to free oneself. Maybe you're slumping your shoulders to protect your heart, or maybe you sit for hours hunched over in a chair reading. Maybe you do both. Yoga can help you release this emotional and physical tightness. By focusing on using my body as a guide to help others, I ended up healing myself. It became easier to be looked at. Still, at times when I had to wear something to be seen in, even if it was just to appear presentable, old anxieties would surface.

Even though I had a healthier, newfound association with my body in public, I wasn't exempt from judgment. As the person standing in front of a room of mostly female students on the Upper East Side of Manhattan—ground zero for the image conscious—I'd receive comments that were meant to be complimentary. It was a double standard between women: the assumption it was okay to make unsolicited lascivious observations to one another under the guise of flattery. These were the same remarks we accuse men of inappropriately making. Knowingly hypersensitive about body, I'd do my best to brush these comments off. It was objectifying though, no matter the intention.

In the case of showing up for court, I was going to lasso my breasts and wear a bra because without shoulders—and I'm not sure how my arms are attached to my body—if I wore a button-down shirt with my close-cropped hair and my preteens in a bralette, I would be called "sir" all day long. That gets old. It could also be unhelpful if I was in an environment surrounded by police and they couldn't get my attention because they were using the wrong pronoun.

While I hadn't drunk the Kool-Aid and purchased a $60 "most comfortable bra" (that's oxymoronic), I did have both a tan and black one, deep in my closet, ready for when the occasion called for it. I thought I'd go with the black one, only because it was on top. Then I moved onto the next layers, choosing a dark grey button-down shirt and adding an old, shaggy, long, well-loved black cardigan over. I'd finish off the outfit with black dress pants and slip-on loafers I found and didn't even realize I owned. I wasn't sure how they got into my closet; they were probably wondering the same thing. The ensemble would make me look like I wanted to work on Wall Street many, many years ago, but instead wound up doing payroll for a department store. I didn't want to look severe or laid back, and a cardigan assuaged those concerns. It was all about the friendly cardigan.

Once home from practice and outfit ruminating, I let Buster out, grazed from the refrigerator, and parked myself on the sofa with the dog. I was mentally spent and was goofing around online to let my mind unwind, when Nancy texted me:

NANCY: Marcy, What's the room # where I'm to meet you tmrw?
ME: They haven't provided a room number. I'm going very early in the hope/s that it's first come first served and I can save you some time...and me. When I know the room, I will text you immediately. You are meeting me

where they handle DATs. If we don't connect by 9:30...hmmm, we should have a plan. Any ideas?
NANCY: Yes. Text is the best way I agree.

That wasn't really an answer, but she was probably more beat than I was. Monday and Tuesdays are her long days in the chair.
ME: You will be there by 9:30, correct?
NANCY: Ummm...if they don't start hearing cases til 10:30, I figured I'd get there a half hr early, at 10

When did we decide they hear cases at 10:30 am? When did we start using the phrase "hear cases?"

ME: I don't know when they start hearing cases. But okay. I'm just going to assume: a) they don't allow phone usage for some reason, and b) my case is heard first and I'm in jail. I will try to text you anything I know...see you hopefully at 10 xo

Feeling a little guilty about this huge favor, I was also equally annoyed by having to repeatedly negotiate whether I needed her at court. I decided to change course in both feeling and content.

ME: BTW...I'm soooo happy you are going to be there. Relieved and feeling loved
NANCY: I'm glad!

It was after 9 pm, a good time to motivate, leave the sofa, shower, and do the things I normally do before bed. When I got up, though, my back said, "Hey, remember me?" I was sore, which is not why they call it Mysore, as in boy am "my sore," but should be. The nice thing about getting old is not having to wait until the next day to feel achy. It happens immediately. While in the shower, I thought about bail. Nancy and I hadn't discussed amounts. I decided I should text her the question, get it out in the open. Before I did, I picked at my face, attacking it for a good solid ten minutes. Worrying about court tomorrow, not having a better outlet for the the double-order of anxiety, manifested itself in a form of self-harm. I didn't feel guilty though. Sometimes, I think the only pleasure left in life is the home facial. Face red, I headed to the kitchen, and made a warm bowl of maple and brown sugar oatmeal. Comfort food. Then I texted Nancy:

> ME: btw, out of curiosity, how much bail is our friendship worth?

The flashing etcetera bubble started immediately, which concerned me. Did she already have a figure in mind? Once I asked a friend, way back in college, if I could borrow a chunk of money. I'm not sure, but I think this is when my car disappeared for six weeks and then turned up parked a block away from where I'd left it. No tickets, but an additional 3,000 something miles on the odometer. I didn't have theft insurance or the money for another car, so I might have been asking for that reason. No one ever figured out why or how my car disappeared and then reappeared, and in my circle of friends, it was an intriguing mystery. I always suspected an ex of mine with keys had something to do with it. She had been suspiciously aghast—"Wait, you don't have theft coverage?"—over the phone, and my car materialized not long after. My friend told me in a beautiful handmade card I still have, that our friendship, while cherished, was worth a hundred bucks.

> NANCY: Hmm...give me a minute til I find my calculator
> ME: FYI your calculator is in the same device you are holding

I decided to leverage my usefulness in Nancy's and her husband's lives. We'd been down this road before. Every time my life fell apart, often necessitating a place to crash, I'd be in their apartment's second bedroom. During one particularly bad stretch of luck, I needed a co-signer on a loft. The building's broker did a rental history check and called me to ask, "Why didn't you tell us you were evicted and a marshal had to come have you removed?" *What?!* I remember taking a long pause and using the most adult voice I had to say that I had never been evicted nor had a marshal forcibly remove me. Even though I proved it was a friend of a friend who took over my lease five apartments ago and didn't get the hint when housing court evicted her, a paperwork error, tee-hee, the building still wanted a cosigner.

Nancy and her husband graciously cosigned the lease for me. In exchange, I agreed to be their bitch for a year. That's exactly what I offered: "I'll be your bitch for a year." Agreed! It worked well for all of us. I had a place to live, and they had endless IT support. I also helped them sell an old car to a man from Russia, even though we lost the title, went to a car dealership and negotiated the purchase of a new one (awakening the skills my mother had bestowed upon me), and found a buyer for the piano hogging up space in their living room. While each of those was a fun, crazy experience, I really loved hearing people test their piano. I'd sit quietly nearby, enraptured by the private recital. It was really charming.

ME: For every minute I'm in jail, you lose a year of asking tech questions.

Sometimes you have to look at a coin to know its value.

NANCY: See I said that on purpose cuz I knew u'd say that!!

NANCY: Ha! Gotcha!

Well, that didn't work.

ME: Like I said, feeling loved and relieved.

Nancy is the only person I asked for help, the first person I called when I got out of the holding cell, the first person I always call. My own family? At this point in my life, I didn't speak to any of them.

If you tell someone you don't speak to your father, which I don't, it's a stand-alone sentence. There's rarely a follow-up question. It's like when I tell people I'm from New Jersey, and then there's silence. If you say you don't speak to your mother, like I don't, people will offer their opinions. I've caught a lot of crap for not speaking to my mom. Though I'd prefer to remain private about it in casual conversation, people usually offer intrusive advice: "You should talk to her, I bet she'd like to hear from you." That's often led to me telling one horror story or another just to pipe someone down. You don't stop speaking to a parent because they're awesome, especially if it's your mom. I also wasn't in touch with my brothers. The last time I talked to my oldest brother, I emailed him to say he was a dick, and insulted his wife. The last thing my middle brother said to me was that I was a piece of garbage. He said it over and over again until I abruptly ended the call. In my family, there was so much water under the bridge, the bridge had long ago flooded and washed away. The tides never receded.

I was going through one hell of a milestone in my life and had zero contact with anyone in my family, extended or immediate. Usually, I found this equally sad and weird. The sadness of my failed familial relationships permeated everything, it was always there. The weirdness in how all of our lives were progressing, growing, and moving in various directions, without inclusion. Nephews and nieces were getting older and having their own first milestones, which I hoped had nothing to do with being arrested, and I missed out on those events. It was safer and healthier for me to keep my distance. It was also, in its way, selfish and isolating. There wasn't a way to resolve the situation where I could live a happy life and have them in it. Thus, I relied on friendships for courage, love and support.

Uttanasana at Wall

← BUTT @ wall
→ straight or bent knees

head on blocks

5-10 minutes

- release, bend knees, roll up to stand.
- or widen feet and squat down.

feet hip distance

not good for bad backs!
(maybe legs up the wall instead)

Wednesday, May 18, 2016 DAT

I'd slept like a rotisserie chicken, turning round and round, as if each side of my body was only allowed to touch the bed for a certain amount of time before it was done. Buster didn't sleep either and was a hot mess of position indecision throughout the night, waking me each time he moved with a noisy "ho-hum" exhale before plopping down. I woke at 1 am, 4 am, 5 am, then again at 6 am, when the alarm went off. Restless with hypothetical possibilities, I told myself all I would be doing in court was hearing the charges. Still, I didn't want to be in a room full of people, even if they were strangers, hearing anything to do with harming a child—an accusation that upset me greatly—attached to my name. I didn't want to be in an environment where charges and crimes were common. To experience lessened anonymity via public negativity. Hope checked in on me, and we exchanged texts. She was in Virginia, getting ready for her daughter's wedding. We were both full of nerves, but on opposite emotional ends. Hers joy and mine fear.

I was anxious about getting to the location, 100 Centre Street, at the bottom of Manhattan. The buildings down there look like they were dropped randomly in place from above. It's below the grid and hard to navigate. It would be rush hour, too. This was a part of town where the subway looked far away from where you needed to go, when it was actually a short walk. Some maps and locations don't match. That's true of Berlin, where wherever you are and wherever you want to go, the distance isn't walkable. It looks like it is on the map, but things are really a day trip away from one another. The opposite happens in Venice, where everything on the map looks far away from everything else, but if you take two steps, you miss three streets because the place is so tiny. Washington D.C. is spread out and not advisably walkable. Boston is completely walkable. Chicago? Nope, don't walk. Paris? Walk. London? Walk, but look in the opposite direction when crossing. In Barcelona, you walk a little, then have a rest and a drink. In Amsterdam, you bicycle. Sometimes, you can't find a correlation between map keys and reality. Sometimes, you just have to go to a place and find out for yourself. First, I would find the court building, then I would find the room. Well, first I would ask which room, because it wasn't on any printed material. Then I would find out where it was.

There was probably a little agoraphobia at play. If I was awoken in the middle of the night to teach an impromptu yoga class for hundreds of students in Central Park, I'd be game. While public speaking is the number one fear for most people, I love it. People. Listening. That's a great idea!! And I can tell them about yoga! Even when I've messed up, it's been glorious. Like the time when I was on a platform, at the front of the room, teaching a packed class how to jump back into chaturanga. During the demo I realized that my core had been preoccupied with keeping gas from releasing. Either I used my abs to land gracefully or I crashed. I had to make this decision while my hands were on the mat and the rest of my body was in mid-air. After nailing a perfect chaturanga, and making a sound that should never be heard in a yoga class, I turned to my students and said, "Like that, except without the farting."

For my 40th birthday I did a bucket list challenge that included going to an open mic night at a comedy club. When friends asked me if I was scared, I said no. I told them it was five minutes long. How bad could it get for five minutes? I've subbed for very popular yoga teachers whose students either left when I came in or death-stared me from beginning to end. To win them over I'd try doing a very complicated and challenging sequence, only to look at the clock and see a mere seven minutes had passed. When an entire class hates you, you're stuck in that room with them for an hour—at least—without alcohol and a two drink minimum. If you want to survive bombing at stand-up, try sucking as a yoga teacher first.

In order to teach yoga you need to like to talk. I was raised by people who've never heard a silence they couldn't comment on. We like to talk. However, talking is not the same as being heard is not the same as being listened to is not the same as doing what you're told. If you have 30 students in a class and 20 percent do exactly what you tell them to do, you've won the lottery. Not everyone gleans information from verbal direction. If you don't get over that quickly, you won't last two months teaching yoga. At concerts when the singer is in a groove and tells the audience to, "Put your hands together," I'm thinking, "Good luck with that." You gotta pantomime the action, or you can just keep saying the same thing over and over again. Or you can yell at the crowd to do it. Some do try that approach.

Yelling at people doesn't work in either environment, yoga or music venues. There are 12 different intelligences. Teaching, I'll start with verbal cues, then add visual ones by demonstrating. Then I'll run over to the students who are most likely to injure themselves and move their legs to the right positions. Without even asking, I'll just grab a leg before it snaps, holding the joint in one hand, keeping it stable, and easing the rest of the leg into the right place. Then I'll run over to the students who are second most likely to injure themselves. Grabbing body parts before liability concerns is a modern-day form of kinesthetic learning. There's a lot of responsibility and fast decisions happening during class, beyond holding the space for students energetically. I don't find it overwhelming. It seems like I should, but I enjoy it too much. However, simply going to a new place for an amount of time I have no control over, can overwhelm me.

Before heading to court, I was sitting at my desk in the bedroom, looking at a zoomed-in map of downtown Manhattan. Trying to familiarize myself with the area, to ease my nerves. Out of the corner of my eye, I noticed Buster. He was across the little hall, in the bathroom, sitting on the bath mat. Usually, he'd be cozy on the bed, watching me until he fell back to sleep.

I got up and walked over to the bathroom, crouching down near the doorway and reaching my hands out. He walked over to me, head low. I rubbed the area at the base of his neck. He loves that. He came a little closer, resting his head against my legs. I put my head on him and continued massaging. He started making swallowing noises. Sometimes he does this when he's just found the perfect snuggle position, and the swallowing sounds self-satisfied. Sometimes he does it when he wants to get my attention, because staring me down hasn't worked. He was doing it now because he was nervous. When Buster's nervous, it'll be a very slow pace of swallowing. Sometimes I forget how connected he is to me. I forget how connected we are. He feels what I'm feeling even if I don't know what I'm feeling. As I massaged him, he was pushing his head into me for security. He knew something was up.

On the subway ride down to Centre Street, I wondered if it was inappropriate to ask other people at court why they were there. In television and movies, the newbies at jail get schooled about asking why their fellow inmates are incarcerated. It seems like a good icebreaker, better than "Where'd ya grow up?" or "Whaddya like to wear before the government-issue onesie?" I transferred to an express train after one stop. The C to the A to the 1 train was my plan. The subway cars were packed. It was standing room only, filled with morning commuters. I was listening to McClure's voice mail from yesterday. I hadn't gotten around to hearing it and now realized it was a gift, because her Southern Kentucky voice was a big hug, asking how I was doing, saying the whole thing was "foolish." For a moment, I had her love and comfort in the car with me.

On the train, I looked like any other person going to work. The regular bra was annoying, but my boobs looked stellar. There they were, all hoisted up for the day. Some time ago, I purchased two pairs of black dress pants during a sale because I didn't own any, and they both fit well. It was too rare an opportunity to pass up, even though I really hadn't any use for them. One pair was a lighter weight and stopped above the ankles, good for warmer weather. The other, heavier-cut pants went past the ankles. I would have never guessed I'd be wearing the lightweight pants for a court appearance. While I did blend in on the train, I didn't feel like myself. It felt like someone else had laid out my clothes for me the night before. I realized I kind of liked it better when I was on these packed trains, with everyone else wearing business casual, and me in yoga clothing, feeling pretty damn good about my career choice. I didn't know I had such an ego about relaxed wear.

Manhattan Criminal Court, 100 Centre Street, is a large building with multiple entrances, all leading to an intense security screening process. There were law-enforcement officers with military gear every couple of feet. They were mostly middle-aged white men who weren't in great shape, but who carried themselves as though they were. Maybe it was because of the weapons they were carrying, or the concerns. I didn't want to see this. I was still fearful of the police, uneasy around them. Their energy wasn't normal. All day long, every workday, they were trying to prevent something bad from happening inside this courthouse. It wasn't personal that they had to look at me as a potential threat. It felt personal, though. What was it like to spend your days trained looking for danger? To gauge whether that lady in the black cardigan was carrying a gun, secretly tucked into her lower back, or just picking her pants out from between her cheeks? Was there a way to protect, and stay focused and prepared, without seeing your community as the enemy? Since it was a courthouse, not an airport, actual criminals were entering, heightening the environment. It was like TSA's big brother.

Crap. I realized I was wearing metal cuff links. I had never worn cuff links, nor owned them. But I accidentally bought a fancy shirt online that required them. At the time I was like, "Grey, goes with everything, cheap, click." When the shirt arrived, I spent an embarrassing amount of time questioning why the cuffs were double in length. Finally, I folded them over and realized the buttonholes matched and that I needed to buy another thing to keep them together. I didn't mean to wear cuff links, but this morning I was, and now they would set the metal detector off, and I would have to remove them. They did look snazzy though, as if I intended to wear such a style shirt when it really was an accident.

When I walked through the metal detector, it made a yawning noise, and I got pulled over. An officer took me aside to move a special device around my person. It looked like a seismic meter, or the kind of thing used by a scientist in a horror movie to confirm whatever unorthodox activity was happening, that would, eventually, gruesomely, kill them all. The officer made a side to side, up and down motion. I pretended he was blessing me. The handheld device picked up the metal on my wrist, and then nothing else, of course.

With the all clear, I grabbed my bag from the end of the conveyer belt, and took the officer's directions to head down the hall, to the left. I made it to the DAT room by 9:24 am. I wanted to get there earlier, but it turned out it was fine. Mine was the third piece of paper in the pile, in the basket. There was an actual basket on an old wooden table. After I dropped my paper in, I thought they'd be pulling from the top anyways, so maybe being the last one to arrive meant being the first one heard.

While I was looking for a seat, there was a woman pleading guilty for stealing clothing. The judge was a woman. The room was lightly filled. I sat to the right of the aisle. The place was laid out like a church. The room was large, with vaulted ceilings. Everything was brown. There were eight dark, heavy wooden pews on each side of an aisle, leading to a chain and wooden fence dividing those waiting for redemption and forgiveness from those who would dole or deny it.

Your honor, the judge, sat high in her pulpit, her desk situated above the people. In a district attorney's area to the judge's right, young, well-dressed cell-phone-watching DA assistants moved folders around and answered questions. They had a couple of computers, and the largest copier I'd ever seen. The DA's area was positioned between the judge and where defendants would stand with their lawyers when addressing the court. It seemed like they were keeping people from directly accessing justice. Each area was equipped with a microphone. On the judge's left stood a section of chairs, perhaps for juries. Behind those chairs a secret door in the wall led to holding cells. The only windows lined one wall of the courtroom, at the top, where light cast down onto the proceedings. The motifs were too religious to be coincidental.

With the proceedings already happening, it felt like I was late to a performance. I immediately needed to pee, but I didn't want to miss my name being called. The two guys behind me were loudly talking and cursing. I wanted to do the movie theater thing where I gave them a half-turnaround disgusted glance, but this wasn't the audience where one should test social norms. The next woman up had multiple long braids down her back. How long did it take to make those braids? Could they stay in for days? That was a nice trick. I didn't see my neighbor, but I also didn't think she was supposed to be here. The judge was threatening the braid woman with not wanting to see her in court again. Lots of fines were being handed out.

I moved to a closer pew. The DAT pile had been taken from the basket. It seemed like you could have a friend put your paper in there and maybe act on your behalf. I checked the time. Nancy wasn't due for a half hour. It felt like I was on an interview, getting to see all the other interviewees apply before me. My pits were wet with nerves. It wasn't as crowded as I thought it would be. Next up was a third-degree assault, with a blond-haired woman appearing before the judge. She knew her number. People seemed to know their case numbers. The blond-haired woman had fought in a club, proving it really is better to stay in at night. It was a pain in the ass for every one to unhook and then re-hook the chain at the fence. Each time, the court was stalled waiting. I bet it wasn't fire-code safe.

All the court officers were wearing bulletproof vests. What about the rest of us? I couldn't wait to see Nancy. I was assuming there would be a moment where I talked to a public defender assigned to my case. The judge looked like the redhead from the show ER—the doctor who used a cane. Looking around, the public defenders and DA-area grunts seemed very attractive. Like 90s TV law show attractive. They wore smart suits and looked well coiffed, exercised and shiny. It was a contrast to the vibe and color palette of the place. I thought I heard my name, but it was another word. My heart dropped. The next woman up also stole. She was told that her case would be sealed if there were no further arrests within six months, and ordered to sign up for a day of community service. Okay, I got it. People who committed crimes and were admitting to them were being taken care of first. Was I going to have to pay a fine or do community service? *Hmmm.*

Given how nervous I was to hear my name called, I could empathize with people who were waiting to hear if they'd won an award. Unlike me, though, they would want to hear their names. There's a whole lot of hearing your heartbeat prior to that. Also, I was positive my name was going to be called. I didn't have to worry about it being someone else's name. I was a shoo-in. There was a slight lull in between defendants. When there weren't proceedings, there were the sounds of papers being shuffled, stapling, things the mic picked up. I was trying to breathe and pretend I was getting ready to teach. That version of me is calmer and confident. I can't say I'm ever truly calm, but I would have preferred to be teaching. Timothy something was called. He was a young white guy with mussy, short curly hair. A lawyer walked him out of the courtroom. Good, you did get a one-on-one beforehand. Didn't it always seem like guys named Timothy got into trouble?

There was a plaque near the basket that said the front row was for attorneys and police officers only. Reserved seating. The braid woman was called again. Kate something. The back of her head was shaved near the bottom. Been there, done that. She was very thin, wearing a black jean jacket and black jeans with the belt undone, her jeans hanging low over a long blue shirt. I would have buckled my belt just for this occasion. She had a tattoo on her right thumb. Would this be me in five years? Or me without yoga? What was I doing here? I didn't steal clothing, have a fight at a club, or even "hit a child." The doors opened, and more attractive attorneys entered. Who knew these people were so stylish? It was almost like a catwalk when they headed down the aisle.

It was nearing 9:50 am. I'd been giving Nancy text updates, and deliberately not asking her where she was so we wouldn't fight. But every time the doors swung open, I looked back like I was waiting for a friend at a movie theater as the lights were dimming. A young man dropped his DAT in the basket. He was wearing grey sweatpants and a green zippered cardigan that was unzipped halfway down the front. I wasn't sure about the sweatpants. I mean, everyone is entitled to their look. But shouldn't you do the best version of your look for a court appearance? When did grey sweatpants become presentable? It was like he was squeezing in his arraignment between working out and an afternoon nap. Maybe it was a young thing. It seems like one day I woke up and suddenly there were people half my age that weren't toddlers or kids. They were in college. I became old when my friend's teenage son looked at me as his mom's friend. Oh right, I was closer to her age than his. He saw me as belonging to her world, the world of adults.

Apatia didn't even tell me there would be a woman judge. It probably wouldn't make a difference. A woman appeared out of the secret side door to exchange paperwork with the DA grunts. The judge asked about "notices" and recommendations for release. Another lawyer came in, headed to the DA area at the fence, grabbed a file and said a name out loud. A young white guy acknowledged the name. The lady lawyer looked patient and kind. I hoped I would get her. It was like I was shopping. I could feel my shoulders high up near my ears. This was both to keep the bra straps from falling (fucking bras) and from tension (fucking tension).

The next guy up was in a brown North Face down coat with a grey hoodie underneath, and light grey jeans. He wore the coat hanging low off his shoulders. I didn't think he was doing that because he was warm. I thought it was a look, to wear your jacket low in the back, like a shawl. His bail was set at $3,000. He had three felony convictions and a slew of other arrest records I couldn't hear because during the reading there was a collective gasping. I guessed this was what they meant by a rap sheet. His appointed attorney was trying to get him out of jail until the court date. He turned around to the back of the court, maybe looking for a friend or loved one. He was older than I would have thought from the outfit. His beard was grey; his left ear was pierced. He had really sad eyes, already pleading his case.

The next guy was wearing a suit and was flanked by two women. It looked like he'd hired attorneys. "Yes," he agreed to the charges of unlicensed driving. "Are you pleading guilty because you are guilty?" the judge asked. "Yes," he replied. "Are you pleading guilty of your own free will?" "Yes." Then the judge asked a longer question I didn't catch. The guy looked to his attorney before making the one-word answer "yes." The judge gave him a fine.

The young white guy who left with the public defender had returned. They'd been gone for what seemed like enough time to discuss what happened. Some of my anticipation and anxiety had worn off. It was feeling real now to be in the courtroom. Eventually, I was going to have my own hallway conversation and hear my options. A big guy in a leather jacket was up. He received two fines: one was $75. He was also driving a vehicle without a license. He had to answer the same questions as the other guy, "…giving up the right to a trial." The judge rattled off a statement fast, mentioning something about being deported.

In order of importance, the things on my mind were really needing to pee, my name being called, and where Nancy was. It was 10:06 am, and they did hear cases before 10:30 am. I knew that now. Maybe these weren't my type of case, but things were being heard. And as I was listening to them, Nancy appeared at the pew's edge, saying, "I just went through a few wrong doors." I was happy to see her and thanked her profusely for coming. I was almost crying. She held my wrist and squeezed it. She sat down and took in the surroundings.

Next up was a very young-looking guy, perhaps even a kid. Substance abuse was the charge. "It's for work," he explained. "I'm a freelance photographer." There was some conversation about police noticing a substance. I couldn't really hear what was going on. What was this substance reference? What did being a freelance photographer have to do with this substance? It was the most interesting crime of the morning, and I had missed the narrative. They picked a court date. I leaned into Nancy and told her I looked like a gallerist. She cracked up, saying "Yes!!" I asked her if she'd brought any reading material or things to do for herself. She had, but she wanted to look around for a bit. It was interesting to her. And it was interesting. I pointed out the public defender I hoped to have—the fashionable yet warm-vibed lady.

At the podium, the defendants who came from jail or perhaps its central booking (this must have been where the sergeant was threatening to take me when I was first arrested) all stood with their hands behind their backs while addressing the judge. Now the lingo was becoming familiar, I could pick out sentences. After the judge asked her routine of questions about defendants being absolutely sure they agreed to the charges, she then ended with, "Good luck to you." She seemed to only say this to people when their cases were over. She said it to a guy with two neck tattoos and time served, maybe for arson. It was nice that she said that. Suddenly, Nancy yelled "shhhh" to quiet the courtroom chatter, and I scolded her. Like me, she thought we were at a movie theater. We moved up two pews to be closer to the action. She was having a very different experience than I was. I didn't want to move because I liked the mojo of the middle pew, but the two guys in front of us couldn't whisper when they spoke. No matter how many times we were asked by the police to keep quiet and stop talking, they went on speaking at a regular volume.

It was 10:16 am. Nancy was sitting to my left with her sweater and bags between us. She's of the age where you carry your nice purse and then you carry along a well-worn, free with your subscription, tote stuffed with crap. She was leaning forward, completely engaged in the goings-on. Nancy moved her stuff to get a better view of the judge. Her posturing was exactly like she was at the theater, wanting a good view of each character when they had lines, moving over this way when the DA had the mic, that way when it was the judge. Then she leaned into me to say that when The Good Wife character was demoted, she worked in a place like this, so she knows all about it. I wasn't familiar with the show. It was like a field trip for her. Having already found the proceedings repetitious, I was moving from anxiety to boredom. I texted my shrink with an update. While I was looking down at my phone, I heard, "That's a violation, not a crime." It was possible I would know the judge's questions by heart in a half hour. Then I could be her understudy. I liked the robe. It was a fancy version of the schmattas Jewish matriarchs would wear at home.

There was a woman, standing with her hands behind her back, wearing a denim outfit. Light blue. Black belt. Timberland boots. Black T-shirt. Hair pulled to the top of her head. She came out from behind the chained area, sat in the same pew as the braid lady, and said "Oh my God." They were friends. Or new friends. Honestly, this looked like a boring job. All that education for this? The judge asked her questions again. It was like the questions you hear at the post office: "Is anything perishable, hazardous, chemical or liquid?" She had the same fatigued look asking these questions. There was no discerning between the judge's intonation and that of a hardworking, under-appreciated United States postal worker. I finally caught the deported statement: "If you are not a U.S. citizen, you will be deported if you plead guilty. Do you understand this?" I remembered asking Frankie about her time as a public defender in the Bronx. "A person's life shouldn't be ruined by one mistake," she'd said. Well, that was a good enough reason for all that education.

Nearing narcolepsy and wrecking my kidneys, I decided to find a bathroom. I got up, readjusted everything that had shifted on my outfit, and headed out. It felt great to move. Outside the courtroom, I interrupted a desk officer from texting to ask for directions. He said the bathroom was on the second floor, take a left, then left again, then walk down the hallway. Or was it take a left before walking down the hallway? I remembered hearing two lefts and went with that. The worst time for me to ever receive information is after I've asked a question.

My friend Pam used to give directions like a long-haired, pajama-wearing apparition, appearing suddenly in the middle of dense woods to white teenagers looking for a key, a ring, a sword, or former hero they were supposed to inspire out of retirement. Once Pam and I were walking in Central Park when a family approached us. They were from another country, visiting, so nice and pleasant, and wanted to know the easiest way to exit east out of the park. Central Park is not designed to get out of, though it's very well designed for entering. When I first moved to the city, I'd try crossing the park by entering at east 86th Street, and after 20 minutes, exiting on east 72nd street, some fourteen blocks south, without any gains west. The park is designed for strolling. It's not a commuter park. Pammy went on and on to this family, detailing precise turns and landmarks, as they stood there nodding along. Didn't she hear their accents? When she paused to inhale, I chimed in, "Go to that tree over there and then ask again." They ran off quick, and I fell over laughing. That's how I deal with directions: remember the first words, then start over.

Bathroom located, I got into a stall, closed the door, and found there wasn't a hook for my bag. Where were my tax dollars going, anyway? The floor was filthy, so I didn't want to place my bag there. In this day and age, in any day and age, people carry things around with them. All bathroom stalls should be designed with some sort of package holder. There wasn't even a place where a hook used to be and someone broke it. It's not easy, especially as a woman, to undress the bottom stuff while holding a bag. I'd brought my messenger bag along because that's my bag, period. I shortened the strap, hung it around my neck, and dealt with it. I've been in stalls in Thailand that had hooks behind doors. When I left the bathroom, I noticed a beautiful winding staircase. I decided against using those stairs since I didn't know if that meant I'd have to be rechecked by security, and I kind of wanted to get back.

When I got back into court there was a different feeling. The vibe had changed. A couple of minutes after I sat down, my name was called by a sharp-looking attorney. We left to talk on the benches outside the double-door court entrance like everyone else. I'd been assigned to Jack at Defender Peeps. He had a perfectly manicured beard with his hair grown out about the same length. He was wearing a Persian blue spring-weight suit with a white button-down shirt. Either these lawyers' base salaries were killer, or tomorrow he was going to wear the same thing, just with a different shirt and tie. Looking at that white shirt, I realized nothing I owned was that white. Buster's chest is that white, and I ask him all the time, "How do you keep your whites so white while mucking up the apartment?" Jack and I sat down. I felt like this guy's college librarian. I felt older than any living organism. I felt like I predated joy and happiness in the world. Most of the hired lawyers were older white gentlemen wearing suits cut from the 80s with large padded shoulders and double-breasted fronts that hadn't closed in years. I was guessing that 30 years ago, the older hired lawyers looked great, too. But boy, had they passed on the baton.

After we sat down, there was a lot of information coming at me. I'd been charged with third-degree assault. Well, at least the "hitting a child" thing had been repackaged nicely. I could now say "third-degree assault" without mentioning the alleged incident. I'd moved from creepy yoga teacher to aggressive yoga teacher. Little victories. We went over what my neighbor stated. Jack said that was her story, and wanted to hear from me what had happened. He was utterly patient. I retold the story in short form, expecting to be interrupted, then I retold it again in longer form when it seemed like I had an engaged audience in Jack. He took notes.

Jack wanted to see the photograph of the doorway that Dewan had sent me. Since Dewan's apartment had the same layout as my neighbor's place, I asked if he could photograph the door from his side, with it open and closed, showing how tiny the space was, especially if you were claiming a kid was behind the door. Jack also wanted to see at least one video of the brick wall with my neighbor screaming at her kids. In order to show him this, I had to log into my storage account and load the video onto my phone. There was crap cell coverage where we were sitting, and my phone kept going into sleep mode. It looked like the buffering would take days.

Jack asked about me, who I was, what I did. Oh yeah, what did I do for a living? Was there more to me than this assault thing? "I'm a yoga teacher," I told him. It felt like a punch line. He smiled a big beautiful smile and perked up saying that was cool. I hoped he would stay focused and not ask me back or hip-pain questions. He wrote down that I taught yoga and that I'd been teaching for more than 15 years. He asked a rhetorical question, "This must then be foreign to you?" He explained what would happen in front of the judge. It was hard to catch all of it. He wasn't pausing at the good parts, making sure I was keeping up. I heard "order of protection," and blurted out, "But we can make that, we can adjust it, to… casual contact." I'd forgotten the phrase. I should have studied my notes the night before because it looked like I had failed the oral exam. "Yes," Jack replied, "we can ask for it to be subject to incidental contact, but I'm going to ask for it to be dismissed, since you are a yoga teacher, and…" he paused, "…you're nonviolent. She probably won't go for that and meet us halfway with the incidental contact." Okay, though I loved the idea of it being dismissed. If Jack was offering up the specials of the night, I'd want the dismissed and not the incidental. I thanked him. I was overly polite.

I couldn't get the video to load and asked if it was okay if I walked away from where we were talking to test for better reception. It felt like I wasn't allowed to leave his side, to be an arm's length away. It felt like I was in custody again. Jack said sure and added that he wanted to now see Dewan's picture of his apartment. As I was trying to get a video to load, I couldn't find Dewan's email. I was losing it a bit. The frustration at my cell phone coverage suddenly being shite opened the door on the day's pent-up energy. The anxiety of getting to court on-time and looking for Nancy, the anticipation of waiting for my name to be called, the terrible night's sleep, not wanting to be there, all of it, had been festering and marinating all along, while I thought I was doing a good job sitting still in the pews.

I was furious at myself, I was furious at my cell-phone carrier, and I was furious at cell phones in general because I could have printed a photo. I was uncomfortable in this outfit, this bra was annoying, my shoes made noise on the floor, and I was walking differently because they were not what I was used to. My clothing kept moving around, my messenger bag kept sliding off the bench and onto the floor, I felt out of place, and I wanted to go home. I was holding my cell phone like I was choking it. Give up the photo. Where is the photo? All my emails are organized in folders and then sub-folders. It was nice and tidy in there, except I couldn't find the email I needed. Since the phone was heavily preoccupied with trying to download a short video, I couldn't get my email folders to show their contents. I knew I put that email in there and I thought I already synced the phone. I caught myself pacing angrily back and forth, stopped, took a breath, and remembered where Dewan's email was. I waited for his photos to download, while stretching my neck left, right, up, and down. I thought about how many protagonists in movies would be dead by now, waiting for the important document to load. Real life takes forever.

Dewan's photos appeared, and I showed them to Jack, thanking him again for being patient. He took my phone and used two fingers to pinch in and out, snooping around the image as if he were investigating a crime scene. Oh right, it was a crime scene. He was really taking the time to look at a door closed and a door opened. I re-explained that this was not my neighbor's apartment, but the apartment below, with the same layout. I added that all apartments in a vertical line followed the same floor plan. I was making useless nervous conversation. I kept adding on, saying that since I'd moved a million times and had gotten furniture through many doorways, I knew that Dewan's doorway was no more than 32 inches in width. Doors are standard sizes. I was positive it was 32. I stood up and dramatically drew my neighbor's size in the air, showing with my hands how she was taller and wider and had about 70 pounds on me. Even though I was animated, Jack was still focused on the photos. I sat down. I didn't think I'd made a clear enough impression. I needed a better visual, and said, "She looks like Pablo Sandoval," referring to the then Red Sox zaftig third baseman. "That's a good image," Jack smiled. Ah sports, the common language.

Jack realized something I didn't, not that I was a detective or this was my field of expertise, though I had spent a ton of time thinking about my arrest. But I didn't put together what Jack did— that if the kid was somehow behind the door and it was shoved open, with such little space, the child would have had more severe injuries than a "bump on the head." She would also have hit her head from behind. Wow, that was a good point. I liked my lawyer. He asked me if I saw the kid get hit. I said I only knocked on the door. Then I went into my explanation, complete with standing up and pretending to have a door open. With my invisible door open, I asked how anyone wouldn't look down at their child if they were right there with the child being injured. I exclaimed for effect, "She never looked down or acknowledged anything happened behind the door." He listened. I was looking for a high five at the most, and at the very least, an agreeable nod.

I guessed public defenders were immune to this, weary even, of the emphatic explaining and of our desperate retelling. It felt like the most important thing, to have someone hear my story and agree. Not the charges, not the aftermath. I wanted him to hear the whole thing and flat-out agree. I wanted everyone to agree that I did not do anything wrong. It's not wrong to knock on a door. It might be ill-advised to knock on a crazy person's door, and it was definitely crazy to be arrested for it. I wanted him to say I didn't do anything wrong. I wanted to be heard. From there, after being listened to, I felt like I could move forward. In the heart, being heard is so close to being understood. Of all the people I'd told the arrest story to, I wanted this person, with an authority on matters of law, not an opinion, to understand and agree. I had not committed a crime. I was not supposed to be there.

I sat down again, and Jack asked me more questions. He wanted to paint a picture of how nonviolent I was. I guessed the whole yoga teacher thing wasn't a big enough selling point. In the moment, I couldn't think of anything else to tell him. My professional life was all I wanted him to know of me. His question felt too personal, and as though he was questioning my version of the events. I told him that when I wasn't teaching, I spent a lot of time reading on the sofa with my dog. There wasn't a whole lot else going on. I read, I wrote, I taught, I walked the dog, I sketched little art pieces that I one day hoped to make. Statistically, I wasn't even putting myself out there enough to run into trouble. Maybe Jack could paint a picture of an exhausted woman who worked six days a week. "Your honor, Ms. Tropin is too tired to bother shoving a door open." He asked if I did any community service or anything else that might help my case. I scratched my head: I. Taught. People. Yoga. Maybe the job didn't equate to a lifestyle for an outsider. I decided to lean on my niche: "I teach restorative yoga, mostly to injured students and the elderly. It's a therapeutic type of yoga." It was kind of the truth, if you swapped out "elderly" for "young people who take too many extreme-styled classes," and if you traded "injured" for "disinterested in joint and muscle health." Jack took notes.

We went over what would happen next. There would be another court date. Jack asked what days and dates worked for me. I offered light teaching days: Wednesdays and Fridays. Then it got technical again. From a set start date (which I didn't catch), the district attorney's office needed a certain number of days (which I also didn't catch) for my neighbor to produce a signed, sworn written statement. I asked if that had to be done in court, or if she could do it at home. I was thinking she wouldn't leave home to do this. But I didn't get a clear answer. Jack went on, and my head nodded along. It looked like I was agreeing and listening, but it was more like my comprehension was bobbing in the waves of understanding, above the waterline, now below it, flailing.

A side thought I was having was how fast Jack was explaining the details of this process. I explain things for a living. You gotta slow down, take pauses, maybe ask the recipient if they have any questions here and there. This explain-a-thon needed commercial breaks. Jack kept going. My neighbor had to agree to what she said in order for the DA to move forward with the case. Jack added, "Usually in these cases…" Did he mean set of circumstances, or actual "cases?" It was kind of a double entendre. Crap, while my head got stuck in that etymology pothole, he had

driven the conversation forward. Now, I had no idea what was usual in these cases.

My brain didn't work for court stuff. It was pretty much stuck in teaching mode, where there are so many questions that my mind can't wander off on its own: Who are the new students and who are the regulars? Who likes a blanket on them, who runs warm, who wants a blanket but not on their feet, and who wants it just on their feet? Who's injured, who's pregnant, who's recovering from something? Who likes a lot of attention, and who would prefer I never even walked near them? Who is unsure of surrendering their trust to me, so I should only touch them with a hand on their shoulder, skipping any big spots? Who likes big spots, and wants to be mauled? Who complains the second I touch them? Who wants me to massage their shoulders? Who should I suggest go to the front of the room, where it's quieter? Who hates the front of the room, and doesn't care how loud it is in the back near the adjoining studio where they play loud music? Who wants the corner spot, and who's a groovy regular I can put near me for inside jokes at the front? Who's already giving me a hard time, and who's already fallen asleep before class has started? Who's crying so later I'll need to casually place a tissue box near them, showing I care without being intrusive? Who's sneaking their phone under their mat and I need to let them know I might step on it? Where should I be when demonstrating the next pose? What is the next pose? How much time is left in class, in the pose, for how many more poses? What's the counter pose to the one I'm teaching? Have they had a difficult yin-type pose so they now need a relaxing restorative pose? I'm parched; do I have enough water? I need to pee; when can I sneak out and run to the bathroom? I need to remember to run to the back of the room, turn the lights down when students are in restorative poses, and remember to turn them up when I'm demonstrating. Did I vary the poses enough from class to class, from last week? Does the student coughing need a shot of water or one of the all-natural throat lozenges I carry around for such occasions? When can I take a second to crack my back? Who needs to leave early? Who's so well-known that I might have to get them out of the room discreetly because everyone deserves at least an hour of anonymity per day? Is the class list on the outside of the door? Do I need to quietly slide the door open to grab it? Do I have a pen to check students off as they leave and make sure no one has come for free? Who are my regulars that I can check off already so they can get going? Who's the student who might try to slip by me? I need to remember to grab my water bottle because I only own one, and I can't figure out how to hydrate without it. I need to remember to leave the room tidy, and goodness, try to remember anything from the last time I saw a student I might have to follow up on regarding fertility issues, medical issues, life crises, a change of careers, moving, breaking up, or getting married. And most importantly, who has a dog that I can ask after? My brain works well chewing on all these things at once. I thrive on it. I like the busyness. I'm not good with this hypothetical stuff that sounds linear, but really branches off in many directions. I can think in the moment better than I can about the future, as the whole knocking-on-a-door-leads-to-arrest experience will attest. I can't mentally keep up with the future.

While we were talking, while Jack was talking and I was supposed to be listening, both courtroom doors opened with a kerfuffle. An officer was escorting two women out of the courtroom. Without any room for discussion, he stated sternly, "If you have taken a picture inside the court, delete it. Now." This guy, he could get people to do things with verbal instruction. He didn't need to rephrase; he didn't need to demonstrate at all. Even I wanted to check my phone. The women held up their phones and seemed to be following through on his orders. Something must have happened. Oh man, I had missed the good stuff. I tuned back into Jack, who was telling me that on the books, third-degree assault carried a sentence of one year in jail. That was on the books. Most likely if this went to trial, which he doubted it would,

I would have to take an anger-management class, which he said was counterintuitive to what I did for a living. I didn't think he meant counterintuitive. I thought he meant paradoxical.

Anger management? Did I have an anger-management issue? For three and half weeks a month, I generally try to pass along as much goodwill as possible, and then for a straight 72 hours, I burn through that goodwill fast. During those three days, I'll get on the subway and think, "Why can't you doe-eyed staring people move to the fucking empty middle for once?" From practicing yoga all these years, I have an awareness of when I'm angry. But like I tell students, "Yoga doesn't stop you from being a bitch; it just lets you know when you are. From there, it's your decision." The decision isn't always easy. Sometimes being bitchy-lite, having an edge, gets you through a day of living in this city faster than being polite. While you're walking up the subway stairs, a slight side brush to the person staring at their phone, clogging up a commuting artery, lets them know what's up. Girls gotta get to class on time. Stairs aren't a library. Those are teachable moments. Do they come from anger? They come from being tired of it all, and from days when I don't want to play nice in the sandbox of life. Wait, did Jack say something about a year of jail?

I told Jack that if the judge asked me a question, I would look to him before answering. "You won't be asked a question, you won't need to talk at all," Jack said, more like a direct command than an assurance. Okay, I could do that. We got up and headed back inside. I followed him down the aisle and up to the fence. Then I asked him what I should do because suddenly—since we didn't go over exactly what would happen next, like every single possible "next"—I was a little stumped. Jack pointed to the pews, indicating I should go sit down. Okay, I could do that, too.

I scooted back through the pews and people towards Nancy, who was now reading. I took out my phone, trying to make as many notes as possible about what had just transpired, when a court officer suddenly appeared and ordered, "Put that away." Without even clicking the screen off, I dropped the phone into my bag. If he had been doing this to everyone in the pews and timing their responses, I would have won. Nancy and I exchanged glances. There was a new vibe from the last new vibe in the courtroom. A stagnant tightness in the air, the beginnings of which I'd missed. I saw that no one had a cell phone out. I also noticed a sign behind the front pew where the lawyers sat that stated there were to be no videos, no photography, and no cell phones. Had they just put that up? It seemed like there was a new sheriff in town, literally, and he was irritable.

The cranky officer, who was instilling his own form of mindfulness via intimidation and briefly worded commands, had a large ice pack tucked into the back of his pants. It was sticking out from his belt. Those belts can carry over 20 pounds of gear. I thought about how weight is relative to time. A bag filled with groceries weighs nothing at check-out, and then a ton after many iterations of subway stairs through an hourlong commute home. I imagined that wearing those belts every day would take a toll. It would also make you less mobile. Heavy belts, combined with what seemed to be a lack of mandatory minimum fitness requirements, might be inhibiting the number one safety mechanism our bodies are inherently designed with: the ability to run. In old cop shows, like Hill Street Blues, television officers ran after criminals. I get liking gear, but it has a tipping point. Like if you can't catch-up to a perpetrator and use deadly force instead.

While waiting for Godot's sister Justice, I took a visual inventory of the cranky officer's belt. First, why was it leather? It should be a ballistic nylon both for weight and for the use of the adjective "ballistic." Leather is heavy and prone to cracking. It's a terrible material for weight bearing. If he replaced the leather belt, the leather holster, and the leather bullet pockets, he could lighten his load by five pounds at least. The wooden baton that the cranky officer was still favoring, that was heavy too. Why not use a polycarbonate and collapsible one? That could save another pound.

The cranky officer was in pain, and he was channeling it into his professional demeanor. In addition to addressing what was just above the belt, there were steps he could take to relieve his back pain, like standing with his legs wider than his hips, doing little standing twists, or occasionally lifting the belt with his hands and doing a teeny tiny squat to relieve his back from carrying the burden. I looked over again, and saw he was leaning against the courtroom wall, placing his hands inside the armholes of his bulletproof vest. This seemed to be the optimum resting position for courtroom officers. I imagined they were bored. All that training, all those gadgets, and here he was, just going around pew to pew, telling people to stop doing inane things.

There were tags on the pew in front of me, names and dates carved into the wood. I could empathize with the anger and frustration of people's situations here at 100 Centre Street. I could understand wanting to express that frustration through defacing public property without better outlets. However, I would not put my own name or tag on the back of a bench. It didn't leave a lot of room for "wasn't me, officer." Perhaps all of us sitting there in the pews lacked foresight, the thread that binds the "alleged."

I thought of my shrink belittling me with her question, "Who knocks on a neighbor's door?" Maybe knocking wasn't a great idea. But it didn't seem as obvious then as it did now. It was glaringly obvious as I sat there in court. But it wasn't like I drove without a license. I didn't knowingly go into the situation risking anyone's well-being or freedom. I didn't run up to my neighbor's apartment full of anger, ready for a fight. I was terribly frustrated after months of trying to do the right thing, pursuing all the normal channels, wanting to resolve the situation. And knocking on a door isn't illegal. When I retold the story, some people acted as though it would have crossed their minds that knocking on a door could lead to this moment, downtown at a courthouse. Like it was there in plain sight, and I didn't see it because I didn't want to see it. But implying that the outcome was obvious also implied that I participated in the outcome. If you drive without a license and get caught, you are responsible. You knew the possibilities, yet you still took the risk. In that case, it's no one's fault but your own. That wasn't true here. Knocking on a door doesn't logically lead to being arrested. "Why would you knock on a door?" Right. It was crazy, knocking on a door. I couldn't go around anticipating that every unknown variable would play out negatively. I was not going to blame myself because this woman lied and the cameras weren't working and I took a photo instead of a video. This was a series of all fail-safes failing.

Nancy leaned in towards me and asked, "Why are they arresting people for possession?" I hadn't been paying attention to the proceedings. I stopped writing (which I'd been doing on the back of my court-appearance invite) to listen in and responded, "I think it's possession with the intent to sell." She nodded quietly in agreement. It sounded like if you'd been caught with more than the maximum amount of marijuana that you were allowed to carry in New York City (25 grams), also known as possession, then they were adding on intent to sell, regardless of intent. Why were we still regulating this plant? Maybe being called "weed" wasn't helping its cause. No one likes weeds. "Herb" sounds like the guy your mother dated after she divorced your father. "Grass" is a weekend suburban chore when you'd rather be stoned. "Pot" is the place you put your waste, or the place you put things to cook before they become your waste. And "marijuana" is too hard to spell and pronounce, especially if you're high. Maybe it's not the name, but how we offer it. Anything that comes after the word "hit," I'm personally cautious of.

A woman entered the courtroom, frazzled and noisy. She wasn't in a suit, and looked a little confused. I watched her head straight to the front pews reserved for lawyers and law enforcement, then stand there not sure what to do. I suppressed a desire to call out, "Bride or groom?" and instead whispered, "Psssst." She looked over and I shook my head, then tilted it towards where I was sitting. She kept walking through the front pews, around the side, up an aisle, and past me, mouthing the words, "Thank you." It doesn't take long to get the hang of waiting in a courtroom.

Cranky officer appeared, walked up to a kid, barked "Take your hat off," then immediately told him, "You can leave." He was looking for a quick reaction time, and the kid didn't make the cut. Cranky officer had an internal timer for doing rounds. A little leaning on the wall, a little walking around seeking out infractions. With zero going on to write about and my e-book in the phone that I couldn't take out, I had nothing to pass the time. I looked over at Nancy, now sitting on my right after I'd returned from speaking with my lawyer. She had her left leg stretched out straight under the pew in front of her, and her right leg lifted a bit, with the foot resting on the pew's back. With her legs cozy, she had scooted forward enough to position herself at an angle so she could rest her elbow on her torso while holding the magazine she was reading. The light through the windows from above was hitting her profile, casting a glow around her. She looked like a postcard of a woman waiting in a train station, circa the 1920s. But instead, she was at a courthouse downtown waiting for her friend to be called up to the stand. Nancy was completely absorbed in her reading. I was envious and asked her if she had an extra magazine. Without really looking, she reached into her tote with her left hand and flopped out a couple of New Yorkers towards me. I have good friends.

Grabbing a magazine off the top, I flipped open to the first story. I was grateful for the time travel that reading provided. The story was by Jessi Klein, called "The Bath: A Polemic." It was an hysterical feminist white-flag piece disguised as a hygiene story. Klein didn't like bathtubs; she didn't understand why as a woman she should like taking baths, and I was totally on board with her. I don't get waiting for a tub to fill with hot water, then waiting until it's tolerable enough to sit in, and then discovering minutes later that the water is cold. Also, you're wet and it's not ideal for holding a device or a book. It seems like more prep than reward. After a bath, I feel like I have to take a shower because I've been sitting in my own basting. It's the same with being in the ocean, except there, it has taken me ten minutes to get all the way into the freezing water, and then I'm thinking, "Okay, I'm wet. Now what?" Supposedly, people enjoy timing duck under the oncoming waves. But I don't care for simulating near-drowning to pass the afternoon. There's a better and more enjoyable way to safely prevent oneself from being pummeled by the ocean: simply stay on the beach.

The article was very funny, and I was trying not to laugh out loud. I decided to slide down a little in the pew to hide my enjoyment. Because of my posture obsession, I had been trying to maintain a perfectly straight seat before this. It wasn't easy. The pews were made of solid wood. It was the kind of wood you'd build a high-end coffin with. The kind of wood you'd carve a gavel with. The pew wasn't cozy. It seemed designed not to be cozy. The back of the pew was angled at a perfect 90 degrees. Our spines have curves, and if I tried to sit up, my upper back, thoracic spine, with its kyphotic curve was hard against the wood, and my lower back with its lordotic curve was unsupported. I could sit like this for a good amount of time, but after a while, my muscles needed a break and I slid forward, slouching. Then I caught myself and sat upright again. Below my spine, my boney ass began protesting, "Why aren't there cushions!?" The punitive quality of these benches was sentencing enough. The second you sat on those things, you were wondering what the heck you did wrong in your life, what events, strung along, led you to this exact moment of unpleasant furniture. Where did this horrible furniture design originate, and why was it still being used? There was enough space for me to lie down and release my back, which was what the pew's hard wood would be great for. My mind was stressed, and now my body was sad. It didn't take much to break me.

I was reading by making sure the magazine was held up straight to my face. Either I'd hold an elbow or I'd lean forward and rest an elbow on my thigh. I would do anything but let my head drop to my chest as if I'd fallen asleep. The head weighs over ten pounds. The cervical spine in our necks isn't designed to hold our heads up for extended periods of time while our heads are tilted downward. Do this habitually, and the lordotic curve in the neck begins to flatten. With the neck angled out, muscles tighten for support, bringing the vertebrae closer together. That's compression. Over time, the neck stays in this position as a cantilever. In yoga, we call this "turtle neck" because visually, that's what it looks like, a turtle's neck. It's also a manifestation of an imbalance in the Ayurvedic energy known as pitta. Here, the overheated internal fires manifest as people being know-it-alls. Whenever I see people with these necks, they are often the first to interrupt, the first to go on and on about their knowledge base, the first to speak, sticking their heads out. It's not just an environmental causation.

With the neck out in front, the body needs to compensate for the weight somehow. It begins to counter this pose by pulling the chest back, increasing the kyphotic curve, limiting one's ability to expand the ribs while inhaling. Next, the shoulders start rounding to assist the chest. While this is going on, you might experience a limited range of motion in your neck because now that it's flat, it no longer turns left or right easily. Most people ignore the aesthetic realization of this misalignment. Some people even ignore the pain and numbing of the fingers when a nerve is pinched from compression. Imagine ignoring pain to the point of not being able to feel your fingertips. Pain is a great communication tool, letting you know something is wrong. It saddens me people ignore it. If I can catch students in the beginning stages of neck pain early, it's relatively easy to fix. I tell them to put the laptop on a stand, hold the phone up to at least chin height, and read without tilting the head forward. The solutions are simple. While mentally and emotionally I was concerned about this arrest thing, my body fought the bench, and I sat up as much as possible. But again and again, the bench won.

Between Nancy and myself, it was like we were having a lazy Sunday at the library. I was so absorbed in my own reading I almost shushed the two men speaking behind me. I did need to look into my sound sensitivity at some point. I turned to Nancy and mouthed that the story was funny. She smiled. We were both kind of ready for lunch. There was a woman with a green hoodie who had jumped up and walked towards the DA fencing. She requested an outside-the-courtroom conversation with yet another magazine-ready lawyer, and another person, too. They had to find that other person, then they all stepped out. She came back now, and plopped down near me. She was exasperated and desperate to speak to someone, to complain. From a feeling of personal boundaries being breached, I could sense her leaning towards me, like a boat that's making a wrong turn. I held my magazine to my face. *I don't want to commiserate with you, honey. We're all here because we got ourselves here, whether it was on the subway or by foot, whatever. We're both not happy about it.*

My phone rang. It was the sound of a duck quacking. I was sure it had been on silent. The phone's volume was loud from when I set it as an alarm for that morning. Why can't I have separate noise levels for my phone's alarm and ringer? There was the sound of court proceedings. And now there was a duck. Nancy was trying not to crack up. I was pretending it wasn't my phone while trying to find my phone in my bag. I'd dropped it in there when the cranky officer asked me to put it away. I had no idea where it was. Now Nancy was inspired to check her phone for messages. I finally found my phone, and switched the ringer off without taking it out. No more duck quacking. Nancy reached into her bag, pulled out her phone, slid it under her shirt, leaned forward, and checked in on her life outside the courtroom. I didn't think she really cared about being caught with a phone the way we "alleged" criminals did. She probably didn't give a shit. At all. She's a doctor. She's not inclined towards theoretical authority.

A woman was called up, and Nancy leaned over to me and said, "She came in long after you did." It had been quite a chunk of time since I'd spoken with Jack. I agreed I should have already been called up to the stand, but I wasn't sure that wanting something to happen entitled me to being annoyed that it hadn't happened. "I don't think it's like the deli counter," I told Nancy, who nodded in reply. I wouldn't have minded if court was more like a deli counter. People had responsibilities beyond this place. The court should let us know how long the wait would be. The justice system is renowned for being disrespectful. It's part of the process, to be processed through with great disdain and humiliation. When you take away someone's dignity, you lose their respect.

I looked up and saw that a lawyer in front of me was playing Words with Friends on her phone. The cranky officer appeared and separated two guys in a middle pew, sending one to the back. I was listening to people's charges. I realized then that the entire morning, when I kept hearing "arsony," it was actually "larceny." That made sense. Before, each time I thought I heard arsony (and as the morning wore on, I heard it multiple times), I thought, "Goodness, I had no idea this was a issue." The courtroom didn't have the best acoustics, what with the high ceiling and heavy woodwork. Things were loud, but muddy.

My name was called. I reacted slightly lower-keyed than a The Price is Right contestant, but with the same urgency. My armpits began their sticky smelling nervous thing, and I floundered around with my stuff. I didn't know where to put the magazine I was reading. The strap on my messenger bag wouldn't cooperate. As I stood, I needed to adjust my whole outfit back into place. It was like getting up after a long flight. Hearing my name spoken out loud made me rush. I walked up to the fencing where Jack was waiting. Then he unhooked the chain, as if swinging open a white-picket fence after walking me home from a picnic.

I entered and stood at the podium to his left. All I had to do was stand there. I held my arms behind my back, mostly to keep from fidgeting. I was looking down at the desk in front, listening. It sucked to be up there. Jack began speaking and he was nervous. His voice was shaky. I turned my head towards him but didn't look at him because I thought it would make it worse. It sounded like this was his first time ever speaking before a judge. I wanted to pause the whole thing and calm him down—get him to breathe, feel his feet on the ground, choose his pacing. He had lost the thread of his argument, which was that I was a harmless yoga teacher. He said I was a practicing yoga teacher. It sounded like he was confusing my profession with something like medicine, where you can put the word "practice" before it, making the job description cooler, when really, it's just another way of saying you're employed. He called the place where I worked Excel instead of Exhale. We were just standing there, me at his side, and it was as though he was tanking an audition. Finally, Jack asked for a dismissal, and this led to an order of protection subject to incidental contact. It played out just how he said it would. I was relieved for him that it was over.

During my time at the podium, I heard about a statement I'd made to the police that I didn't actually make. When I got back to my seat, I was pissed, fuming. I never made a statement to the police, and I didn't like the idea that they'd made one up. I thought it through for a moment, and decided to get Jack's attention, motioning to him that I wanted to speak outside. When we got out of the courtroom, my fuming turned into a teenage whine. "I never said that," I insisted. I might as well have added a foot stomping. Jack was a little confused. He held out my file and opened it to the page of my statement. He was about to reread it to me, but it was fresh in my head, and it wasn't true. I was there. I didn't make a statement. I interrupted him, "They're saying I admitted to shoving the door open and saying I didn't know I hit the kid. They're quoting me saying, 'I didn't know I hit the kid.' I never said that, I never made a statement." Jack waited to make sure I was finished, then he said, "Oh, your statement, I never pay attention to those." He paused. I stood across from him with my arms crossed, feeling cross, looking straight into his eyes with an expression that said, "What the what?" It was less a question and more a call to arms. Jack continued, "Cops usually make those up. I never pay attention to them."

I wasn't on board with his enlightenment on the matter. Or with police fabricating statements. After each statement on a police report, there is a short warning regarding such an issue, should the temptation arise: "False statements made in this written instrument are punishable as a class A misdemeanor pursuant to section 210.45 of the Penal Law, and as other crimes." Does this not apply to police officers? "They never even read me my Miranda rights," I said. Jack shrugged, "I'm not saying all cops are bad, but most of the time, they make statements up. I see it all the time." "False statement" was yet another term I'd heard before but not in real life, not applied to my life. Okay, false statement was now a real thing. So much for innocent until proven guilty, blah, blah, blah. They were not going to get my signature on that. And since it was there in a file, I guess they didn't have to. I was just guilty. The End.

We headed back in. I was supposed to wait for paperwork. I would receive a small white piece of paper that had the date of my next court appearance. We'd chosen July 6, with Jack conferring with me to make sure I wasn't going out of town for the Fourth of July weekend. Nope, I wasn't going on vacation. Life was kind of all about being arrested right now. With the paper in hand, Nancy and I left. We were hungry and hyper to be moving about and touching our phones.

When we got out of the courtroom, Nancy told me, "I have to pick up my property," and pulled a small ticket out of her purse. We headed to a half-moon desk in the middle of the ground floor where the police were stationed. "They confiscated my emery board," Nancy explained. When she's annoyed, she appropriates an 18th-century Jane Austen manner of speech. She was using the term emery board instead of nail file because she found the whole thing tiresome. It was taking the officer a long time to find her property. I was dying to get home, get my dress clothes off, get to Buster, get out of there. "If they don't find it soon, I'll get a new one," Nancy offered.

We started chatting about what had happened. She asked about the next court date. I tried to remember what Jack said. There was a time frame for getting a sworn statement from my neighbor, and the next court date was to see if the DA could procure one. Nancy asked why there had to be that particular time frame. " I don't know," I said, "Maybe the right to a fair and speedy trial?" "Ohhh yeahhh," Nancy agreed. Somehow, I'd pulled a piece of the Sixth Amendment out of my head. Then Nancy asked if my trial would be by a judge or jury. I didn't know the answer, but I recalled this phrasing, also out of nowhere: "You have the right to a trial by your peers…You know, the Bill of Rights?" I sounded cocky. Nancy said, "Yeah, I do, I just never thought…" she trailed off. "You'd have to apply it to real life?" I asked. She looked me up and down, like a visual sniffing, dismissing the idea of my being the kind of person who needed such protections in one vertical glance. It was shocking and upsetting to her. She knew I wouldn't shove a door open.

Like most women after a long day, I got home and removed my bra, tossing it on the bathroom floor, grabbing whatever yoga clothes were near, and taking Buster out. We walked across the street to the trail. It was a beautiful day. I was happy to see my dog. I was happy to have the DAT behind me. I was happy to be in the woods, even if they were a stone's throw from traffic. I was happy to be in cozy clothing. Light was shining through the trees and onto Buster; my little dog had an angelic halo. I paused to take a photo.

After the hike, we were walking back into the building and I stopped to check the mail. I had a small package, and was tucking it under my arm just as I heard my noisy neighbor and her husband arguing, or talking as usual. It sounded like they were in the hallway three flights up and getting closer. Maybe coming down the stairs. Crap. With my hand on the key chain (stamped "Be Here, Be Now," which was starting to become more of an annoyance than inspiring reminder), I froze. Oh, I was in the moment. I was very much in the fucking moment. I was paralyzed in the moment. Buster looked up at me. Not two hours after being assigned an order of protection, I was going to be testing its terms. I didn't know what to do.

My first thought was to put everything back in the mailbox, and close and lock it. Then I could time it so I was busy getting the mail when they came down to the lobby. It was a great idea, for two seconds. What if they, too, wanted to get their mail? I thought maybe I should leave. But that was ridiculous. I couldn't leave every time I heard my neighbor approaching common areas. This whole order of protection was more of a quagmire than I had anticipated. Then I realized I could start filming. This time, I took out my phone and made sure to tap the red "record" button. I filmed my closing the mailbox, locking it, retrieving my key, switching hands, walking up the stairs, unlocking my door, and entering my apartment. Once I closed the door, I deleted the movie. Hopefully I wouldn't need to keep recording myself entering and leaving the building. It felt like I was the one who needed protection.

COBRA

5-10 min

STRAIGHT ARMS

★ Pelvis on mat

- don't press down
  on hands
- don't prop up,
  let butt relax
- legs relax

feet turned out

modify arms on blocks

★ release by lying completely down.
  roll over, knees to chest, couple
  of breaths. Roll to the right,
  sit up.

not trying to push up, hang out w the pose.

(less, do less)

feet not
flexed b

194

Thursday, May 19, 2016

I woke at 5 am to teach, and then headed to practice. Once I got on the mat, I felt exhausted. Everything went well from inhaling my arms into the air until I folded forward, the third pose. My hamstrings and lower back screamed. Internally, my muscles told the story of yesterday: the frustration of waiting in a courtroom for half the day, imposing on a friend's time for support, being charged with a crime I didn't commit, hearing a statement I didn't make, getting an absurd order of protection, and making a date in six weeks to repeat the process.

While my mind was bewildered and catching up, my body was locked-up emotionally. I couldn't move myself through space mindfully. I couldn't be present in my body. I couldn't do anything. I made an effort, modifying, getting through some of the primary series. Then I raised a white flag and went to the finishing room for some last poses and savasana. But when it came time to rest, all I could do was stare at the ceiling. My new favorite past-time. Since my arrest, it was hard for me to close my eyes and let go. Afterwards, I told my teacher I was emotionally and physically spent, and headed home. Where did people find the time to know how they felt? I was running from responsibility to responsibility before landing on the mat and realizing I was a wreck.

Friday, May 20, 2016

Friday I sorted through the recordings I had made of brick walls with my neighbors screaming. No clip was longer than a minute, so I didn't have hours and hours of people screaming. The videos could be separated into two categories: loud, or yelling at the kids. Unfortunately, there weren't perfectly sampled episodes of just my neighbor yelling at her kids, which was a weird thing to feel badly about not having. She had done it, and was still doing it, but after three months, the thrill of recording the yelling, along with not wanting to violate the order of protection, kept me from further filming.

If there was a trial, though, I would need this evidence. All the shots from my phone were in a folder of downloads on my computer that gets sorted once in never. I tackled organizing all the other clips, as well. There was me telling Hope's dog Ginger that she was cute, and her barking in agreement, "Who's cute? You're cute!" "Bark Bark Bark!" There was an attempt to capture my dog's impressive ability to jump straight up in the air, about two feet. Buster does this when he's overjoyed. On cue though, I wasn't able to recreate the vibe by saying "jump, jump, jump!" I ended up with a shot of him walking up to me, lying down and rolling over for a belly rub, which I gave him, because he's done a better job of training me than I've done of training him. There were a couple clips of men masturbating on the hiking trail, which I deleted. I took those in case the men followed me. It was quite the library: dogs, brick walls with screaming, and exhibitionist disorders.

I caught my friends up on what happened in court. Some people told me not to worry. I felt like they were saying, "You're white, nothing will happen." It was there. The notion of not worrying was in itself a form of white privilege. The shock of it happening was also a form of white privilege. Innocent people do get falsely arrested. Most white people don't think they will. But once you're arrested and charged, it's not far-fetched anymore. I was conflicted about my own shock. I didn't know how to deal with being arrested emotionally, physically, or politically. It felt terrible, and I went with that. Did it feel worse because I wasn't raised to fear the police? Nope. My mom liked calling the police on her children. On my end, I was always hungry because my mother refused to go grocery shopping. There were a lot of big blowout fights about food. She'd tell me, a kid, that if I wanted food, I could walk to the supermarket. It was only a mile, but a mile along a road without sidewalks, traffic going in both

directions, over train tracks, past an empty field on one side and a trailer park on the other, through a busy parking lot, to the store. Hunger was my problem, not hers.

Once, my hometown police brought me to their station as a scare tactic when my mom played victim, using a ploy similar to the one my neighbor had used on me. Instead of asking me what was going on at home, the police lectured me on how good I had it, living in such a nice house, a nice town, going to a good school. An officer put his face inches from my mine to yell these sentiments at me, adding that juvenile delinquents like myself were put into homes. I was a juvenile, but thought by delinquent, the officer meant late, and since I had my father's DNA for punctuality, I had no idea what he was talking about. I also didn't care for being screamed at, especially at such close range, and told the officer he had bad breath. What was waiting for me at home was scarier than being at a police station. Tough talk finished, they drove me home. I ended up getting a job at a fast-food restaurant, at the age of 12, so I could eat. Thank you, Roy Rogers, for your weekend day shifts, endless fries, ten-minute-old burgers, and paycheck. While I wasn't raised to fear the police, I was inadvertently raised to see them as inefficacious participants in my mother's manipulations.

People said, "Don't worry, if your neighbor doesn't show up, the case will be dropped." It wasn't true, but if I said it wasn't true, then I would deny friends the hope they had for me. This thinking also didn't acknowledge she could show up. She might. She might also sue me. She might be convinced to pursue the case, or the district attorney could do so regardless. There wasn't a script. I hadn't been worried like this, in a what-if holding pattern, for a long time. I asked myself if I was worrying too much. Was I contriving the fear of a criminal record, or was it really a possibility? Did I secretly think it was going to all work out well? If I did, would that be a form of denial? How should I think about my arrest? Was I using this experience as a vehicle to finally write? Did I want it to go on and on so there was more of a story? Could I sustain living with so much stress if it went on and on? Until there was a dismissal, I could go to jail, no matter how statistically implausible that seemed. There wasn't a place mentally where I could rest. One minute, I was sure it would be dismissed and it was just a matter of time, and the next minute, I was berating myself for not being realistic. "Don't worry" didn't apply here. It was as helpful as being told to relax. You can show someone how to relax, but telling them really does nothing.

Walking Buster back to the building after a short stroll, I ran into my super. He was back from an impromptu vacation, after being recently separated. We started catching up. He wanted to let me know the security cameras were working now. Then he mumbled something about speaking to management and telling them, "This is why I need them working." Did this mean that when he first showed me the apartment, and I asked him about the cameras, that they weren't working? My Super probably intended for his update to make me feel better, but it intensely had the opposite effect. It also reminded me of management. *Right, them.* How much did they know? How much did they need to know? It occurred to me then that my building manager never responded to the email I sent her right before being arrested. The one where I said my neighbor, their tenant, was threatening to kill me.

This was a company that rotated who they were trying to evict from the building by pretending not to receive personal checks. Then they posted notices on doors, declaring tenants had three days to pay this amount and showing how much a tenant's base rent was. It was a shitty way to do a shitty thing. From all the door postings, there was a paranoia in the building about how to pay rent. Some tenants chose to go directly to the management offices and receive a paper receipt. I ordered mine online through my bank. Paying rent shouldn't have an air of mystery to it. Usually when you send money to a company, things go well. But because sending a check in the mail backfired, some tenants felt vulnerable. It was our homes, stability, and safety management was fucking with.

My super was being uncharacteristically chatty, maybe from guilt. It wasn't management that had prevented the cameras from working. They were difficult to deal with, but notifying management about them not working—and making sure they did work—fell under his job as the super. He was in charge of maintaining the building. Had those cameras been working, I wouldn't have been charged with third-degree assault. My super said third degree was nothing. If third-degree assault was his nothing, what was his something? He wanted to show me where the camera's monitor was, and how it was set up, but I needed to get ready for a show. A friend and I had purchased theater tickets back in January, and I was really looking forward to the distraction.

I put on black skinny jeans and a black T-shirt. We were in the nosebleed seats of the theater, and I felt like that meant I could look casual. I didn't want to try and dress up again. I wanted to be comfortable without looking like I'd taught a class beforehand. Walking to the subway, I ran into Dewan, and he held my hand while we exchanged updates. He was upset about the third-degree assault. I thought I should start keeping a tally of those who thought it was something, and those who thought it was nothing. Right now, it was tied. I thanked him for the picture of his door and also told him what the lawyer had said. Since I'd just told my super the same deets, I was a little flat in the second re-tell within such a short turnaround.

Part of having been arrested was being arrested in the moment of my arrest. I kept telling the same painful story over and over again. Instead of presenting it to a group of people, an audience, it was like I was doing individual shows, one at a time. It was challenging to revisit how wrought I felt. Maybe I needed a longer break between performances. As a yoga teacher, I have endless patience for repeating alignment cues. My arrest story wasn't even close to being as fulfilling. It was also different from telling an anecdote where there's the possibility of being rewarded by laughter. Laughter is happy currency. Forget om, the universal sound; laughter is the platinum card of noises. Empathy can be forged, but a big laugh can't. I know my friends' laughs. I know if they're going to do it silently but with their mouths open, if it's a repetitive "ha," a belly-rolling thunder, or a laugh where they'll fold over and can't breathe, fearing for their lives. You don't get any of those from an arrest story.

After the show, my friend and I headed to a divine hole-in-the-wall noodle place and I told her the arrest story. We were already saturated with entertainment, so I did it like sending telegrams in between bites. "Was preparing for my workshop." Stop, chew. "Neighbor called the police." Stop, chew. She was curious about the third degree. How many degrees were there, and how did they decide? I didn't know. I wasn't prepared for follow-up questions.

Saturday, May 21, 2016

Getting ready to leave for work, I buckled up Buster's harness for a walk. Usually, in the middle of the day, around the block, I wouldn't bother grabbing my phone. Now, I always had to have it on me for the "what if." As we were heading back home, I saw my neighbor entering the building. She was wearing a black leather jacket over a red shirt, and black pants. Her hair was pulled back tightly into a ponytail, and she had large sunglasses on. It was like she was staking out the building, incognito. I slowed down and let Buster smell everything he wanted to. If I kept letting him do this, it could waste hours, and all I would have to do was look down and watch him. It was a good plan. He was smelling a building corner, up and down, left and right. He walked over to where the garbage was placed for pickup that morning and surveyed the leftover stains and smells. He was doing great. As long as I didn't pull on the leash, it wouldn't occur to him to go inside until his next meal. When I thought enough time had passed, I looked up. The front of the building was clear, and we headed in.

When we were leaving the building, there were some odds and ends on the table near the stairs: a small toy, a cell-phone cover, one of those flat combs people used to keep in their back pockets during the feathered-hair trend, and some rope. It was kind of like the setup for a game of Clue. Nothing of great interest, though. As I was going through the glass doors, I could see my neighbor was at the table. She was looking at the haul. How did those four objects occupy her interest for so long? Buster and I wasted a lot of time outside. Was she waiting for me? Was she going to contrive a confrontation? I needed to get out my cell phone to record, but casually. With abysmal acting skills, I pretended I'd heard a noise from my cell, pulled it out of my pocket, had my mouth move as if I was reading a message, and again made sure to hit "record."

I was stopped before the second door entrance, and Buster was looking at me with great concern about his future living with this crazy lady. I was recording the floor and talking to my dog. The building's security cameras were recording me recording the floor, talking to my dog. "Do not try to smell that woman," I told Buster. I was nervous. I needed to drop my dog off and get to work. I would need to walk by my neighbor to get up the stairs to drop off my dog to get to work. The space between her and the stairs was less than four feet. She could call the police on me if I said one word to her, or lie and tell the police I'd said multiple words to her.

We headed through the second door. I was looking down at Buster, fake smiling, saying really sweet things to him. Can you instigate a fight with someone who's telling her dog he's a "goober?" No eye contact. No mistaking a glance. Let me get up the filthy, sticky, over-painted, damn stairs, lady. I was trying to get Buster to move faster without it looking like he was being pulled, and he was not happy about it.

Two nights before this, I had held the door open for my neighbor's husband, reflexively, and Buster had wanted to smell him and say hello. Did the order of protection extend to my dog? Usually, when we got into the building, I would take off his harness and leash. It was easier on his short legs and long spine to bound upstairs untethered, taking the steps two at a time. Then he would stop at the top of each landing and wait for me. I'd never trained him to do that; he's just a great dog. With his leash on, he was stalling at the first step. My neighbor was behind me. I once hydroplaned a '96 Jeep Cherokee, with zero airbags, across five lanes of traffic, spinning in out-of-control circles, smashing the front-end into a concrete median, completely totaling the thing, and was calmer.

Buster does not like being rushed. He's a diva. He was resisting going up the stairs with his harness and leash on. He needed more time to find the right angle. I'd turned my head ever so slightly to see my neighbor from the corner of my eye. Size wise, she definitely had a lot going for her against me. Being so close, I felt the stress of her possibly calling the police, and the fear she might physically harm me. If I had hit her child, I don't believe she would have resisted annihilating my physical presence in the world. I heard this woman yelling all day, at her family. If I could articulate that into a legal defense, it would make sense.

I was about to carry the little fucker when he finally got going. It felt like I was climbing the stairs with ankle weights. I wasn't going fast enough, and my chest wouldn't expand for a full breath. I had started to panic. Around the second set of stairs, my heartbeat was in my throat. I could hear my neighbor climbing the steps behind me. I held the phone at my side, still recording, but now upside down. I got to my door. I was shaking, the key couldn't go in fast enough. Then it couldn't turn fast enough. Then the doorknob couldn't turn fast enough. Then the door couldn't open fast enough. And then we were in, the door closed. I leaned on my knees to breathe. I heard my neighbor passing my flight, going up to hers, entering her apartment, and shutting the door. What was that about? Had she been waiting for me in the lobby? Why was she waiting for me in the lobby? I sat on the floor and rested my head in my hands. The building was quiet. If she was calling the police, I would hear her. But instead of listening, I had to get to class—kiss the dog, grab my bag, and run out.

The next time I saw Dewan, I didn't tell him I found out, for a fact, that if a female police officer isn't available, they don't have to get one. Loopholes. It's all useless opinions after the "fact"—the "should" and the "should haves." I had already knocked on the door, I had already changed in front of the guy, I had already been violated in my home. While we were talking, I got worked up about the idea of suing the police. Dewan said I should sue, and I wasn't going to sue, but I heard myself saying, "I'm going to sue those pricks..." like a daytime-soap star. It was a nice verbal release. Lawsuits take a long time. It would just prolong the experience with even more negativity. It wouldn't even feel as good as letting go of some tension with a dramatic declaration. It wouldn't make my apartment home again. Suing wouldn't undo the past. It was not an eraser. Suing entangles your life with paperwork, lawyers, and court dates. Wasted time. In order to sue, I'd need to keep up a momentum of anger, see myself as a victim, and hold myself frozen in place, in life, until the resolution. I couldn't move on if I sued, neither physically nor emotionally.

Monday, May 23, 2016

Every day, I was waking up with back pain. It eased itself out by mid-morning, and it wasn't about my handmade Swedish bed. I was broken. Sunday there wasn't Mysore practice (in ashtanga, you skip practicing on the days with new and full moons). Instead of doing yoga, I hung out at home until needing to teach three classes. Having taken yesterday off—and a burden of unyielding stress—I went to practice with slow expectations, stepping onto the mat, my feet near the edge, swinging my arms as if nervously contemplating a jump off a high cliff into frigid waters. As I went along, I kept telling myself to take it easy, modify, and know I had a whole week to practice. The thing to remember about having a dedicated practice (sadhana) is pacing. If you go a hundred percent every day, you'll end up breaking down your body instead of building it up. Rather than pushing through, I was stepping back, lowering a knee, focusing on long ujjayi breaths.

Sometimes I'll tell students, "There's no gain from pain. That's what your high school gym teachers told you, and they were failed athletes." or, "Unless you're sponsored, stop at pain." Then I'll apologize if there are any gym teachers in class. I don't ignore my body when it needs food, water, sleep, or to back off physically. I can't always accommodate myself, but I don't pretend I'm above it. There's a thick line between pushing yourself to see what you're capable of and being an asshole to your body. I wasn't great at team sports. It never felt important enough to run faster because someone with a whistle was yelling at me. It's character building to be the bench warmer on a non-contending high school team. You have to have a strong will to keep going to practice, knowing you're never going to play in a game. Or a terrible home life to stay away from.

I was standing at the front of my mat, waiting to do the half-wheel drop backs, rocking my hips side to side, rubbing different areas, wooing my lumbar spine into the idea of opening. It must have looked like either I was trying to get it to rain or something was up. When my teacher came over, I told her my lower back was cranky, especially in the morning, and I had no idea why. "Well," she replied, "there's a lot going on." Oh right, the arrest thing. Then I put it together and realized my back had started hurting the morning after my court appearance. She spotted me carefully, then gently eased me into the forward bend afterward. It was in the forward bend, during the longest ten-breath count ever, that I had time to think and feel. The order of protection allowed for incidental contact, but since my neighbor lied to get me arrested, I had been on guard, prepared for her doing something to get me arrested again. I was living in fight-or-flight mode at home, waiting for the next bad thing to happen, bracing.

Prior to my arrest, I was used to a fairly chill existence. This amount of stress, it was like drinking. If you have a high-powered job, your tolerance for stress is high; you can drink a lot of it. At my job, I walk around a room barefoot, saying whatever I want, teaching however I want, dressing however I want, with an occasional hiccup. Then I go home to my dog. My tolerance is maybe one lite beer of stress. I know what to do with stress, but I don't know what to do with a constant flow of it. I couldn't tap out of being under so much stress, and it didn't seem to be ceasing. Would other people find it stressful that they could be arrested simply for entering or leaving their apartment building? Would most people just brush off a possible encounter with the neighbor as highly unlikely?

When I took Buster out in the morning, a tenant had spilled something down the stairs. The spill covered each step, flight to flight to flight, through the lobby, and out the doors. Most likely, it was from leaky garbage followed by some brash inconsiderateness. The porter would have cleaned it up, but this tenant didn't ask him, so I went to find him. While I was looking, I thought how easy it would be to run into my neighbor and say, "Hey, be careful." And then she could have me arrested. She could have me arrested for being thoughtful. Yeah, this was why my lower back was hurting.

Tuesday, May 24, 2016

I was watching Ginger while Hope was away for her daughter's wedding. It can't get easier than a 12-year-old dog that's happy to see you and only needs to go out twice a day. Since Ginger can't do stairs anymore, and there were two cats at Hope's place for company, Ginger stayed there overnight, and I came and visited. Sometimes I could take her out with just the two of us, but most of the time, I had both dogs, each with their own directional desires. I'm no dog walking pull-over, but it was challenging. I tried hooking their leashes together. We'd start off walking very proper, one on each side. But Ginger only goes in a grassy area, and Buster wants to smell everything. There were some incidents where my legs got cat's cradled in the middle of the leashes, and I had to use all of my yogic balance and flexibility to not end up hog-tied.

Dogs don't have any regard for linear movement. They're not concerned about strollers, cyclists, corner-cutting cars, skateboarders or fast-moving dark clouds, unless any of those things are their bark triggers. Each dog brings to the leash its own special set of issues, and there were moments when Ginger and Buster pulled at exactly the same time, in exactly the opposite direction, bringing the leashes to form one straight, taut line in front of me, where I could let go and bounce my finger on the middle, before hauling everyone back in, saying "Stay with the tour, guys, we're going this way."

We were heading to the Morris-Jumel Mansion, where I knew Ginger liked to "go." She was walking ahead and stopped at a large tree near the entrance. As she was starting to squat, a man exited the gates then turned back around towards the mansion. I could see his arm moving repeatedly in front of him. *No way.* He was masturbating. Since moving to the neighborhood, I'd been asking women friends, "Are you ever, say, on a nice nature path, not secluded, and then feel an overwhelming desire to mount and grind up against a tree, or stick your hand down your pants?" So far, the public self-love craving seemed to be a predominately male pastime.

I was about six feet away, with two dogs, one taking a big dump, and the guy wasn't stopping. I started to praise Ginger loudly, "Good girl, good job, good girl." The guy didn't seem to notice or care, so focused on the task at hand. There wasn't enough room between the parked cars for me to avoid him via the street, and since I wanted to go into the mansion's grounds, I wasn't turning around. I was about to yell out an angry, "Hey!" when, appropriate for the location of what was once George Washington's headquarters during the Revolutionary War, the cavalry came in the form of two guys yelling, "Put your cock away!"

With the guy's attention distracted, I took the opportunity to walk around him and through the mansion's gates, aligning myself with the men whose pants were zipped. It was quite nice to have them there. They were absolutely livid. Unbeknownst to me, there was a kids' group on the property. The men's yelling for the other guy to zip up wasn't working. Then there was some racket coming from the mansion behind us. We turned around. Bursting through a door, in white painter's coveralls, all six foot something, long-haired, blond, heavily bearded and broad-shouldered, came one of the maintenance men, who was going to effect change. It was like Thor appearing out of nowhere. The masturbator stopped and put it away. It really does help in these situations to be a large and imposing figure. Someone needed to call the police, and unshockingly, it was me.

While we were waiting for the cops, I walked the dogs around the grounds and ran into the lady gardener, who said, "Ewwww, you got flashed dick." Then we walked back to the front. Technically, I didn't see anything. With all the self-love and urinating on cars around the neighborhood, I'd learned to look away at the first sign of low-waisted hand movement. The police weren't really interested in coming, and eventually, the guy walked off. I wondered about all the calling 911 and police interaction I was suddenly having. I didn't think it was random; my energy must have sucked. I needed to stop calling the police. I set it like a goal, with a mental picture of a factory sign that read, "Days Without Incident." Starting tomorrow, the timer would reset to zero.

Thursday, May 26, 2016

I had the afternoon off and had been listening to my neighbor and her family yelling at each other all day long. They never stopped. Someone was always yelling at someone else. Or the babies were crying, when my neighbor wasn't screaming. Even everyday home goods that don't usually make a noise did. The oven was slammed like a van door; the refrigerator, which was lined with rubber, made a thud when closed. Some noise is common, of course, but none of the other neighbors came close to this kind of skilled sound-making. In any place I'd lived, stayed, or traveled, I'd never heard so much daily living noise, so loudly, so very, very loudly. If it wasn't so miserable being their neighbor, it would have been fascinating. It would be like a Philip Glass performance that never ended (instead of never started). Most of it I was learning to tune out. I didn't have any other choice. I couldn't move. I had asked for help, and nothing helped. I had been arrested. I was stuck. Maybe I could get to the point where I tuned out the family entirely. It gave me something to do, a challenge. It was not as though the more upset I was with the noise, the worse it felt. Getting arrested hadn't made them louder. I was not looking for it to feel worse, as is often the case when one is wronged. I wanted it to get better, and there was nothing I could do.

Dewan was still calling, fighting the good fight, contacting 311 and management. Living below them was a nightmare. He and his girlfriend, who was now his fiancé, couldn't do anything at home and stayed away as much as possible. There was constant jumping on the floor to the point where ceiling plaster had cracked and rained down. Their bathroom got flooded. They couldn't sleep because furniture was being moved around all night.

Regardless of income or type of building, we were entitled to the same legal statutes of peace and quiet as the tenants of high-end rentals. There shouldn't be a quality of life difference because there is a price difference. Every person paying rent signs a lease. The terms on my lease weren't lesser than the terms on anyone else's lease. It was probably the same wording. In our building, though, we couldn't get those words to mean anything.

After my parents divorced and before my mother found real estate as her calling, we were financially challenged. My mom came home one afternoon to find me wearing dirty older brother hand-me-downs of jeans and a t-shirt and said, "Get cleaned up. Just because we're poor doesn't mean we have to look poor." What was she saying? Poor people don't care for hygiene? Poor people: a double entendre, money being associated with demeanor. It was on her directive that I wear old clothing to play in the yard in the first place.

It might also be the case that tenants in my building were wealthy, but preferred their rent-stabilized apartments. Still, there was a resolved nature to how the building was being managed. Was the problem that I wasn't playing along, or that the other tenants weren't rising up? Dewan and I weren't the only ones who were miserable hearing these people.

The previous evening, I'd gone to my articles club. Instead of a book, we would read an article. Most of the ladies who attended had families, crazy workweeks, and not enough time for a book a month. I found my way into this club by paying a shiva visit to a friend whose mother had passed away. You're supposed to bring food to a shiva, and by the time I got there, there was quite a haul. Baskets kept arriving by the hour; there were plates and tables set up on every surface and along the hallways. The fridge was packed. It seemed like every bakery and niche food hall on the Upper West Side was sponsoring the event.

It's not easy to walk into an apartment and see so much food, so much delicious food, and focus on the reason you're there: death. I had to stop at the doorway to center myself, spot my friend's dad, and make a beeline for him, sitting down to chat. I told him an anecdote about his wife from a dinner years ago, consoled him within the proper amount of time for being a fairly new friend of his daughter's, and then grabbed a plate.

It had been some time since my last shiva visit, and I couldn't remember the decorum. Was it okay to fill my plate because all this food was a burden and they wanted me to eat? Or should I pace myself like a well-adjusted adult? In front of me were cookies, lox, lox smear, more cookies, every single kind of olive in the world, and more fancy foods that I forget to treat myself to. I piled it on, but made sure you could still see my plate. I decided to do subtle returns, where you go back, put something on your plate, stand there and eat it, then refill your plate again, and casually walk away. This way, it looks like you've only gotten seconds. I learned these tricks going to art gallery openings for dinner in college.

Looking around, there were a bunch of chairs setup in a half circle. I sat down, placed my plate on my lap, dove in, and was in heaven, which felt wrong for a shiva. After a couple of bites, I needed to talk to someone about the food. I turned to the woman eating next to me, whispering, "I know this is tacky, but this is the best spread I've ever seen at a shiva." The woman paused from her own plate, mouth full, and said, "Oh my god, it's amazing. I'm going back for thirds." We became friends, and I got invited to her new articles club.

The article we discussed was about data mining. The person hosting had a converted triplex rental in Harlem with a terrace. If you climbed up to the roof, there were 360-degree views of Manhattan and the setting sun. It was a little different from my pad. Every place I'd been to for this articles club has had its own special "holy crap you live here" thing, which reconfirmed my decision to never host. If we went to my apartment, it would be a different kind of inflection on "holy crap you live here." Articles club evenings also had good spreads. It was an intimate group of women, eating, drinking, catching up. It couldn't have been better weather or a nicer evening to be on the patio.

When we got around to talking about the article, there were a lot of dystopian future fears. Were our cell phones being tracked? Our computers and conversations? We discussed how we carry these gadgets with us all of the time. We shared stories of unsettling occurrences, questioning whether someone was indeed watching or tracking us. The stress of the conversation increased my arrest stress. I was having trouble engaging in the dialog without inhaling the energy of it. It also seemed to be related to what I was experiencing, but I couldn't figure out how.

Allowing myself to be arrested was difficult. Meaning, I had to talk myself into it at every second, because any sign of conflict or questioning meant I would be resisting arrest. No one wants to be arrested. Do the police understand this? You have to woo yourself into the idea. I used fear tactics on myself: don't give them a reason to harm you or your dog. Being arrested is horrible, but surrendering to it is upsetting and humiliating. In order to be arrested, especially in my case where I was innocent, I had to allow an awful experience to unfold. I had to allow strangers, regardless of the badge and uniform, to disable me and take me hostage. Whenever I see videos of people getting pummeled for "resisting" arrest, I think, "You try it, officer, try giving up your freedom in the blink of an eye." Without yoga, I don't know if I would have had that moment near my closet door, when I got very calm and present to the situation and its possible outcomes. It scares me what could have happened. Hearing all this dark-web tracking stuff at my articles club was not helping. I decided I needed to talk about my arrest. I needed these women, who are smart, warm, amazing people, for support.

Even though I wanted to talk, I went back and forth about whether or not to tell the arrest story. Would it be selfish of me to possibly hijack the conversation? Was it appropriate? I decided I needed a question answered, "Was I entitled to be stressed about the experience?" It seemed like the idea of being tracked was extremely stressful to these women. Where was my experience on their scale? I had a really difficult time allowing myself to be upset about it, and I think this is where yoga was doing me a disservice. I was inhibiting myself from feeling because it's my responsibility to have great wisdom about stress, to be above all these silly human emotions. It wasn't working because my body was taking the brunt of holding it all in, and I was acting out, snapping at people on the subway, being short with friends, wanting a student's trust faster than they were willing to hand it over. I struggled with the idea of wanting the sympathy of these women.

Then there was an opening to speak, and I asked if it was okay to tell a story about something that happened to me recently and maybe I could tie it into the conversation. They listened. These ladies had their plates full, with not a nook of the plate showing. They had big jobs, with after-hours texts, reports, paperwork, and emails. Some had partners, children, and mortgages. They were in it, life. They were adults in ways I never seemed to get around to myself. I wanted to know, given what they deal with on a day-to-day basis, if what I was dealing with seemed stressful. Was I not handling it well, or was it indeed a situation warranting how horrible I felt? They all said it was stressful, very stressful. Reply all, confirmed, stressful. It was great to have their reassurance, to include them in. Then it was time to go back to my apartment and deal with hearing the neighbors yelling.

Later, processing peoples' reactions at home, I thought about Esther's offer to pay for a lawyer. I wondered if she thought I couldn't afford it, or why she would do that. When I had the

chance to ask, she said, "Because you're a good person."
Sometimes as a private yoga teacher, and more so earlier in my
career, I'd feel like I was the help, instead of helping people. I
don't really know how students see me, even those like Esther who
I've known for a long time, and her comment made me well up
inside. She did it because that's what you do when a person is in
shock and they can't move forward. You get them out of the
situation. You help.

Friday, May 27, 2016

Most of the time I was spending around people was as
their yoga teacher, and I couldn't say how I was really doing, or let
on. Falling apart isn't what draws students to a teacher. To
constructively (rather than destructively) channel a space for not
doing "great," I'd started using naps as my drug of choice.
Napping gave me a break from thinking about the arrest and
offered me rest. Stress is tiring. It helps to have a sleep enabler by
way of a snuggly mutt.

After Hope and I took the dogs on the trail in the morning,
Buster and I hit the sofa. It was hot out, and I hadn't slept well the
previous night. When I don't sleep well, my dog doesn't sleep
well, and then I really don't sleep well. I wondered what I was
doing to keep him from a good night's rest, because he's great at it
by himself. I first started reading, and stretched out. Buster
squished his long body between me and the cushions. It was hard
not to feel judgmental about wasting the middle of the day on
something I also do at night, but it did have advantages over drugs
and alcohol. It didn't affect my performance, and people couldn't
tell. People don't know if you've spent the entire time before
meeting them curled up in a ball with your dog, snoozing. You can
hide a nap, narcotics are trickier.

I fell asleep and the doorbell rang, and then my neighbors'
doorbells rang. This happens in buildings without doormen: a

delivery person, ConEd or a con artist will ring every bell to gain entry. Stay-at-home parents, off-schedule, and home-office tenants become the building's ad-hoc concierges. At the first bell, Buster used my belly to leap off the sofa, and I made a human yelp noise. He began with a couple of barks, then went into his high-pitched reverse barking routine. His eyes were wide, his tail was up, and he didn't know what to do. Since moving into this building, with the constant ringing of doorbells, I'd had a lot of time to observe this reaction. It was wearing on me. The doorbells, including mine, kept ringing, and then someone buzzed in whomever it was. As much as I hate the abuse of ringing bells, I wasn't happy it was often resolved because one of my neighbors allowed access without inquisition. Blindly letting anyone in because they were being persistently irksome negated the whole buzzer-as-security function. Did they have a conversation about intent prior to hitting the buzzer? Or did they just hope it would play out well?

Now that I was up, I decided to put the crazy furry thing losing his mind in the bedroom. There, you're safe. I opened my front door a crack. Then I closed it quickly, grabbed my phone, and cracked the door open again. I was annoyed that my nap time had been interrupted, and being annoyed story-topped my personal safety. Things hadn't worked out well for me when I knocked on my neighbor's door, but that didn't seem to inform this moment.

Whoever was in the building was now knocking on doors. It sounded like no one was answering on the first floor. Then I heard many feet go up the first flight. Was it a group? What was going on? They stopped on the second floor, below mine, and began knocking on those doors. Then I heard scraping noises. Were people trying to break into apartments? I put on my baseball cap and left my apartment barefoot, wearing old, black cropped yoga pants, a sleeveless white T-shirt, and no bra. I probably looked like the one breaking into the building. I walked down a couple of steps to peer over the banister and see what was going on. It was cliché stupid.

Around the bend of the stairs, I started recording two guys with my cell phone. The sound I heard was an actual scraper, a metal putty knife used for removing paint or spackling. They were trespassing in the building, and were now trying to get into apartments. From their demeanor and appearance, they didn't exactly seem threatening. I shouted out "Hey!" from the top of the landing. They told me they were there to work on the fire escapes. However, they couldn't get to the fire escapes from outside the building. They were inside, hoping to go through someone's apartment for access. Part of me thought this was perfectly normal, given how management hired workers and dealt with building improvements. Another part of me thought it was the kind of story a victim retells from their hospital bed while the greater public is like, "I would have never believed them."

In order to access the fire escape from my apartment, you had to walk through the whole place to the back bedroom and then out the bedroom window. Except I'd put screws on either side of the window frame, so it only opened about ten inches. With my small head and lack of shoulders, I could get through that. But if you weren't my size, you couldn't. These guys were bigger than me, and looked like it had been awhile since they'd had any intimacy with a bar of soap. They were not going to be allowed into my apartment, or probably anyone else's apartment, to crawl out onto a fire escape, even if that was what they were truly there for.

I was now standing on the landing between the two flights, and between two choices. I looked up, towards my apartment, and walking away from what was happening. It wasn't really my concern. I looked back down, to the guys, who were going to keep knocking on doors, because they felt entitled to bother other people at home. Until this moment, I hadn't realized how angry I was about the arrest. There was a shift. I'd spent so much time pushing my anger out of the way, mostly to move forward, that I couldn't feel it until I could see it. Not being able to tell the police to get out of my apartment, not being able to tell them they weren't arresting me because the woman had lied, was seething in my muscles. I had an endless daydream desire of wanting to say no to them. I would relive the moment when they were about to enter my apartment, all five of them, and then fantasized closing my door, and locking it instead.

Being in police custody isn't safe. There aren't reliable statistics for exactly how many people die each year in police custody because it isn't reported. Some states slyly don't report this, and some refuse outright to participate in reporting. Often, deaths are deemed suicides or due to medical issues. The guess, the rough estimate, is that there are nearly a thousand deaths a year among people who are being detained. We know this from news reports of the deaths of victims like Sandra Bland and Freddie Gray. Then there are all the others outside of the media spotlight whose lives disappeared. What happened to those people before they died, we will never know. More painfully, friends and loved ones will never know. It's terrifying. My anger about being in police custody had topped off. There wasn't room for any more. The shock had moved on and turned into something else. I didn't like having been arrested. It reminded me of surrendering to abuse as a child, submitting my body to emotional and physical pain, telling myself, don't make it worse, do nothing. Realizing from a very young age that the best play is the long game, waiting until interest is lost. It can make you bitter, though.

I guessed that out of the tenants who had access to the back fire escapes, exactly none would want two guys to come in, with painting and scraping tools, to go through their homes, and out their windows. Except these guys didn't even have any painting gear. One guy had the scraper, and a dust mask. The other, smaller guy just had pink wireless headphones. While it was likely they were there to scrape the fire escapes, they didn't have any paperwork or know the names of my building manager or my super. I asked them to leave the building, and they refused. The entire time, I was recording them. I threatened to call the police, and the scrawnier guy said go ahead. He then made a phone call. I was infuriated. I managed to get them down to the lobby, but they still wouldn't leave. I argued that since they didn't have access to the back fire escape, they shouldn't be in the building.

Instead of trying to get to the fire escape legally, they opted for making themselves at home in the lobby. One hopped on the table near the stairs. This wasn't how I would go about a long day's work ahead of me. It was a stalemate. I called the police. After that, I explained to the guys how it looked to me, two men ringing bells to gain access, one of them with a metal tool, both of them trying to get into apartments, and then refusing to leave. The scrawny guy made another phone call and handed his phone to me saying someone on the line wanted to talk. Through his phone I heard the word "hola?" repeatedly. I pushed the red circle on the screen, and the call was ended. "I don't speak Spanish," I told him. I wasn't doing a great job inspiring them to do the right thing by being a jerk myself.

While waiting for the police, they started discussing my arm tattoos. From what I could gather, they liked them, and thought the work was good. *Great, thanks.* We started having a merry-go-round conversation, where I would tell them they were trespassing, they would disagree, I would ask to see any paperwork, they would say they didn't have any, I would ask them to leave, they would say they were there to work, and I would point out that staying in the lobby isn't a form of working. Finally, I changed it around and asked why, if they were allowed to be there to work, they tried to ring every buzzer to get in. The scrawny one said no, he didn't have to buzz, he had a key, and he didn't have to show it to me. I said I had a video of him agreeing that he rang every bell to get inside. He thought for a moment. He didn't remember what he'd said to me. His cohort asked him what was going on because his English was limited. To me, he only said, "I sorry" while holding his chest.

I took Spanish in eighth grade, and barely passed. I can manage a brief exchange with an amenable taxi driver or inquire where the bathroom is, but that's it. Whenever I see a person belittling someone because they don't speak English, I want to ask them if they are fluent in two languages. If you're not bilingual, you shouldn't expect the person talking to you to speak their native language and yours too just because your native language is English. Yet, here I was being a bitch about the language issue. The awareness was there. I knew I was being the aggressor, making things worse. I also knew I wasn't walking away. In that moment, I was the ugliest version of myself. I would have felt ashamed if I wasn't so angry. As I was standing there waiting for the police, I started to want to go home, back to Buster, who was still in the bedroom. So much for his personal comfort. What the hell was going on with me? Obviously, these guys were arrogant, but not aggressive. Who cared? It wasn't my building.

The nice thing would have been for them to leave the building. The cohort responded that he didn't ring every bell, only the back-of-the-apartment-building bells. "Are you 41?" "No." "Are you 21?" "No." "Are you 31?" "No." "You got the apartment numbers wrong, idiot." I was behaving like a small town bully. Scrawny admonished me for saying his friend was an idiot. It felt like every minute I kept this exchange going, I was giving into the anger. I was going dark from the inside out while I was simultaneously causing what was happening on the outside. This was my doing, and I didn't stop it.

I called the police again, and the 911 operator told me that I'd called three minutes ago and to give the police more time. It was good to know the police were on top of response times, but my call log said it was five minutes ago, and from personal experience, I knew the precinct was a short drive away. In the lobby, it was me and either two entitled trespassers, or two workers who weren't working. It had become comically awkward that I was standing with them, arguing like playground foes, while waiting for the police. Standing there in the lobby, blindly enraged, I wanted justice for my false arrest by having actual illegal activity accounted for. But regardless of how I was acting, the guys weren't leaving.

The cohort walked over to the mailbox area and found the name of my super and his contact number. He told his friend this. His friend started to call my super. I took out my phone and called him, too. I knew he wouldn't answer the phone unless he knew who it was or unless a person called more than once. The scrawny guy couldn't get through. My super answered in two rings for me. He was *my* super. I told him what was going on, and he said, "No, that's not how it's done." He said he didn't know about any fire-escape scrapers due in the building.

While I was on the phone, the police arrived. The guys started talking and then I interrupted saying, "I'm the one who called." It was my turn first. I explained what happened and how my super didn't even know they were supposed to be there. They thanked me and said they would handle it. I explained to the female officer how it looked, two guys coming in, knocking on doors, trying to get into apartments. She thanked me again and scolded me, saying I shouldn't have stuck around, I should have stayed in my apartment and waited for them, to avoid a confrontation, and for my safety. I told her she was right—but those guys started it—and sulked up the stairs like a petulant teenager being sent to her room.

Days without calling 911: 0

An hour later, there were scraping noises on the fire escape. The good news was it blocked out the yelling neighbors. Then it all stopped. Inexplicably. For a moment, the building was quiet. The neighbors weren't screaming; even the little squirrel-esque barking dogs from another building were quiet. There was only the sound of two air conditioners, reverberating off the five brick walls in the air shaft, like noise-cancelling machines at a shrink's office. It was peaceful, maybe for the first time since January. I wanted this back, the way the building was before. I wanted the ability to hear my thoughts, to let my mind wander to its creative corners.

During my yoga teacher training, we were taught that as long as your eyes are open, you're taking in and processing information. We learned to teach students about drishti, a focused and concentrated gaze, to foster stillness in their minds. Did something similar happen with sounds? Did the mind keep processing endless noise, endlessly? Even if I mastered tuning out my neighbors, wouldn't some part of me still be absorbing their screaming? Without the yelling, I felt relaxed. It had been a long time since I'd felt this way.

The scraping started again. I was online about to purchase dog food, hemp protein, and noise-cancelling headphones. But I'm not a big fan of owning things and rarely make casual purchases. The cheap headphones had inconsistent reviews, and the good ones cost a month's food budget. Also, did I really want to walk around my place wearing cans all the time? What if I wanted to hear all the noises my dog made to communicate with me? Or my phone, email, or text alerts? I went to my tool bag, found some old earplugs, and put them in. They were little orange foam inserts, the original, minimalist noise-cancelling devices. Then I lay on my bed and closed my eyes. I didn't want to sleep; I wanted to think. Because the scrapers were on the back fire escapes, I had the window and shades closed. The lights were off. The walls were plaster, and it was cool in the bedroom. I lay there wanting to think of something other than neighbors and responsibilities. Something other than what needed to be done next. It was my one day a week off.

One of ladies from articles club sent a sweet message saying she couldn't stop thinking about my arrest. She wanted to know if I'd thought about suing the neighbors. I got where she was coming from. What do we do with our frustration and anger? In America, we become litigious. Is suing the modern-day duel? We can't legally take ten paces then turn and shoot, thankfully. We can't physically fight until someone surrenders or dies. I'm thankful for that as well. We also can't burn the other person's village down in the middle of the night. That's probably a good thing. How do we deal with being wronged? Forgiveness? Though I am a yoga teacher, I find forgiveness to be mental flimflam, an emotional con. What I wanted was to drain the negativity from my body like twisting a sponge dry. I wanted it out of my muscles, my nervous system, my constant thoughts, my possible future, my life. Trying to get even has it costs. It can take time, money—or time and money. Retaliation wouldn't bring the arrest to the surface where I could skim it off the top and into the crapper. It would further tattoo the experience into me, pushing it deeper. I didn't want to hang out with my arrest one more day than I needed to. I wanted the case dismissed. Winning, getting even, would happen when I no longer felt anxious and worried all the time. When I no longer felt powerless. When I was in a place to make a good decision about moving. I really needed to get out of my apartment building.

Around 3 pm, air conditioners turned off, the scrapers were on a break, and the yelling returned to the forefront. I decided to compose an email to my building manager. As concisely as possible, I explained how the neighbors had me arrested, how they were still loud, and how nothing was being done. I asked when something was going to be done. I wrote that social services should be contacted because a little girl had a bump on her head and her parents got her to lie to the police about who did it. I attached an old video of the air shaft wall and my neighbors having a speakerphone conversation as if the whole building was conferenced in. You could hear the third caller perfectly. Each word. In my apartment. The email gave me something to do, an outlet, a moment of control. Then it was back to the noise and waiting. There were six weeks until the next court date, when I would find out if my neighbor had signed a sworn statement. If she had, the case would go on. Until then, there was all that time, all those days wasted, waiting.

Later, Buster and I were heading out for a walk, except we couldn't. In front of the building were two blue tarps, laid out like picnic blankets along the sidewalk, covered with paint chips. Holding down the tarps were bottles of paint thinner. The guys from this morning had been scraping the fire escapes without scaffolding for their own safety, a canopy to prevent debris from hitting bystanders, or any protective anything. Looking through the glass doors, I saw it raining paint chips and paint thinner. People were trying to pass with strollers and bags of groceries, their heads not covered, looking up to the building in shock and annoyance. Paint thinner is harmful in three paragraphs of ways on the back of a container. Improperly used it can cause skin and eye irritation and is highly flammable. This would never happen below 96th Street, where the more affluent zip codes reside. What they were doing was not funny dangerous. It wasn't anecdotally dangerous. It was very real dangerous.

I called 311, which took the complaint and then transferred me to 911 because it was a hazardous site. No work permits, no shelters, no shields, nothing. I banged on the glass to get them to stop and then ran out while carrying Buster. Even though they'd paused from scraping, the drips from paint thinner were still falling. I got to the corner, put Buster down, and turned around to look back at what was going on. As I was standing there, my neighbor Jim approached. He was also pissed. He had left his toddler's bedroom window open in the morning, and was concerned about lead paint particles. We stood there, looking at our building in disbelief.

Parents living in an apartment on the ground floor and front of the building approached us. They too were pissed. The smell was coming in even with their front windows closed. Those fumes were toxic. Every apartment they'd been scraping next to would have those fumes. I only had one window facing the fire escape and could close the bedroom door. It would be nice if on any given day my entire apartment was usable regardless of neighbor noise and construction. No one knew about the scrapers, or where they were working next. Either your place would be a superfund site when you got home because you left the windows open, or it would be hot from being closed all day and a superfund site because the fumes would still seep through. It's not like apartments are airtight with the windows closed. If they were, there would be a higher turnaround of tenants. The guys scraping didn't have a plan. They were moving around the fire escapes like shoots and ladders: up, down, across, up again. They should have started at the top and worked down. It would have been easier on them, and tenants would know whose apartment was next.

After a walk, I carried Buster back into the building. Once home, I emailed my building manager to say what was going on and included two photos. I called my super to commiserate, and he said, "Listen to me, I asked [my building manager] about putting up notices on Tuesday for tenants saying what was going to happen, so people could close their windows, and she said if they have a problem they can call the management office. Listen to me, they don't give a shit." I thanked him for listening. But hadn't he then lied to me earlier when he said he didn't know anything about scrapers coming? What was the point of contacting anyone? No one seemed to care. The police didn't do anything about the falling debris and paint thinner. There was no stop work order. No interest in the people walking by. I get wanting to save money on a project, but the building could have put up one sign notifying tenants and the scrapers could have worked on one area at a time. They could have also hung a tarp from the top so it lay against the fire escapes and directed their waste down. It's always seems like it's more work to do a terrible job, than a good one.

Since 311 transferred me to 911, Days without calling 911: 0

Later on, I received a response from my building manager. Instead of an update on how management was handling the situation, she told me that I was harassing tenants and to wait for court papers. Even though she requested that I not speak to her anymore, I wrote back asking for clarification. Was I going to hear from a lawyer regarding the neighbors, or what had she meant? I asked her to please explain. It was the first time I'd ever heard "You'll hear from our lawyer." Normally, I would feel sad and devastated by this rejection, but this woman had been miserable at her job. I was calcifying from stress, and I knew other tenants were complaining. She couldn't tell a tenant not to speak to her. She managed the building. Dewan had warned me when I first moved in that management would appear friendly and then be adversarial when it suited them. What was he talking about? What could possibly go wrong?

I started getting concerned about whether emailing the building manager about my neighbors was a violation of the order of protection. I also wondered if the building manager was giving Dewan the same response. He called the building manager regularly, leaving voice mail messages, and still contacted 311 with complaints. His catalog of documentation was now a binder. I personally hadn't spoken to the building manager in six weeks regarding the noisy neighbors. That got contentious quickly.

Sunday, May 29, 2016

I hiked with Buster early, headed to Mysore practice, and then had a full day of teaching. It says a lot about one's home life if you're relieved to be at work. When I got back to let Buster out between classes, I ran into the super and chatted with him in his urban garden at the back of the building. Being a contractor and all, he turned the basement into a darling three-bedroom apartment, and most of the front into a catchall for tools, along with living quarters for the porter. While the front of the basement was below ground, the back was ground level. He paved that area, adding flowers, seating, grills, and large coolers for long parties.

Standing along the side, to avoid the fire escapes, he told me management had called and offered him the job for $2,000. His own estimate, including insurance, permits, labor and materials, was upwards of $4,000, and $6,000 if he wanted to make a profit. Management said no and hired the two guys. I looked up and watched the ticker-tape parade of paint chips falling to the ground. Whatever minimum care the scrapers might have been taking in the front, they completely did away with in the back. It looked pretty horrific back there. The building walls were wet from paint thinner, and some chips stuck like glitter. The super looked on, emotionless. He said, "These guys don't know what the heck they are doing and don't have insurance or nothing." I looked at him, then up to the fire escapes, and then down to the mess. Was everyone going through a little hell living here?

I remembered to tell the super about the court-paper threat, and he thought that's exactly what it was, just a threat, to have me back off and keep me quiet. I wanted to believe him. He said that for the building manager to send paperwork, she had to go to her boss's office. For a moment, I took that literally. Momentarily confused as to what was the big deal of walking over to her boss's office to get paperwork signed? I'd been there and it wasn't a big workplace. Then I realized he meant get approval for filing paperwork, not the physical activity. Go through the boss's office, not to. His theory didn't feel like a warm cup of chamomile tea. It didn't soothe my nerves. While management didn't like to fuss about being good landlords, they did like to fuss about being terrible landlords. It was plausible that telling me to wait to hear from their lawyer was simply a threat. However, I don't find hypothetical viewpoints comforting. I got arrested. I already won the improbable lottery. Buster started getting fussy, and I left the super to watch his backyard get trashed.

Tuesday, May 31, 2016

I spent the rest of the weekend navigating the harassment of the fire-escape scrapers and carrying Buster in and out of the building. If the scrapers saw me entering or leaving, they'd yell profanities or make jokes about my appearance. They even made snides about my dog, though I think that had more to do with how much I struggled carrying him in and out. With the debris falling, and the potential for little paws to get tarred and feathered, I had to pick Buster up about ten paces out from the front door and rush the building, as though the world outside were on fire and our safety depended on being inside with only seconds to spare. I was reverse fleeing. To the scrapers, it probably looked like a vaudeville act, or something my dog's namesake, Buster Keaton, might have choreographed: me holding a near 30 pound mutt in one arm, who, with no prior negative experience to inform the moment, was positive wriggling around would better serve his safety, while I put a thread through a needle, key in the lock, and slammed my body into the door to get it opened, before dropping my dog or falling backwards. I need to be the Hindu goddess Lakshmi with her multiple arms, or Lockshmi in this case, to get the door open. It was a losing battle.

The endless commentary from the scrapers, who were like younger versions of the old Muppet guys, didn't help. It was similar to how I feel when parallel parking and that random dude shows up to keep yelling, "Cut the wheel." It's okay not to be good at everything or to take a long time to do a menial task. If I've managed to maneuver the car prior, to drive it without repetitive directives, there's more hope than allotted by those pedestrian life coaches. While I could see the humor in my entrance dance, it was still a hazardous construction site, and no one was doing anything about it.

By Sunday, they had moved to the back of the building again, and I could walk in and out without having to carry my dog or hear insults. Originally, it was stressful entering my building because of the order of protection against me. Now I had falling paint chips, paint thinner, and feedback. I dreaded coming and going. Just when I thought it couldn't get any worse, they eventually started painting the fire escape with black enamel, turning the sidewalk, garbage cans, and side of the building into a Jackson Pollock painting with haphazard splatters. It wasn't just a drag for me. All the tenants were coming into the building angry. Even if they stopped painting when you wanted to enter, they were applying the enamel generously, and it wasn't hard to get dripped on. It seemed like if they wanted to paint the fire escapes, they should have painted the roof of the building instead, and the fire escapes would then have been covered in paint.

I've been house painting since I was a kid because my mother saw her children as free labor. Like the little girl in Schindler's List whose small fingers were perfect for cleaning bullet shells, I was entrusted with what's called "cutting in." Cutting in is the worst, absolutely nightmarish part of painting. It meant going along all the edges of everything, without getting paint anywhere but exactly where it's supposed to be, framing out a wall, so an older brother could have fun using the roller inside my perfect lines. I wasn't given blue painting tape, which might not have been invented yet. Nor was I given a proper trim brush that's angled and short haired. I had cruddy old brushes from suspect previous lives and developed ways to keep them usable. If they were needed the next day, I would put the brushes and rollers in plastic bags and store them in the refrigerator. This saved me from the long and tedious process of rinsing them.

To make sure wood floors stayed pristine, I used those annoying subscription postcards from magazines below each stroke on the molding. With painting, you either take the time to do the prep work in the beginning or deal with cleaning up afterward. Usually, it's the same amount of time no matter whether you park it in the front or back. The difference really is in regard to health and how much gets ruined. My house-painting expertise helped me score a gallery assistant internship while in college that later turned into a real job. There I'd spend two years painting the same walls every five weeks. In other words, I knew how to paint. These guys did not.

I got dripped on once while entering the building. Paint was on the back of my calf, and I didn't realize it until getting ready for bed. Then I had the Sherlock Holmes joy of taking a fine eye to my apartment, retracing the evening backwards, reenacting my previous movements, and cleaning up black paint. I'd lucked out by sitting cross-legged most of the time—thank you yoga—and the inside of my upper thigh got the worst of it. After my days of making art and endless home projects, this didn't bother me so much. I'm highly tolerant of art mess. It wasn't the first time I'd tracked materials through my home unknowingly. I used to weld steel sculptures, and if I forgot to blow my nose afterward, I'd end up being caught off guard later by a huge, black-gunk-spraying sneeze. In our live/work space, my former loft mate got paint on Buster, oil paint that never dries. I then had to retrace Buster's movements like a professional tracker. Paint is a noun and a verb.

I wasn't looking to have a perfect suburban home life in New York City. I didn't have unreasonable expectations of renting in a multi-unit building. I knew I wasn't the first inhabitant of my 100-year-old apartment, which had been repainted so many times the rooms were probably a half inch smaller on all sides. What was happening with the scrapers I had initiated. If it made them feel better to harass me, I took it. I didn't like it, but eventually, the fire escapes would be finished and I'd never see them again. But the brazen malice of management, that remained.

Thursday, June 2, 2016

I had a tattoo session on my back. With the black outline finished, I was nervous and excited to get some color into the piece. From careful observation, tattoo clients fall into two species: the ones who put on headphones and never talk or move, and then me, never shuts up and wiggly. It's hard to be quiet when you have a peerless interesting person all to yourself. My tattoo artist, Emu, is about as groovy a lady as you can find. She's also as insightful as a shrink, but more fun to talk to. Aside from the whole pain and being naked thing, it's a treat to have an audience with her. Our last session was hours and hours, and we covered a lot of topics in that amount of time. As I headed to our appointment, I thought my arrest story should come in handy. Chitchat is a great pain-distracting salve.

On my way out of the building to meet Emu, I saw my neighbor, her husband, and two of their kids in the lobby, talking to the paint scrapers. I pulled my cap low, held my head down and sprint-walked out. Every time I saw her, I thought I was going to be arrested, and I really wanted to get to the tattoo session instead. Getting tattooed is something you either do or you don't. If you don't, and you don't get it, don't feel entitled to ask a person who is tattooed to explain it to you. I personally don't have a good answer except that everyone should have at least one hobby that wastes a lot of money.

Before Emu and I get going on my back, there's a little "Hey how ya doing, how'd the last session heal?" chat. Then I go into the bathroom and turn an old flannel, my designated tattoo shirt, around so the buttons are in the back. If we're working on my lower body, I'll wrap my waist in a piece of fabric I got in Thailand. I wear it like it's a sarong with the back open, and it's the closest to wearing a skirt that I get. Most of the time, I'm in variations of almost naked, lying on my belly with my butt crack covered, arms in sleeves, my back exposed.

In the beginning, when she started the piece, Emu had to train me like a puppy on how to get my back tattooed. First, don't be a pain in the ass. This was the biggest challenge for me. Second, get over being naked. This was the biggest challenge for me. Eventually, I'd get over the nudity part and find it a bother to go to the bathroom to change. Sometimes, though, I'd still be a pain in the ass, and eventually I wore Emu down on that one. You can show a girl she's being neurotic, but you can't stop the neurotic from showing.

As I was telling the arrest story, lying on a massage table, the rocks on my shoulders being filled with solid black, Emu was pissed. "Wow, I can't believe that," she said. "Someone can make something up, and you get arrested." I was a little concerned that if the story upset her, she might inadvertently get a little spicy with the machine and its pointy needles. Maybe the arrest story wasn't a good idea. I needed this woman to be chill. The session lasted into the late afternoon, and then I was dopey and tired. While I was on the subway home, Hope texted me a cute photo of Buster, to confirm she'd let him out for me earlier. And to say he pooped! Now I could go home and relax.

But my subway ride back became one of the most challenging aspects of getting tattooed. I lived an hour away from Emu's tattoo parlor in South Williamsburg. Commuting home meant taking two trains, usually during rush hour. I was in pain, and the part that had been tattooed was glopped in ointment and wrapped in plastic. The entire ride, I was craving being reclined on my sofa with the dog and a cup of tea. At 145th I switched to the local train and saw a guy from the neighborhood.

He was a handsome young blind man. The last time our paths crossed, it was early in the morning. I'd just woken up and was in the dog walking bubble where you know people are around you, but you pretend you're still inside your home. My blind neighbor had just exited his building ahead of us. He took a couple of steps before getting his walking stick stuck in the short fencing around a tree. It happened mid-stride, not allowing for a quick stop. Before my mouth could open for "Look out!" (which wouldn't have been helpful anyway, seeing as he couldn't see), he toppled over the fencing and into the tree. I helped him up, and saw he had a huge bleeding gash on his head. Then I was shamelessly grateful that he couldn't see because I'm squeamish. It allowed me to be audibly concerned while looking away.

On the platform I walked up to him and introduced myself. Then he took my arm and I eventually led him onto the train, off the train, up the stairs, and toward the right direction home. This is me, I thought, the person who's exhausted and in post-tattoo pain, but still helps people. It had been hard seeing myself through the eyes of the paint scrapers the past couple of days. Or through the eyes of the management company, or through the eyes of my neighbor. I've lived all over the country, and have never been that neighbor. I like community. Now I was the person charged with third-degree assault, emailing management with complaints, and always calling the police. As Hope advised me on one of our walks, "I think if there's another situation that arises where you need to call 911, just don't, lay low." Agreed.

As I was approaching my building, one of the guys who lived on the second floor was trying to get his mountain bike with thick fat tires and a bulky battery for cruise control, through the front door. It looked like the door was winning. *That freakin' door!* I ran up and held it open. Maybe today was the turnaround day. Maybe the cloud had passed. Maybe I was the cloud, and now I'd made the decision to be the sky. Maybe my horrible mojo was changing. Maybe I should play the lottery. Buy some flowers. List something over list price for sale. Eat ice cream. Maybe today was the day I stopped trudging the energetic bottom of the muddy lotus and headed up the stem, towards the bright and colorful petals, from where I could sit and watch the rest of my life unfold, above it all.

Bicycle neighbor and I chatted about wheels. Those fat tires were popular. Bike frames and tire thicknesses go through trends. The setup he had looked kind of cumbersome, like he might as well get a scooter. While we were joking, I went to grab the mail, and there was a white envelope, thick with papers inside. The return address was that of a company with two last names divided by an amber sign. A law office. I was opening the letter while walking up the stairs. Why delay good news? The letter contained eviction papers: a "notice to cure." The building apparently needed to be cured of me. Once inside my apartment, I gave Buster the quickest of hellos and then read the seven-page summary.

The papers said the assault charge was grounds for violating my lease agreement. It was business. Getting me out meant they could raise the rent by some 20 percent for a "vacancy" lease, plus percentages on renewal and "repairs." This was like turning tables over in a restaurant. My neighbor probably told the same story to the management company that she told to the police. The summation was a dramatized account of the previous three months. In this new version, I was harassing tenants. I was such a nuisance to the building that tenants had threatened to withhold rent unless I was evicted. Moreover, the letter charged, I spent my time calling the police on tenants who weren't home, filming tenants who were, harassing tenants some more, and fostering a stressful environment for all occupants. I received no points for being the only tenant who broke down their cardboard boxes for recycling.

The best part of the summons described that fateful Monday in April. It stated that my neighbor wasn't home when I complained about her yelling and screaming, and that she had just come home when I knocked on her door, asking her to stop talking loudly. When she closed the door on me, the statement read, I then kicked the door open, hitting her two-year-old daughter. I made a mental note to somehow get a photograph of my neighbor's front door showing it wasn't damaged. My neighbor now feared for the

health and safety of herself and her children. There was no mention of her husband. I didn't think there was going to be an opportunity to change the building manager's mind. She had the email I sent to her right before being arrested, where I said my neighbor was threatening to kill me. Without my phone in record mode, without the security cameras working, all they had to go on was that I was the one who got arrested.

Even though it wasn't true, I imagined myself trying to kick my neighbor's door open. Could I kick a door open? My building wasn't like an old-timey saloon with SROs on the second floor and doors made of thin masonite with simple keyhole locks. Our apartment doors were fireproofed with steel panels. They are thick, solid, and heavy. It would probably be painful to attempt, and I'm rather disinclined towards bodily harm. However, like problem solving how to commit suicide in a holding cell without shoelaces, I wanted to think through this accusation. There are declarations—I'm going kick that bitch's door down—and there are realities. Aside from never having the desire to kick my neighbor's door open, I considered the notion.

I decided to try it out in my apartment rather than being caught in the hallway on camera, or worse, by a neighbor, pretending to kick open a door. First, I measured the distance between my door and Dewan's door. It was seven feet. The measurements should have been exactly the same on the floor above. Using my living room closet door I spaced out the distance. There would need to be enough room to get some sort of momentum going. I gave it a casual try. In super slow motion I could go exactly a step and a half. After that I needed enough leeway to lift my door-kicking leg. The tricky part was extending the leg to land my foot properly. It seemed like I would just run my knee into the door before my foot got out ahead. I'd have to practice this maneuver hundreds of times before I could nail it. Even so, in all likelihood, once my foot hit the door, it would jam stop, and I'd ricochet backwards, fall down and break my hip. Not to mention some writhing in pain and screaming.

Had no one thought this through? Not the police? Not management? Not their lawyers? It was ridiculous. People didn't kick doors open anymore. They'd moved on to shouldering forced entrances, putting their weight behind the endeavor. Maybe it looked possible on Starsky and Hutch. Maybe we needed to stop forming opinions based on crime serials. If I wanted my neighbor's door to open, the easiest thing to do would be to knock, which is what really happened.

The summary also said I had been harassing my neighbor for the past couple of weeks. It was the exact amount of time there had been an order of protection. Someone had a fly on the wall of the courthouse. I was poring over the summons, and there was a part of the whole thing that was hilariously over-the-top absurd. Then there was the other part where this was really happening. I was reading about myself, they were talking about me, it wasn't a fictional character, it wasn't about someone else. The summons got approved and went through many channels before it was mailed. They were going to try to evict me. I knocked on a door. Twice. Judging from the version of the story that the management company sent, it seemed like my neighbor had the intention of signing a sworn statement for the DA.

Every day I tried to navigate the situation from as much space as possible, and then it kept getting worse. Now I was being evicted. I called Nancy. She was in the car driving to Connecticut. It was a great time to catch her, and left us with about two hours to talk. Over the years, I had kibitzed her through this drive dozens of times. I read her parts of the "notice to cure." When I got to the door kicking, she cracked up. Okay, I knew it wasn't possible, but the fact that this was so amusing to her made me want to debate that I could kick down a door. I had to wait for her to stop laughing before reading on. Eventually, I left Nancy in the parking lot of a big box store, and we picked up the conversation a couple of hours later.

To pass the time, I'd marked up the "notice to cure" with notes, and read up on the legal aspects of a "cure." Because I was upset when I was reading the papers, I thought they said I was being evicted by June 15 (in less than two weeks), when in fact I had been given until June 15 to "cure" the violations of my lease and tenancy. After a failure to "cure," then they could elect to terminate my tenancy. Since the accusations were embellished lies, I wasn't able to resolve any of the issues. I couldn't cure this. Maybe they were only trying to scare me, I lied to myself. Believing that helped me to function for the rest of the day.

Friday, June 3, 2016

It was a perfect rainy day. Not hot, not cold. Ideal for resting after a tattoo session. I woke up, let Buster out, ate breakfast, read the news, cleaned the tattoo, went back to sleep, woke up, drank tea, played with the dog, and tried to relax. Then, around noon, Jehovah's Witnesses knocked on my door. Instead of calling the police or asking them to leave the building, I said, "No thank you, ma'am, have a lovely weekend." Have fun ladies, knock on all the doors you want, I'm out of the "get off my mountain" business. If a nearly 150-year-old theology needs to go door-to-door for membership, they have their work cut out for them.

Later, I emailed my attorney Jack about the summons:

On June 2, 2016, 7:10 pm, Marcy Tropin wrote:

Hi Jack, We met on May 18 for my desk appearance. Unfortunately I've been mailed eviction papers by my landlord because of the tenant. Can you please advise me on how I should proceed, what to do!!

-Marcy

And Jack responded:

On June 3, 2016, 8:22 am, Jack wrote:

Hi Marcy, I reached out to our housing attorney… regarding the eviction papers. He should be reaching out to you soon. However, please contact him this afternoon if he doesn't reach out to you this morning. His extension is… Also, since I'm an arraignment attorney, Perry will be handling the remainder of your case. He can be reached at ext… Have a good day.

Because anything could get worse, Jack used email to break up with me. The good news was that Defender Peeps was a one-stop shop for all my attorney needs.

Saturday, June 4, 2016

A first floor neighbor was moving out. He told me that the rent was too high, and he was going to the Bronx. I liked him. He wore belted slacks over his belly, had doormats he kept methodically clean, and was a gentleman. I doubted he thought I was harassing him with our casual conversation.

Nancy emailed me and said a friend of hers was coming to town and she wanted to gift him a pound of weed for when they were at the house together. She asked if I knew a seller. I sussed out the details a little more. Why did he need a whole pound? That's a lot of weed. She told me he smoked daily. Still, a pound? I thought maybe she didn't know what sizes weed comes in. I didn't know what sizes weed comes in. But a pound sounded like too much. I asked how long he was going to be in town, and she said for a week. Okay. Not only did I not want to help purchase and then carry around a pound of weed, in addition to already having my third-degree assault arrest, I also didn't want my friend to lose her medical license. I searched "legal amount of weed" because I thought I read somewhere that the law had changed, and I came across a colorful spreadsheet entitled "New York Marijuana Penalties." For possession of 8-16 oz., first felony, the penalty was one to four years in jail and/or a fine, while for the second offense or felony, it was three to four years, with a mandatory half-year jail sentence. I sent this information along to Nancy with a note:

On June 4, 2016, 10:46 am, Marcy Tropin wrote:

Please check the link. Please find another great gift idea. Don't be white, it can happen to you: http://alwaystestclean.com/marijuana_penalties/New-York-Marijuana-Penalties.pdf

And Nancy responded:

On June 4, 2016, 1:49 pm, Nancy wrote:

Well, that made for some interesting Sunday morning reading. My, my….they're certainly a bit chintzy on the amounts they consider not so significant, aren't they? Sobering indeed! Well, maybe a scented candle for his bedside??? XO, Nancy

Later, Nancy's friend explained to her that a pound of weed is an insane amount to purchase. Especially for a week. A couple of joints would have been fine. A pound of lox, a pound of grass-fed beef, a pound of fat, a pound of coffee, a pound of fancy dark chocolates from the Belgium place, a pound of weed: same weights, different amounts, different attributes.

Sunday, June 5, 2016

When I left for my 6 pm class in midtown, Buster had withheld delivery of his second poop. Ah, the elusive second poop. My entire world revolves around the delivery of this package. It can happen any time between 11 am and 10 pm. Since being arrested, the arrival of my dog's second shit was causing a shitload of worry. I was having these daymares where I was arrested for violating the order of protection. I'd imagine being arrested outside the building, where police were waiting for me, and then I couldn't let Buster out. I'd plead with the police to please let me take my dog out, telling them it was a simple run around the block, asking why the dog should suffer. The police would refuse. I would start to cry, begging, and then they would take me away.

Aside from keeping myself from becoming homeless, my real responsibility, my one responsibility, was to make sure my dog had a fabulous life. He's a sweet, snuggly little guy, and means the world to me. At the end of the daymare, my anxious fear would turn into anger. Would my dog suffer because some bitch lied? In reality, I was sure I could text my friend Hope, and she would let him out. I didn't know why my mind needed to keep my nervous system in fight-or-flight response with these horrible hypothetical scenarios. Once they got going, though, it was hard for me to snap out of them. My dog was fine: he was on the sofa, or burrowed in the bed pillows, sleeping. He had toys, water, and safety. My mind was uselessly replaying scenarios of powerlessness.

I was teaching my class, knowing I had to haul back home to Washington Heights and let Buster out, and the feeling that the police were waiting for me kept resurfacing itself. Over and over again in my head, the scenario played out between teaching poses. It was the weekend. Weekend train delays would make getting home more dramatic, adding fuel to the hypothetical.

It ended up taking me three trains, on the same line, to get back uptown. If you can make it here, you can make it to anywhere! I was exiting the subway, playing out the merits of adding more rain attire, walking towards home. Then a police car driving down the road towards me turned on its flashers, made a student driver U-turn in the intersection, and pulled into the bus stop across from my building. I paused. Police sightings still made me fearful. The reality of them outside my building, after the endless arrest scenarios in my head, didn't help.

As I was trying to shake off the cruiser across the street, I saw my neighbor up ahead. She was just outside the building, giving a guy a cigarette from her pack. All those hours inside her apartment with little children—did she at least open a window to smoke? Now she was standing on the top steps leading to the front doors. She was blocking the entrance. With her there, the order of protection, and the police across the street, it was a perfect stress storm. I started to panic.

My mind was racing through the day's events. I recalled leaving for work and passing one of her children. Did I miss something? Or did something happen that I didn't know about because it was made up? I was walking towards the building, wondering if the police were there for me. Things started slowing down. I had to get into the building and let my dog out. I had to get by my neighbor to do so. I couldn't say, "excuse me." I wasn't allowed to speak to her. Should I try standing opposite the building and waiting, or would that seem confrontational? As I got closer to the front door, I could feel myself walking through each second. I began disassociating, my thoughts separating in two like they did when I was handcuffed:

PANICKED: Get the phone out! Start recording!
CHILL: No. She already thinks you record her all the time. Get your keys instead.
PANICKED: Really good idea!

CHILL: Don't worry, the building has exterior security cameras. So does the one next door.
PANICKED: Actually, that's not comforting at all. How do we know they're working?
CHILL: Close the umbrella, fold it small, put it away, otherwise it can be misconstrued.
PANICKED: Right, it could be perceived as a weapon.

I closed my umbrella and felt the rain soak in.

CHILL: Look down, no eye contact.

My chin dropped as I approached the front door. My neighbor shifted to the left. I put the key in the door and entered. My heartbeat sounded like the theme to Jaws. I was choking on fear and had to swallow to breathe. All I wanted was to get my dog on a leash and get him outside. The faster I desired this, the slower it felt like I was going. Then I was inside walking through the lobby, towards the stairs. I kept telling myself to keep going. As I climbed the stairs, I heard the second door open and multiple feet shuffle along the floor. The footsteps behind me could have belonged to anyone, but I was sure it was the police coming for me. My neighbor was waiting for the police, they were going to arrest me again. She made something up. I'm going to jail. I couldn't talk myself down as I tried to talk myself up the stairs and get to Buster. It was becoming harder and harder to keep moving. I became intimately aware of what being scared stiff meant.

With my new paranoia, that even Kafka would find intense, it felt normal, mentally logical, to worry that people were coming after me. I needed to get going, but my legs were under water, moving against an invisible current. I couldn't go any faster. Maybe I needed more air. I expanded my chest for a deep breath, and the effort tired me out. By the time I reached my door, I was winded. Breath and the nervous system are connected. If I could get my breathing back to normal, I could calm myself down. Or so I'd been telling students for nearly two decades.

I was struggling and juggling too many fears. I was also trying to get my key in the door, but it either looked like I was moving in slow motion because I was having a panic attack, or I was moving in slow motion because I was having a panic attack. I got in and closed the door behind me, whispering to Buster to come. He stayed on the sofa. Buster and I have our own language, comprised of noises. I rarely tell him to "come," instead I use sounds like R2D2 would make. The other truth is that my dog's not much of a team player. *Get off the fucking couch and get the fuck over here, my love!! Beeedooooo!!* I crouched down with his harness, and he bounced over. Wait, the rain. I dropped the harness and grabbed his raincoat. I was putting his head through the opening, trying to close the Velcro straps under his belly. But my hands weren't working right, like they were on low battery. I had to cheerlead every movement: keep moving, keep going, get the leash, hook it on, leave, get him out.

Before I opened the door, I could hear the heavy stomps and radio static of officers coming up the stairs. They were about to reach my floor. I stuffed my wallet and phone into pockets and got the key ready to relock the door. If I could get this mutt outside the apartment, then maybe I would have some room to negotiate letting him out. I just wanted to walk my dog. All the horrible scenes I'd been playing in my head about being arrested again were spiking my anxiety. It was like I manifested them into happening. This was the opposite of a how you were supposed to use visualization. I was shaking. I let Buster out at least three times a day—something that used to be a joy and that was now stressful since the order of protection. I hadn't been able to find a reliable dog walker to help. Right there, I wanted to surrender, to stop trying to hold it together, to sob, to say out loud, "I can't do this anymore."

241

Buster made a Godzilla noise with a yawn, letting me know I was taking too long. My dog needed to shit. With consistent outings, I earned his trust when he was a chocolate smoothie, projectile splattering, bad bellied, very much not housebroken, puppy. The heavy steps and radio static stopped. They were in the hallway. In a rush I decided to open my door before there was knocking, but I heard knocking as I was opening my door. Confused, I looked at my door for a moment like it was making that noise on its own. There was nothing there. The officers were across the hall knocking on a neighbor's door. The sound of my door opening caused the officers to turn around abruptly, hands on hip belts. Every one stopped, except Buster, who casually strolled over the length of his leash to wiggle his butt and smell a boot. I apologized, and scuttled us down the stairs and out into the rainy Sunday evening.

31 days until the next court date.

Monday, June, 2016

It was the 15th anniversary of the first yoga class I taught. I was back from practicing, hungry, cooking breakfast, when my phone quacked. I ignored the impulse to check it, and let it go to voice mail, saying out loud, "That's what voice mail is for." I would not be wooed by repetitive noises. It wasn't like the caller knew I was standing next to the phone. There was a message I listened to while eating: "Hi, this is a message for Mrs. Marcy Tropin…" No one I want to speak with uses 'Mrs.' or my proper name. "It's Noah…I work with your criminal defense attorney…" Another phrase I never thought I'd hear in real life: "your criminal defense attorney." It was a message regarding my eviction, and Noah asked me to return his call at my earliest convenience. *Okeydokey.* This would require adulting. I told myself to be careful with the humor and give simple answers. Calling lawyers, my new hobby.

I went online to the Defenders Peeps website to see if there was any info on Noah. Their "about us" section, while professional, could also pass for a dating site. All the headshots were fabulous: perfect lighting, no hot spots, eyes level, clothing that lay even without wrinkles, everyone with perfect posture. Seeing a picture of who I was about to call would ease nerves. It would dilute the strange in stranger. My entire childhood, I was told never to speak to strangers, especially if they were in a muscle car and offering candy. Then I became an adult, and it was one blind phone call after another. Where was the training for all this?

I returned the call and got Noah's voice mail. Ah jeez. I leave notoriously bad voice mails. I often freeze after the beep, with my mouth gaping open. My first time driving across the country from California to New Jersey, I stopped at a Wendy's in Des Moines. I needed to stretch and eat, and this was before I developed a conscience about my health, and the health of the things I was eating. I walked through the double-glass doors, and the place got quiet. For a moment, everyone turned and looked at me, the whole establishment pausing. It was 1997, the world was still both digitally and provincially not a web. While the restaurant patrons were all blond and peachy white, I was a bit of a contrast with my baggy, art-stained clothes, big Jewfro, and jaundiced sheen. Aside from looking out of place, I didn't exactly have the appearance of someone who had a place to live.

Cutting right towards the bathroom, and to the beat of "One of These Things Is Not Like the Other," I decided to use the pay phone first. The line is from a song I learned while watching Sesame Street as kid. Technically, it's to promote memory function. Somewhere in those developmental years I borrowed the first bars to self-soothe when feeling out of place, and it's carried on into adulthood. My next stop was Chicago, where I'd crash at my friends Alyson and Marie's place. Alyson had moved there after finishing her MFA a year earlier. We became good friends while attending the same art school. Marie was an old college buddy of hers. Eventually they'd fall in love, buy a house, and have two equally smart and funny kids, making visiting them even better. Chicago was a day's drive away. Now would be a good time to check in, and perhaps tell them this was where to find the body.

I got Alyson and Marie's voice mail and leaned into the wall, pulling the phone close to my mouth. I was a little uncomfortable, and it was about to shine through in a recorded message. My voice was low, comically fearful, and I was using a lot of "ums." I told them I was at a Wendy's in Des Moines, and the place was really weird. Except I pronounce it "Dess Moyn Ez." I used Ebonics. I don't recall if, prior to driving through Iowa, I'd ever had the opportunity to say the state's capital out loud. It was an unusual interpretation of the spelling, sounding less like the Native American name for "shit faces" or the French term for "of the monks" and more like I was stopping at an Hasidic furniture reseller on the Lower East Side. My friends kept the message and played it, often, for years. I hate leaving voice mails.

I was listening to Noah's "away from my desk" recording while making exaggerated throat-clearing noises, the kind of sounds you'd use to get a crowd's attention before making a toast. I kept thinking that the first impression of me to the staff of this place, to every new person who got involved, was that of a person who'd been arrested for shoving a door open and "hitting a child." As a survivor of abuse, it was horrible for me to be associated with violence.

Add to that first impression the details of my "notice to cure." Defender Peeps lawyers would be reading about how I snuck around my building, photographing and filming tenants with "the intent to harass," fostering such a stressful environment that one tenant gave up her lease (that had to be the Airbnb neighbor I helped management to evict, and it was now being used against me). Not to mention a building-wide rent boycott. All that lying, in a formal document. I was feeling like I needed to overcompensate by being a stellar legal client. I wanted to sound upbeat and easygoing. I left as normal and friendly a message as possible. Then I put the phone down, sliding it to the far end of my desk, like pushing away the plate when you're full.

Just before 6 pm, Noah called back, and I missed it. I looked at the voice mail, and it was over a minute long. Goodness. I called back rather than listening, and caught him still at work. He was friendly over the phone and just as verbose as he was in voice mails. This had been the case with my case: the lawyers did all the talking, and over-explained. There weren't breaks. Once they got going, you had to wait until the very end. I'm not a fan of men over-explaining. It reminds me of my dad constantly asking, "Do you know what that means?" He had a penchant for using phrases from Spanish and Italian, like "Capo di tutt'i capi," which he said meant "father of fathers," a mafia reference he was enamored of. He'd say the phrase for the zillionth time and ask me for the zillionth time if I knew what it meant. He did this with big words, too. He did this to me all the time, but never to my brothers. He also questioned my sources, asking "Where'dya hear that?" It was beyond his own intelligence that I might have some of my own. By the time I was 14, I'd traveled and read more than he ever would. While Noah was talking, I was telling myself to listen. He was not my Dad, he had a law degree, and he was trying to help me.

Noah was saying he'd looked up my case file, but couldn't find one. He asked if I'd gotten a letter in the mail saying the case was dismissed. Wait, what, no way, dismissed. I hadn't checked the mail yet and visualized that inside my mailbox was a crisp white letter, with a big red rubber-stamp mark, the outline of the mark smudged here and there, with the word "dismissed" in all caps. Noah asked what I'd received, and I said a "notice to cure." He was relieved, and said, "Oh, you're not being evicted yet." I guessed that meant he was looking for my case in the housing-court files and it wasn't there. Ahh fooey, nothing had been dismissed. Then Noah explained what a "notice to cure" was while I listened, curled over into myself. There was a lot of information coming at me, without any "ums" or "uhs." He had said these things so many times that he doesn't need to think; it just flowed. It flowed like a power wash, and I was bending into the constant stream so it bounced a little. It wasn't too long ago that I didn't know anything about being arrested. Now "eviction" had been added to my course load, and I couldn't keep up.

Noah requested that the pages be sent to him. This I could do. I had them photographed and filed already on my computer, with labels, not just the date of the photo as the title. They were ready to send. I'd been very organized about my arrest. I was a helpful and competent client. Hopefully—the secular version of praying, like sending out a "To Whom It May Concern" into the universe rather than a DM "Dear God"—he could prevent me from getting evicted from my apartment, where I didn't even want to live.

Noah mentioned he would be out of town through Monday, and I said reading my "notice to cure" would be fun commute-ride material. I used the joke to segue into seriousness, telling him these documents, this after-school-special version of events, wasn't me. Laughing, he told me he didn't judge—he just needed to read the pages so he would be prepared. Yeah, yoga teachers say that, too, but I've said or heard, "A student in my class today…" to another teacher more times than I've said or heard "bless you" after a sneeze. Students do things and exhibit behavior teachers aren't trained for. Under the guise of "spirituality," which is absolutely not shorthand for "it's all good," students do wacky shit.

There are students who refuse to separate from their six-figure purses, wrapping them in towels and keeping them at the corner of their mats, or putting them directly in front of the class, on a windowsill. Thus, dedicating their practice to drowning in the

Kool-Aid of materialism. I once had a regular student who'd bring her little dog in a small carrying case and hide it on the prop shelves. There are students who have inversion wardrobe malfunctions; mostly boobs falling out and flashing the class. There are students who go commando in their well-worn leggings. (A good test is to hold the seat of pants up to a light. If you can see the bulb, I can see everything a doctor sees). There are students on mental cocktails. Men who wear high-cut running shorts with tiny, built-in underwear that the boys fall out of. One of the more unpleasant alignment cues I've given is to tell a man his junk has fallen out of the drawer. With how miserable they seem restrained, it's hard to believe men can't feel the difference when the boys sneak out, and take the initiative to call them back home.

I've witnessed fighting couples. Erections. Open wounds, bleeding. Students who've just come from the salon and are raining little hairs. Ladies who've gotten their cycles during class (and I know it before they do). Women who don't want to ruin a fresh pedicure or manicure (or both) and who practice, the entire class, with toes and fingertips up. New face-lifts and students who are medically restricted from folding forward. Rather large new boobs and ladies who can't lie on their bellies because it creates too much of a backbend. I had a private client sneeze something like a digested sandwich out of his nose and be the one to tell him, "Hey, I think something's on your shirt!" while tempering my gag reflex. I've heard phlegm-clearing sounds (and I'll stop there on that one).

I've been sneezed at, sweated against, and puked on by a newborn I was holding while mommy practiced. I've been accidentally slapped and kicked in the head more than once (please don't bend your knees while being spotted in handstand), had my back yanked out, and my knees hyperextended. I've been pushed, pulled, grabbed, and petted. I've been told off, thrown out of a brownstone on the Upper West Side, and cursed at. I've had my music player stolen (the owner of Exhale graciously replaced it).

I've been hit on (but never by a person I wanted), and stalked. The standout, though, was the woman with the red ball.

In my heyday, during a packed Sunday-morning class, an older lady came in with her red ball. It wasn't one of the bouncy ones that kids get when they're screaming in toy stores, but a fitness-type ball, like a smaller version of a dodgeball. She placed it near her mat. Sometimes, students bring in props they'll use for savasana or to address a health issue, and I need to wait and see how it plays out. While it was strange, I had to get going and teach. *Whatever.*

We got to the backbending section of class. Students were on their backs, preparing for bridge pose, with legs at right angles, knees bent, feet under their knees, hips lifted, arms underneath, and hands clasped. Instead of doing what all the other students were doing, because that's what you're supposed to do in a group class, the lady put her ball under her butt. Okay, she wanted to do that, though a block would have worked, too. *Whatever.* It was a beginners' class, chill enough that I could keep an eye on her and her red ball while teaching.

I was getting ready to call out another bridge pose when the lady raised her legs straight up, the ball still under her ass. That wasn't a great idea. Balls are round, and she could have rolled off. Then she started swinging her legs violently. They were going side to side, scissoring front to back. It was like she was land drowning on her mat and trying to attract help. I was frozen at the front of the room, my mouth open, eyes like saucers, watching those legs and thinking that if she over-swung, the ball was going to shoot out from under her butt and hit a student. Then she would come crashing down, hit another student, or the same one, and definitely get injured herself. It's normal to spend a good amount of time as a yoga teacher preventing students from injuring themselves. I'm not a neophyte to dangerous physical feats or wildly inaccurate interpretations of verbal directions. Over the years, I've developed some good reaction time in that department. Usually, it's because students are not in their bodies and they aren't aware they won't be able to use their elbows…ever again. This was the first time, though, that I'd have to prevent a student from being dangerous to herself and others by bouncing on a ball.

I walked over, sat on my shins at the front of her mat, casually postured, and told her she couldn't use the red ball. I explained that it was dangerous. In a stealth blur the lady went from lying down to spryly seated inches away from my face. "First," she said, holding up a hand with one finger so I knew she was on "one" and was about to list a sequence, "You don't talk to me that way. Second…" (Now two fingers were raised. How many points was she going to make? It was only an hour-long class.) "…I'll do what I please." She raised a third finger, and I stood up.

We were done with backbends, and I called out a child's pose. It's the perfect counter pose for backbends, and it left me enough time to quickly sneak out. I quietly opened the door, then sprinted to the front desk and told the sweet, young manager on duty that there was a lady rolling on a ball. *Help!* Then I ran back, casually entered, and resumed teaching. The manager slipped in and talked to the woman and they both left, along with the red ball. I marveled at how smoothly it went. After class, regulars stayed around, and we joked about the whole thing with unflattering retells and general snarkiness. So the truth is that everyone judges. It's a great release. Sending Noah the "notice to cure" meant it was heading out into the world for review. That sucked.

Noah and I ended the call. I checked the mailbox in case there was a dismissal notice in there. There was nothing.

Tuesday, June 7, 2016

On social media, Emu had posted a close-up of two hands and an arm, all with variations of the same small design. The caption said they were by beloved Japanese tattoo artist Hideki. The design looked like a colorful squid, but was balanced, spiritual and weighty. It wasn't cutesy or faux-tribal. I took a screen shot to keep as inspiration for "filler" ideas. Those are smaller tattoos placed in-between larger pieces to fill-up awkward free space. Like playing Tetris on your skin. During our last session on my back piece, I hunted around Emu's arm for her little squid, asking "What's that about?" She was good friends with Hideki. He did the "hoju" squid-looking tattoo for her some years ago, during a difficult period of her life. She explained how you get one during a crisis. I think she said there was wishing involved.

Immediately, I wanted one. It wasn't envy, but more a feeling of this needs to happen. I told Emu I'd like to get one, and she said, "Sure, we can do one of those." It's probably intensely annoying, when you're in the middle of working on a piece that starts at the base of someone's neck and goes all the way to the back of their thighs, for the person to be shopping for their next tattoo. I had about another year and half to go, at least, until my back piece was finished.

Still, I had nothing to do, and the hoju had me absorbed. I'd messed up by asking Emu, though. I wanted Hideki to do the piece. Suddenly, desperately, it had to be him. It felt important to have the authenticity of a Japanese artist doing a traditional Japanese design in a traditional Japanese method. Hideki uses hand-poking, called irezumi, to apply tattoos. This is for when the pain of a needle is no longer exciting. It's also beautiful to watch. I thought the magic wouldn't work otherwise. Never mind the back piece. I needed to make an official wish. My life was consistently getting worse and worse. It was hard to corral the bad energy swirling around me. I needed a higher power to intervene on my behalf.

Still preoccupied about it after the tattoo session, I emailed Emu asking for more information. And she replied:

On June 5, 2016, 5:57 pm, Emu wrote:

Hey Marcy- So I looked up the hoju—or wishing jewel—and if you [search] for "cintamani," it gives you an explanation. It's a pretty cool symbol. OK, talk to you soon. Cheers, Emu

From what I read, the hoju grants blessings and wishes, especially to those who are suffering. Or, it can be understood as offering clarity. It brings lightness into the darkness. I romanticized that you make a wish while getting the tattoo. I could wish for my arrest to be dismissed and my eviction resolved, though that would be two wishes. I'd need to suss out the wording prior so it was a single concept. This was a great idea. Instead of hiring a lawyer, moving, or buying noise-cancelling headphones, I should get a tattoo. I found this plan completely reasonable, full of logic, and on par with my spiritual approach to life. I would go old school on my ordeal.

Getting this little squid design became a thing for me. It was a mosquito bite on my thoughts. It needed to happen, by Hideki, as soon as possible. The problem was that I needed Emu to refer me. I couldn't walk into a shop where Hideki worked. His studio was private. He also wasn't on social media. An introduction was necessary. People ask me for help all the time, and my comfort in that role inhibits balance. I don't like reaching out, but in the end, I used the email from Emu about the design to sheepishly ask if she wouldn't mind referring me:

On June 6, 2016, 2:10 pm, Marcy Tropin wrote:

Emu,
Thanks so much for remembering. What a great wormhole to go through!!! There's even a Bhagavad Gita version of the gem called syamantaka.
Favor!!! After having a groovy session on my back with you, I came home to eviction papers. My

landlord is going to try to use my arrest to get me out. I was thinking that evening about how you got your hoju tattoo during your own shitstorm. Since I've moved into my apartment, it's been raining crap.

Is there a chance your friend Hideki would do a hoju on me? Anywhere, any colors, anytime, any size…please.

Hope this doesn't sound idiotic or insincere. It's hard to write out in an email why one feels a connection to a piece of art and an intuition about an artist without it turning into a thesis paper.

Completely understand if it's not possible!!
-Marcy

And Emu responded:

On June 7, 2016, 12:18 pm, Emu wrote:

Holy Crap!! What a fuckin' bummer. I'm so sorry buddy. Maybe it's the universe getting you out of there, it has been crap since you got in. I will reach out to Hideki and ask him—I'm sure he will say yes—when he does I will pass on his email contact. Hoju will be good, especially by him. -e

It worked, and I got to email Hideki directly. I took a long time to compose my message, reminding myself he was doing a favor for Emu and that I was representing her. Hideki doesn't do small pieces anymore, he doesn't need my money, he doesn't need my business, and he doesn't need to hear about any of the drama going on in my life. If he agreed to do a hoju on me, I was going to let him put the piece wherever he wanted, in whatever colors and size he wanted. I'd come with a pile of cash and snacks, and say nothing. I would be the most amenable piece of canvas he'd ever worked on.

Wednesday, June 8, 2017

My eviction had one positive: it was nice to have a different subject to talk about besides my arrest. I'd had years where things kept piling on, but there was something about being in my 40s that made this pathetic. In my impetuous 20s, living before thinking, this sort of thing was expected and interesting. Two decades later, I was the friend you casually ask, "Hey, how's it going?"—and there's a maelstrom of updates. In less than three months I'd become a sad story. It was also hard to give an update and then maneuver the conversation into an upbeat, "And how are you?" People kept telling me that my eviction was a sign. A sign I should move. I like signs. There's a big sign motif in the whole Moses gestalt that I was taught as a kid. It's not a brush fire; God's talking to you. The eviction didn't feel like a sign to me, except maybe a sign that my landlord was an asshole.

I ran into Dewan, and we shared updates. Management was trying to evict him, too. We commiserated. He didn't really care. He'd grown up in the building. He knew how the management company operated. He was used to this. Years ago he made sure to get all the lease paperwork in his name, legally. Now that his parents had passed away, management was trying to intimidate him out. After 30 plus years, they greedily desired to turn his two-bedroom apartment over. In buildings where there are long-standing, rent-stabilized tenants, this is common.

Management wouldn't do any repairs in Dewan's apartment. He had to go through external channels, like calling an inspector. I didn't know if I was impressed by how well he was dealing with the landlord, or sad for him because he was so used to this kind of treatment that it no longer fazed him. We bonded about when the neighbors were their loudest. It was on Fridays, and we couldn't figure out why, but we were each ecstatic that the other person knew this, too. We also agreed the neighbors had gotten worse. Maybe my being arrested had inspired them. Dewan told me he was never home anymore. I told him that on Sundays, the neighbors weren't home. "It's peaceful all day," I said. "Try it."

Friday, June 10, 2016

It had been relatively quiet. My neighbors installed an air conditioner in their living room window, which faced the air shaft. Aesthetically, it broke up the black garbage-bag window shades. I can understand not having money for window treatments, but it must be hard to live in a space where black bags cover windows. Why not use white kitchen bags? At least they would diffuse the light with a soft glow. With their AC on and their windows closed, their yelling was muddled. I could tune them out and turn them into background noise. Every day, I was getting better at hearing them yelling while still living in my apartment, and I congratulated myself on this.

In the mail, I received my June rent check along with a letter from management. The company's name and address were in enormous bold type across the top of the page, and then my name and address underneath there in normal type. Under that was a checklist for the reason my rent has been returned:

- Insufficient funds/payment stopped: Please replace with cash, money order, or certified check.
- No signature: Please sign check.
- We cannot accept checks from anyone other than the tenant(s) of record.
- Your lease has expired.
- We have begun legal proceedings against you.
- Your account has been in arrears for the past_____.
- No personal checks accepted. Certified check or money order only.

- Full payment only: total due $_____.
- Due to excessive returned checks on your account, personal or business checks will no longer be honored on your account.

and, lastly

- Other:_____.

I got "other." In the area with printed lines for handwritten comments was a name and contact information embellished with a large asterisk and a note that said, "We are unable to accept any rent payment at this time."

There's a legal time period for "curing," and it didn't seem like management was planning on waiting it out. I was being "cured" fast. It was hard not to feel victimized. I knocked on a door, twice. For that, I might have a criminal record and be forced out of my home. It was a bit much. I thought using online banking to make rent payments was foolproof. It should work perfectly, except in instances where the check was returned back to me. It wasn't supposed to come back to me. I looked at it, waving the paper in the air and asking, "What do I do with you? Open an escrow account?" I took a picture of both my check and the letter, and emailed them to Noah. All this rejection. They didn't like me; they didn't even like my money.

Saturday, June 11, 2016

Friday was the 21st anniversary of my bicycle accident, the event that led me to yoga. On June 10, 1995, I was a young art student cycling down Grand Avenue in Oakland, California. I'd just finished my shift at Noah's Bagels in Berkeley. My backpack was stuffed with two dozen onion day-old bagels to drop off at my friend Alyson's place on the ride home. It was a beautiful Saturday afternoon. I was about to pass Linda Avenue when a bus overshot the stop sign. Back then, buses were actively adversarial towards cyclists. As the bus went half its length past the stop sign, I slowed down to see if it would cut in front of me. Then it stopped, and I stood up in my saddle to start cycling again. That's when an oncoming car made a sweeping left turn.

The driver probably didn't see any traffic ahead, turned hard left, and didn't see me until I was in front of their car. The driver didn't even have a reaction to seeing me and never hit the brakes. Without the good fortune of standing on my pedals, I probably would have been pinned under the car, or maybe even driven over. Once the car hit my bicycle, I flew backwards, headfirst, into the windshield, smashing the glass. This is why you wear bike helmets, because of other drivers, not because of your own personal cycling skills. Even after I hit the windshield, the driver didn't apply the brakes. If they had, I probably would have been thrown forward off the hood, hitting the pavement. Instead, I rolled off the car and onto my feet, and was left standing in the middle of the intersection. I couldn't have planned a snazzier dismount. Even the Russian judges would have applauded.

From the intersection, I watched the black Lincoln Continental keep driving up the street, then stop on the side of the road. Through the back window, I could see the windshield was a spiderweb of cracks, the center caved in, where my head had hit. I looked over at the bus, still there at the stop sign. I looked down at my left leg. It had a cut that was bleeding. I walked over to the bus driver, who initially refused to open his window, and then, after I motioned to my leg, he cracked it open to hand me some paper towels. No one got off the bus. To this day, this bothers me. Not one person left the bus. I was holding the paper towels against my leg when the driver of the Lincoln walked towards me. A short, 86-year-old white lady, who spoke as if she were answering a trivia question, with a matter-of-fact logic about nearly killing me, "Oh honey, I didn't see you. I was wearing my dark sunglasses."

She was wearing those drugstore wraparound sheets of black plastic you can place over eyeglasses, rather than getting prescription sunglasses.

I was wandering around the intersection when a man ran over with his cell phone, maybe the first cell phone ever made. He was telling me he'd called the police but I was finding the thing he was holding to his ear—about a foot long, five inches thick, off-white, with a long silver antenna—absolutely hysterical. Even back then, it looked like a parody of a cell phone. When EMS arrived, four paramedics launched out of the ambulance and asked who was injured. I raised my hand. The first to get to me was a woman so upset I'd been walking around—with a possible head injury—that she was almost yelling at me. Then I felt hands grab major joints and take me from vertically standing to lying on the ground as gracefully as if we had practiced it with the Bolshoi. From the ground, I saw a friend of mine from college appear. She was driving past with her boyfriend, and said, "I hope this looks worse than it is." They asked if there was anything they could do, then threw my pretzeled bike into the back of their pickup truck for me.

I was somehow on a backboard. Pieces of foam were being strategically placed against my body and fastened down. Then I was loaded into the ambulance and driven to the emergency room. I'd been in an ambulance before, and if you haven't, and you're conscious, know they're going to chat you up per protocol. It felt like a third uncle catching up at a ten-year family reunion asking, "What's your full name? What's today's date? Where were you born? Where do you go to school? What do you study?" One of the many benefits of verbally engaging a person in shock is keeping them from having a "what the fuck just happened" freak-out. Being in an ambulance rushing through traffic really brings an event into context.

I was rolled into the emergency room, and they immediately took X-rays. Somewhere in there, a nurse asked whether I wanted to call anyone on my behalf, and I gave them Alyson's number. I don't know what I would do in that situation now, because I don't have anyone's number memorized, and if my cell phone were smashed, there wouldn't be an easy way to get contact information. But back then, I called friends. We all called people regularly, and knew phone numbers. Getting the X-rays was painful, but I don't recall why. I remember afterwards being in a double room. The door was in the middle and one patient had a section to the right, with curtains. The other patient, to the left, was me. Since I was duct-taped to a gurney, there wasn't much to do. The only part of my body I could move was my eyes. I looked at the clock on the wall across from me. A nurse came in and said as soon as they received the X-rays back and knew I didn't have a spinal injury, she could release me from the tape. Now I was freaked out. I also had to use the bathroom.

I told myself I didn't have a spinal injury and I was going to walk to the bathroom of my own volition, any second now. I was watching the clock. It was all I had to pass the time. I gave myself the challenge of waiting a whole hour. But after the large hand had circled around, and then some, and the X-ray results still weren't back, I gave up. The next time the nurse came in to check on me, I asked her, "What are my options for peeing?" "Well, honey," leaning on the bed as she spoke, "we can hook a tube up to your bladder and drain it." I responded faster to anything ever said to me in my life with, "Orrrrrr?" "Or I can get a bedpan," she added. I opted for the bedpan, and the nurse left to retrieve one. When she came back, she undid the middle taped areas and pulled my shorts and underpants down. It occurred to me then that Alyson, being the good friend she is, was probably en route and might show up at any moment, like this moment, when my pants were down.

For some reason the 90s version of feminism had a lot to do with being hairy. Not shaving was a feminist protest statement. For me, it was a very big statement. I'm a pale woman, and my lady hairs are solid black and curly. I wouldn't say I had a bikini line, I'd say I was upholstered in between my legs, down my thighs, and almost up to my belly button. (This was gratefully resolved early in my teaching career when I bartered with a private client who owned a spa and used every single session for laser hair removal. God bless you, Eugenia!!). If Alyson were to walk in at that moment, with my pants down, I didn't think our friendship would survive it. Sure, we'd say "hi" on campus, but as a visual artist, she might never get the image of my overgrown lawn out of her head. I needed to get this over with as soon as possible, for the sake of my kidneys and our friendship.

Unfortunately, when the nurse brought my pants and underwear down, she saw my first-ever tattoo, of a turtle, and paused to let me know her nephew was thinking about getting a tattoo. "Oh yeah, that's cool," I responded while strapped down, immobile, and awkwardly half naked, "What's he thinking of getting?" After a couple of exchanges, the pan was placed, a sheet was laid over me, privacy was given…and then I couldn't do it. My body refused. Thus followed possibly the greatest disagreement I could have with myself without the forced intervention of antipsychotic meds. Whatever long-forgotten training I'd had as a child not to wet the bed, it was a strong and mighty foundation, with zero cracks. The fear of pissing myself would not let go, no matter how much I argued, "There's a pan, just do it." Finally, I closed my eyes and forced myself into the moment. Once gravity presented itself, and I heard the ting of liquid hitting metal, I relaxed, and was relieved.

The nurse came back, removed the pan, pulled my clothing up, taped me back down, and left. Moments later, Alyson appeared from around the curtain, saying, "Hey!" The nurse returned to ask if I wanted anything to eat, and I said, "No thanks." Then Alyson made a subtle noise somewhere between her nose and the back of her throat and I changed my answer, "Wait, what do you have?" When the nurse's selection hit "tuna sandwich," I heard another low-honking sound from Alyson, and told the nurse I'd love one of those. In college, as broke artists, we were all about free food, no matter the circumstances.

The X-rays eventually came back, and I was fine to go. Except I wasn't fine. My neck no longer moved. It wouldn't turn or tilt. I'd spend most of my 20s in constant pain until I found yoga. What saved me, though, were those two dozen bagels, the food of my people. One bagel for each vertebra, 24 in the lumbar, cervical, and thoracic spine—my spine, which would have been destroyed had the bagels not been in my backpack at the time of the crash and had they not absorbed the impact. I always thought there was something predestined about my accident, like it happened because I was meant to teach yoga.

To celebrate the anniversary, I had insomnia. Having my rent check sent back felt very real, even more so than the summons. That was just paperwork. Sending money back meant they really wanted to do this. I was depressed and anxious all day except when I taught class and was too busy to think. I walked with Hope in the morning, but it felt like I was just trying to be better company than how I really felt.

After class, I walked towards the subway with book-stealing Goldie. I started to tell her about my eviction, then crumpled when she asked a lot of follow-up questions. She was upset, and the heat of her being angry at my landlord and my neighbor was inadvertently directed towards me. It was kind of like when drivers yell at other cars and it's their passengers who receive the hate. Goldie wanted to help, and her questions were well-meaning, but I didn't know the answers to a lot of them. I didn't know what was going to happen. I didn't know the future. *I don't know, so don't ask me.* At the time I couldn't handle suggestions, though that has never been my forte. No, I didn't know if my neighbor had hired a lawyer or if she had done this before. No, I wasn't hiring a lawyer. Yes, it didn't make sense intuition was informing this decision. Why did empathy have to come with so many questions? I wanted to be able to update people without dealing with their own personal reactions. I wanted a hug or a hand on my shoulder. That's what I needed.

Goldie reminded me to cover up my tattoos in court. *Yeah, yeah, yeah.* To wear a long-sleeve shirt. *Yeah, yeah, yeah.* She told me to wear a tight-fitting shirt to show off how small I was. I was guessing she wasn't referring to my being slight of chest. Then she said I should wear makeup. It reminded me of when I was little, and my mom and I would drive out to my aunt's house on Staten Island. There, my mom and aunt fought, and my cousin and I would play. Back then we had normal, fun, kid-playing time thanks to our budding imaginations. There was a lot of garage-sale adult clothing to pretend with and stuffed animals to act as co-conspirators.

Less often than we visited them, my aunt and cousin would drive out to New Jersey for the weekend. There, my mother and aunt fought, usually over the thermostat. These women would go at each other with no verbal holds barred, right in front of their kids. My aunt would threaten to leave, while my cousin and I held onto each other, crying. As we got closer to our preteens, my cousin would arrive dressed in a fancy outfit. My aunt had contrived a competition between the girls, but had forgotten to get my mother or me involved. The pressure on me to wear more "feminine" clothing would happen later. At my mom's house, within minutes of arriving, my cousin and I were dirty from playing in the backyard. Playtime in New Jersey happened outside, away from my mother's museum-style decorating. I learned how to remove grass and mud stains during these visits, trying to make sure my cousin wouldn't get in trouble for messing up her outfit. I developed a technique of sneaking outside with a sponge and a small kids' cup filled with dish detergent diluted with water. The best way to remove a stain is to "dab out" and never "rub in."

My aunt was not a friendly woman, though she pretended to be. Back at her house, she'd tell me I was pretty, if I only wore a little makeup. This statement never made sense to me, what tense was she speaking in? Was it a compliment or an insult? I thought she and my mom looked ridiculous with their blue eye shadow. Why place blue there, above your eyes, and red shading on your cheeks, never mind the process of putting a pointy object near the base of your eyeball to draw a black line? I stood up to that woman from a very young age, and I'm very proud of it. I absorbed her constant making fun of me with acerbic snides, defended by the putdown, "I was being funny Marcy, you have no humor." Then she would give me a shove. Perhaps you can knock some sense into a person, but it doesn't get them to laugh while they're being ridiculed. All of my aunt's ire for not looking "pretty" by her definition. Maybe sexualizing little girls is normal, but I don't think so. I also don't think using funny as a weapon is a great enabler. But the more laughs my aunt got at my expense, the more inspired she was to continue. Even when my cousin joined forces with her in our teen years, I never gave into their peer pressure to look the way they wanted me to look.

Standing across from Goldie and her concerns, the hullabaloo of Columbus Circle weaved around us. I think what was happening here was a reduction in my friend's confidence in me. That if I'd gotten myself into this situation, then I must not be that bright. Intelligent people don't get arrested by their lying neighbors. I could no longer be trusted. It could no longer be assumed that I would make logical decisions. I was getting this kind of advice because friends were concerned I was going to make the situation worse. Why does concern often feel so annoying?

Instead of answers about procedures, lawyers, time frames, paperwork, and probabilities, the only thing people really needed to know was that it sucked. That was all anyone needed to understand. I'm really unhappy. This sucks. Goldie sweetly asked if I wanted her there for the next court date on July 6, and I said no thank you. I was concerned about falling apart. I had it in my head that if my neighbor signed a sworn statement, that would make the charges official. If she didn't participate, the case would fall apart. So it was either me—or the case—that would fall apart. If I did, I wanted to be alone. "You might not," Goldie said. I felt close to unraveling already. I was being held together by dog hair, Clif bars, and afternoon naps. It wasn't holding up. I wasn't holding up. I didn't say any of these things to her. My head hurt. The next weekend, I was planning to visit Alyson, Marie, and their kids in Chicago. After I purchased my ticket, it occurred to me I might not be allowed to leave the state. I'd never had to worry about these issues or ask these questions regarding my freedom. The arrest had changed my relationship, my ownership, of personal decisions. Like being strapped to a gurney.

At home, my rent check was on my desk. I'd been paying rent since I was 18. I'd never not paid rent. It's something I like about myself, being fiscally responsible. Being nonviolent was also something I liked about myself. All those perceptions, those ideas of who I was, I no longer had control over. They were seen through other people's eyes now. The character I had thoughtfully built, the integrity I wanted to be associated with…why was that so easy to undo? If other people didn't see me that way, could I still see myself that way? It felt bad enough now, and there was still the option of my going to jail, where it would really feel bad. It seemed like every week there was a new surprise.

Also on my desk was a pink postcard letting me know there was a certified letter waiting for me at the post office. My guess was that it was from the management companies' lawyer. I hadn't told anyone about it, not any lawyer-type person. I was simply not going to get it. I didn't have to. I was going to be a child and pretend it wasn't there. Like vegetables on a plate, the notice would be pushed around my desk until it was hidden under some other stuff. If I was asked about it, I could use the Reagan defense and say "I don't recall." I'd received enough bad news for the year. I was tired, it was late, and tomorrow would be the same as today, another day of waiting until July 6.

Tuesday, June 14, 2016

After teaching my lunchtime class, I rushed downtown. I'd scored a session with Hideki, and I was excited and giddy. I couldn't believe I'd gotten an appointment so quickly, and I couldn't believe I was going to his private studio. I'd always wanted to go to a secret something in New York City, so long as it didn't have drunk revelers, loud music, casual sex, or crowds. That rules out a lot of scenarios, and since I don't gamble, that rules out all of the scenarios.

My directions were to go to a gate and ring a bell. I didn't know if I should look side to side beforehand, or just ring the bell normally and try to blend in. I'd gone to gates before and rung bells. This wasn't any different, but I was not going to talk myself out of feeling mysterious and special. I exited the train at Delancey Street and immediately walked with great purpose and speed in the wrong direction. There are some subway exits that flip my internal city compass. I couldn't figure out which way was up, and I'm finally at the age where I don't care, even as a resident, about asking which way Central Park is. (Don't reference "north" in New York City, it doesn't make sense to us. It's either "uptown" or "downtown") I found the gate, pushed the bell, and was buzzed in. Woohoo! I walked up a flight of stairs and through another door. That was it. That's all I wanted to do, knock on a random door and gain entry to a groovy place on the other side. Now I had to get tattooed.

Hideki's studio was very clean, and quiet except for beautiful low-playing guitar music. There were two small rooms, one you entered where business-type stuff happened, and another room for tattooing. I was taken aback at how peaceful it was. It didn't have the unnecessarily edgy, testosterone vibe I'd experienced at other parlors, even though a man was the proprietor. I took off my shoes and shook hands with the assistant and then with the artist. It was hard to contain my excitement about getting my hoju and about getting the tattoo without the nudity and mental stamina my back piece was requiring. It was like I was on vacation from my back piece, or cheating.

I was wearing the t-shirt and Patagonia yoga pants that I had taught in, with my designated tattoo flannel on top. This shirt had been worn to every tattoo session because of its versatility. I could open it down the front, or roll up the sleeves, or spin it around, depending on where the tattoo was going, and still be clothed. It was a lightweight cotton, fine for any weather. It was baggy enough to put over finished wrapped pieces, and it hid ink and blood well. My outfit was covering everything but an ankle piece. Hideki was probably guessing I didn't have many tattoos. It was a nice moment for me when I took off the plaid shirt to reveal my covered arms. Hideki went from being perched on his stool, arms crossed, asking where I wanted the hoju, perhaps settling in for me to take a long time deciding, to suddenly smiling, his expression changed. I was pointing, "There's some room here, or maybe on my hands." He wouldn't have to spend much time placing the tattoo. There wasn't a lot of space left.

While he was looking at the work on my arms, I mentioned Emu was working on my back. Did he want to see? I turned around and took my shirt and bralette off in one swoop. I was facing a mirror and watching Hideki look over the artwork on my back. I pulled down my pants a bit and said it went all the way to the back of my thighs. Showing a tattoo is different than showing your body. Hideki neither cared nor was interested in my physique. He was completely absorbed in looking over Emu's work, nodding and making little noises to himself. Then I put myself back together and turned around. He motioned for me to hold out my hands, took them in his, and turned them over and back. He was a man of few words, which might have been an

English-language thing because when he needed to tell his assistant something, long flowing Japanese came out.

So far, I was doing a great job of shutting up. On my left hand, near my wrist, are lines from a piece that goes up my arm, an ode to the painter Agnes Martin. I didn't want anything else on that hand, but waited to see what Hideki said. He decided on my right hand and asked me to lay down on the massage table. From my new vantage point, I saw the ceiling was wainscoted with light-colored tongue and groove, maybe bamboo. The space was spa-like with the exception of a large bare LED bulb in the center of the ceiling. I was zoning out on the slats of wood and how cozy they felt, wondering if I should have wood on my ceiling. My right arm was on a tattoo armrest. I'd mentally separated from my hand; it wouldn't be mine for a while.

Hideki held my hand and was moving his fingers between the metacarpals, then moving my wrist up and down. The process felt authentic, and similar to what an acupuncturist would do before placing needles. *This is going to work. This feels right.* I was about to zone out when Hideki asked me if he should stop smoking for his yoga practice. He had just started with Mysore and knew I was a yoga teacher as well as an ashtanga practitioner. I sat up and told him of course, but I also said it would happen naturally as he deepened his practice. Asana purifies the body, and it becomes very difficult to drink, smoke, or eat poorly the longer you practice.

I laid back down and was about to zone out again when he asked me a breathing question. I sat up and taught him how to breathe properly. He was holding his chest tightly, not letting his ribs expand. I laid back down. I was about to zone out and he asked me another question, so I sat up again and was explaining something, when his left shoulder went into spasm. Right there, it was twitching and he was in terrible pain, holding his shoulder. I began to work the pain out with my hands and asked him if it was too hard. "No, I like hard," he said. *Oh buddy, don't underestimate my hands.* Shoulders can be pulled forward from tight pectoral muscles in the front. When I'm working on a tight shoulder, I first dance around the scapula in the back. Then I have to dig into the pec, the heart chakra, with its emotional tangles. This can be quite painful. I found the knot in Hideki's chest and pressed deeply. He begged off, smiling.

Harder bodywork isn't better. It doesn't mean you're "getting in there." Often, it's simply, needlessly, more aggressive. People are angry about their bodies being stiff and want healers to fight their muscles. But you can damage a muscle by going too hard, and it doesn't make the releasing go any faster. From where Hideki's shoulder was being pulled, I guessed he was doing chaturanga with his elbows out. It's a common beginner's misalignment. I explained the proper form, but felt like my descriptions weren't turning into visuals for him. I got off the table and demonstrated a proper chaturanga on the floor of the first room.

Once the alignment was understood, I got back up on the table and lay down again. I was about to zone out, when I felt a soft brush against my skin. Peeking over, I saw Hideki was going to place the tattoo directly on my hand. The soft brush was a fancy marker. Usually a design is sketched beforehand, during the tattoo artist's unpaid free time. Maybe he had done many of these before, or their design was simple enough, or there was magic to them being drawn onto the skin. Whatever it was, I was loving the process. It was fascinating to watch. If I could chat him up, I would want to know how he was making each decision, on each line. But I knew better than to interrupt the process. I knew better than to keep lifting my hand every 15 seconds to have a look-see. When people ask me technical anatomy questions during bodywork, I want to put a "we'll be back soon" sign on my forehead. Once I've gotten into working on a client's body, I'm connecting to their energy. I'm in a place mentally where I can't put together a thought. I've said some of the stupidest things to clients while I've been trying to remove pain from their bodies. It's not a great way to win over someone's confidence, but I'll agree that it's hard to shut up.

I looked around the room; there were some stickers on the ceiling, near the light, large photographs of finished back pieces lining the walls, and all that soothing wood. I closed my eyes, finding a peace in my body that hadn't been there in a long time. I was happy. As painful and expensive as tattoos can be, I love getting them. I love meeting the artists and seeing their work areas: the drawings for other clients pinned up here and there, the dog-eared art books, stickers from travels and all the different hand-crafted machines hanging in rows from hooks. Drawers with bottles of color. Drawers with various-sized needles individually sterile wrapped. Maybe an incense holder, a picture of a beloved pet, a cup of coffee, a bottle of water, a wallet and phone thrown into a corner where they will be hunted for later. If there's conversation, it's always good, and if it's quiet, there's plenty of work on the tattoo artists' own bodies to peek at. I love the thimble-sized plastic cups that are used to hold ink and the big glop of ointment nearby. To keep the little cups from tipping over, artists will touch the bottoms to the ointment, so they stay in place. I even like watching them do this, making a row of cups that will eventually be filled with the colors for a tattoo. The whole setup process is captivating, and for a couple of minutes I forget the eventuality: I'm the canvas for all this crap.

Hideki had finished drawing. I took my hand back as part of my body and looked at the design. Something felt off. I didn't say anything, just took a picture of the drawing with my phone and rested my hand down. The lines of fire around the jewel weren't right, but I wasn't going to mention it. Internally, I was conflicted. Then I felt Hideki rubbing off a line and redrawing. He felt it too. When he was done, I looked at my hand again, and the design was perfect, like it was meant to be there. There was a black outline sketch of a hoju that would permanently be with me in a short while. Hideki set up his materials to tattoo the outline. In terms of pain, the outline sucks the most. This has something to do with the needle used. It's also because the artists aren't staying in one area that can numb out. They're moving around, and every spot is new. Now I started second-guessing how easy I thought this would be, to have my hand tattooed. It wasn't like I wouldn't feel anything.

Hideki set up the black ink and began. He was doing the outline with a machine. It was painful, but nothing like having my back worked on. I smiled and said as much, relieved. I could have fallen asleep. After he was finished with the outline, I held my hand up. There it was, my very own hoju. Next, he would fill in the piece with color.

Hideki had asked his assistant for a cup of water, which he poured into three smaller cups on his work station near him, something that looked similar to a surgeon's tool tray. Usually, tattoo artists just have one cup of water nearby, so I was watching how this would play out. Hideki explained how the middle part of my hoju would be charcoal ink, and how that was made. I was watching him hand grind the black ink for my piece. As an artist, this was a huge treat for me, watching pigment being made. I remembered some advice to give to him about beginning a yoga practice as intensely as he was. I warned him that around week two, he might get flu-like symptoms. That was the body detoxifying. I tell students this so they'll keep practicing and won't give up. Depending on how much a body has been wrecked, this can be a huge turnoff when people start yoga. "It's part of the process," I told him, "just get through it."

For the colors, Hideki was mixing his own pigments with water. I filmed this a little with my phone. It was absolutely mesmerizing, watching colors being made that would eventually go into my skin. He didn't ask me which colors I wanted, and I didn't say anything about what he was mixing. There was an orange, a yellow, and a teal, and two kinds of red. In the cups, the colors were bright and clean. Hideki didn't seem to mind me filming. There was a timelessness to his craft. When it looked like he was finished with the colors, I laid back down.

I was about to zone out when Hideki started to ask me a question. He seemed very serious. I thought, this is it, the ritual part of the piece where he will ask me what I am wishing for. What intent did I want to instill in this hoju? I was working through a short sentence in my head. Something about home and safety. Not just this moment in my life, but moving forward. It was like I was about to address a battalion on an auspicious day. I totally forgot to prepare for this, and it was important. The whole reason I was getting this thing was that the piece called to me, it reached out through social media and said, "Me, get one, now!!" And here I was, without any forethought, yet again. Hideki paused after an inhale—I was trying to clear my thoughts because I would have to do this off the cuff—and then he said, "Why no food before practice?" Oh, he had another yoga question. There wasn't going to be a symbolic time-out for a wish. "Right, okay," I said. "You don't want to eat before practicing mostly for two reasons..."

Question answered, I settled into zoning out again, but as I was closing my eyes, I saw him pull out a large, long metal thing in a sterile wrapper. It wasn't like the needles that I normally see. It was more like what's laid out in a movie to let you know torture is forthcoming. Before I could phrase it in my head constructively, respectfully, or maturely, I blurted out, "What the hell is that?!?" In terms of results, you wouldn't even need to use this thing. Simply the presentation would suffice. It was silver metal, shiny, almost the size of a chopstick, with small pricks at the bottom. It was the Japanese needle. Oh yeah, the poke method. I'd also forgotten to prepare for being poked. I definitely would not have known to prepare for poking by an ice pick with prickles on the end. This was the authenticity I craved. I signed up for this. In my head, I was berating myself for not doing a visual of the experience last night. I should have given my nervous system a heads-up. Then I mentally moved on to prepare for it being a little more painful than one of those electric tattoo machines I was used to. I didn't know why one long metal stick would seem more menacing than a tool that makes the same sound a dentist's drill does, but the unknown fosters fear like nothing else.

What was nice about the chopstick was that it was quiet. And I was there mostly because I have a thing for peace and quiet. That's how I got into trouble in the first place. Arrested, and blah blah blah. So there was a plus to the poke method. Hideki held the large needle in one hand and then, like he was lining up a shot with a cue stick, he rested the front end against the finger or thumb of his other hand for steadiness. He began poking the chopstick into my flesh. It did not, to my immeasurable relief, hurt more than a machine. It did, however, feel as though I was being prepared as food. The poking sounded like a banana being chopped. I tried to push this imagery out of my head. I decided to ask a question: "Why do American tattoo artists use a machine?" Hideki thought for a moment, looking off to the side, then said, "Machine is faster and…" I chimed in, "Oh, of course, that's it." He smiled and we both went about our business, mine staying still and quiet and his poking ink into my hand. I thought of how pleasant it was being in his space and how happy I was to have him do this tattoo for me. Then I made a wish.

Wednesday, June 15, 2016

I had a nice walk with Hope in the morning, took a depression nap after, and then couldn't do anything. I ended up lying on the sofa playing sudoku on my cellphone. I told myself it would help prevent Alzheimer's disease. My body felt weighed down. Continuously hearing my neighbor's yelling, going on four months now, had beaten me. I had lost the battle. On one side of the air shaft was my ship, with Buster, and we were a solemn group. On the other side of the shaft were my neighbors, and they were celebrating. Their yelling, like the sounds of corks popping

271

and toasts being made. While on my ship, I emotionally baled water and made repairs. It was demoralizing, hearing my neighbor yell to her dark heart's content.

Then Noah called about my returned rent check. I took notes. He was explaining what was currently happening and telling me what to expect would happen, and I thought I had a grasp on it. We were not going to do anything for the time being in the hope that management would get sloppy. If we did send something in response to their "notice to cure" and returned checks, it would inspire them to do their job. This seemed like a good game plan: wait, and wait for the other side to make a mistake. I was to keep sending my rent, and when the checks were returned, deposit them into an escrow account.

Noah explained that it was common for big management companies like mine to accidentally deposit rent checks for tenants they were evicting. If they did deposit my check, they would have to start the eviction process all over again. After the "notice to cure," the next thing they would do was send what is called a "notice of termination." If for some reason they didn't send the notice to terminate, then after a couple of months of them not accepting rent, we could send them a note about how they should deposit my rent and claim it was prejudicial that they weren't. The "notice of termination" would let me know they were going to terminate my lease. A month after that, they should be sending another notice called a "petition." I thought that was the order of things. The "petition" would mean I met with Noah because it was tied to a court appearance. We were also hoping that my criminal case would be dismissed on July 6 to support my housing case before these notices even appeared.

I gathered two things from our conversation. The first was that I didn't really have to do much but send rent checks, and the second was that this was a very long process and wasn't going away soon or even months from now. Noah asked me if I'd had any contact with my neighbor. Contact with the person (or the family of the person) who had an order of protection against me? Nope, I had not. After receiving all this swell legal advice, I found the contact question silly. Noah wouldn't ask that if he hadn't had clients break their orders of protection, or if there wasn't an order of protection in my case in the first place. I was guessing some of his clients just didn't get the gravitas of the situation. As was the case with Goldie's questions, I wasn't in a position to be granted confidence. I hadn't had any intended contact with my neighbors since my arrest on April 11, though at times they were hard to avoid. I was in a jail, both in my apartment and mentally. I didn't have the freedom to do anything about anything, lest it be construed as harassment. It was like living on the top of an eggshell and hoping not to fall off.

It was also like living in my childhood home. One of my brothers is older and taller than me by some two feet, or so it had felt when were kids. Our bedrooms were separated by a hallway. Mine was down one end of the hall, the bathroom was down the other, and his bedroom was next to it. I spent huge chunks of my childhood alone with this guy and his mood swings. Mostly, I stayed in my bedroom as much as possible. The challenging part happened if I needed to eat or use the bathroom. To eat, I could quietly sneak downstairs. But the bathroom, and things needing to be done in a bathroom, made noise. I'd wait as long as I could possibly hold it in before opening my bedroom door. Then I'd try to make it down the hallway without attracting attention. More often than not, he'd appear out of his bedroom, shirtless, in our mother's old lounge pants because he didn't want to mess up his own clothing. He suffered terribly from OCD, but back then we didn't know that was a thing and it had a name.

My brother would come down the hallway and there were two common scenarios. There was "the claw," and there was the take-down move. Both had the same desired effect: to cause me physical pain. "The claw," I believe, was his own invention. It meant he was going to use his right arm and hand as if they were robotic. He'd announce it like it was a separate entity from his body, like a pro wrestler's name was being announced, as if it had a mind of its own, separate from and not accountable to him. After the introduction, he would walk towards me, making machine-like noises whenever the claw moved. It would end up in front of him, like a snake. Then he would have it—since it was my brother doing this—grab onto a part of me, his hand squeezing tight, like a claw. Whatever he grabbed onto, he held onto, as hard as possible. The pain would be so intense I'd fall to my knees, pleading for him to stop. He would be standing over me, laughing as I begged, "C'mon, let go, leg go." But the more I cried out in pain, the worse the pain became, the more it continued.

My brother knew some martial arts and wrestling. He liked to practice the moves on me. So if he wasn't using a grip so tight I writhed on the ground in agony, he was simulating disarming an opponent. About halfway down the hall was the entrance to another bedroom. I'd usually get taken down around there and thrown into the extra room. Then he would twist my limbs while I tried to get away. One of my legs would be pretzeled inside his legs, and I'd slam my hands repeatedly against the floor because I was in so much pain I couldn't even yell. I remember it hurt each time my hand hit the floor, and that the feeling was almost a welcome distraction to the pain of my bones being bent against one another.

Again, my pleading caused him to laugh and increase his force. This went on for most of my childhood. After a while, and I wish this had happened sooner, I came to realize he would lose interest if I didn't scream, squirm, or contest him. I learned to have "the claw" wrapped around my arm, and just stand there watching it. I learned to look bored while my leg was twisted. I learned to tolerate a lot of pain, and stuff my anger down. As an adult, needing to pee or eat, things that are often easily resolved, would trigger the terrified little girl who hid in her bedroom.

My neighbor having the freedom to do whatever she wanted, and my being scared to leave or enter the building, mirrored this abuse. Instead of worrying about getting myself to a bathroom, I was worried about addressing Buster's needs. It was the same feeling of being stuck inside a room, with no authority figure like a parent, police, or management to help me. I wanted Noah to know I was going to do exactly what he asked, and not violate my order of protection. Having him and his team help me helped me more than I could thank them for. Someone finally had my back.

I was in my bedroom writing while my dog was on my bed, wanting his lunch early. I heard my neighbor yelling at her kid and her kid yelling back. It was noise pollution. It was like secondhand smoke. I thought when I moved into this apartment it would be for a long time. The renovation was hell, but so are all renovations. Then bedbugs pushed me into sleep-deprivation mania. After that, between the bugs and the arrest, there was a period when things were normal and I was happy. My apartment was cozy for a minimalist, and nearly done. It was rent-stabilized and I didn't have to worry about crazy yearly increases or, at the time, being evicted. I could stay put until I chose not to stay put. And at that point, I wanted to stay put.

Before this apartment, I had lived in my last place for two years, and then the owner listed it for sale. Before that, I spent less than a year living with an awesome loft mate—then he fell in love and moved out, and I couldn't find anyone else to fill his shoes. Before that, it was two years in a ground-floor apartment in the East Village, and then the lease wasn't renewed so the place could be gutted and the rent raised. Before that, it was a couple of months in a loft in the Bronx, and the crime element scared me away. Before that I was in LA for about a year. It went on and on and on. I couldn't seem to stay put. I wished it was wanderlust, but it was more about not having the time to make great decisions— and also being a renter. When I moved into the apartment in

Washington Heights, I really thought it was the end to whatever patterns had been fueling so much change.

If I was found guilty of third-degree assault, I might get a new place to live: jail. I would also be evicted and tenant blacklisted in New York City. Even if the outcome seemed unrealistic or preventable, the stress of it was happening. The stress was real.

Tuesday, June 20, 2016

I was back from a long weekend in Chicago—days of porches, kids, baseball, old friends, and junk food. I'd consumed so much junk food I started to think of the weekend as a retox. I enjoyed the pleasantness of entering a home from the outside, rather than climbing flights. Car trips, driving, the privilege of choosing who to share your ride, unlike public transit. Grocery shopping along wide aisles. Lawns. Upstairs and downstairs. Little ones and giggles. The inimitable familiarity of old friends. After a certain age, you don't get old friends anymore. Old friends start young. Keep them, try to, and cherish them.

As I landed in New York, my return plane came to a stop, and there was that bong-bong sound like they used to make in malls. The "fasten seat belt" lights went off, and you might as well have heard a starting pistol. New York City is the only place, from Tokyo to Los Angeles to Beijing to Salt Lake City to Paris to London to Boston to Denver to Thailand, where getting off a plane feels like a fire drill. I got caught up in it, like usual, and ended up standing hunched under the overhead bin. Why couldn't I resist the mayhem of people exiting small spaces? After the plane, I was on a bus back to Manhattan. There was a guy standing over me, even though it looked like he could lean back a little and enjoy some personal space of his own. He was on his cell phone. He was so close to me that I could read the number he'd called. I was watching him talking as I was watching the vapors of my vacation evaporate. Welcome home.

Before leaving Chicago I made it to the airport with enough time to catch an earlier flight. Though the gate was quiet and the plane wasn't full, I had to pay an exorbitant fee to change flights—all worth it to see my dog sooner. While I loved being in Chicago, I would push a pillow against my side when I slept, to recreate the feeling of having Buster there. While the pillow didn't have his constant donkey-kicking, or dramatic "I just can't find the right spot" circling, it helped, as I missed my little dog.

Once at my building, I grabbed the mail, and there was a letter from the management company's lawyer. I was happy that Noah told me to anticipate one. I opened the door to greet a dog who was as equally happy to see me as he was annoyed I'd been gone. Not sure what his problem was? He'd had a fantastic time at Hope's. I was doling out the love, and he was acting betrayed. So much for shelling out the bucks to see my loyal companion sooner.

I opened the letter. It was the "notice of termination" papers. They said to surrender the apartment by July 2. They might as well have added "high noon." *Wah Wah Wahhhh.* I was being run out by my neighbor and landlord. I surveyed my apartment. I could sell all of it before the end of the week. Just get out of here. Get out of New York. I wanted to go somewhere where no one knew me, and fall apart. But there was the issue of needing to not miss the July 6 court date, or a warrant would be issued for my arrest. Reality, always getting in the way of life.

Heading out for an evening class, I opened my apartment door and found a dead water bug. Was this another burning bush? A sign? Leave, leave, leave! After class, the night sky was lit with a strawberry moon, reminding me that there are other places and other versions of my life that I could be living. One that included being alone while commuting, alone while living in a structure, alone with my thoughts, and alone with my dog on a hike sans masturbators. I could do better than this. Better than: bedbugs, screaming neighbors, the bathroom flooded from above every other month, one false arrest, court appearances, a fear of entering and leaving my building, and living sequestered in the back of an apartment. Like the characters from Lost, I had to get off this island. Like the characters from Lost, I couldn't.

Wednesday, June 22, 2016

Noah emailed asking for the "notice of termination" letter. This made me feel better, and for a moment, I didn't know why. Then I realized the obvious: he was a housing lawyer, and he was on it. I looked at my notes from our phone call, confused because I thought this letter wasn't supposed to come for a couple of months. Around 5 pm. I leashed Buster to head out. There had been a lot of noise in the stairwell, the banging of things, and my neighbor's husband on speakerphone. When I opened my door, there was a young boy having trouble climbing up the stairs. Intuitively, I thought he was headed to my neighbors' place, and waited for him to pass. He was holding onto both banisters, pulling himself forward, panting. Why was he so haggard? He couldn't have been more than 12. I was watching him like a disgusted coach, thinking, "C'mon kid, push off the back leg."
When I had the all clear, I start walking down and caught my neighbor's husband as he was walking up. He was wearing khaki shorts and a bright green polo shirt. We were about to cross one another on the second floor when he stepped back to let me pass. I looked down and flung my arm up the way you do when thanking a driver who's just let you merge in front. I longed to be able to enter and leave the building without strategizing and without fear.
Walking out, I saw that boxes were propping open all the front doors—the single one with the brown frame and the two glass doors at the front. Outside there was moving truck. A moving truck? No. Way. The building's porter was watching from the

basement entrance. I asked him who was moving out and he said it was the noisy neighbors. Really! Then he called me toward him to confide in me, but he was missing most of his teeth and wasn't one for compensating with careful enunciations. It sounded like he was saying that their tub was being repaired. I asked if they were moving back in after that, though it seemed strange to move a family in and out for just a tub repair. My tub was reglazed twice, because the first attempt was a crap job, and I made sure to shower beforehand. It was a simple day of mild inconvenience. The porter told me no, they weren't moving back in.

I started taking Buster around the block, shooting a "thanks" back behind me. I could feel myself standing very tall, not from decades of yoga but from busting with good news. I texted Dewan but was vague, saying, "Dearest Neighbor, I think they are moving out right now. -Marcy." Then I called the super to get the scoop. He told me the building manager came that morning and said my neighbor was being relocated to another building a couple of blocks away. That was it. "No fucking way," I said with a smile. It turned out they were complaining about the condition of the apartment so much, particularly the bathtub, that management moved them to another unit. I saw the apartment before they moved in. It was perfectly fine. I texted Dewan back, "Confirmed. They're out." I wanted to be vague in case something happened and the texts were used in court. Even though I trusted Dewan, I still had the arrest and eviction thing going on.

Back inside my apartment, I was walking around with my arms in the air, like I was doing a victory lap. Sometimes, when a favorite sports team has a dramatic win, I'll raise my arms up, but this was even better. This was a win for me personally. The people who'd made my life miserable—along with the lives of other tenants, because it wasn't just me in this building—were leaving! Hands reaching to the sky, buzzing around, I was overjoyed. I was raising my arms for winning the war after being crushed in the battle.

I stopped to peek through the curtains at their living room window. I'd kept my shaft-facing windows covered since the "notice to cure." Even though my apartment viewed brick walls, it got great sunlight. I had been metaphorically, and literally, living in the dark. When I looked up, the black plastic garbage bags were gone. The air conditioner was gone. All that remained were the glass window panes with two horizontal paint lines in the middle from when someone painted the frame and didn't really care about the quality of their work. I could see a bare bulb in the apartment's ceiling. They were really moving out. I could come and go without it feeling like I was in a Mission Impossible episode. My arms still raised, I was smiling. Suddenly, I liked everything, and I was in the mood to do whatever came next.

Thursday, June 23, 2016

Dewan and I exchanged congratulatory texts back and forth all night. If you didn't know what we were referring to, awful neighbors, it would have sounded like we were the lone survivors of a terrible tragic event. We joked about how the neighbors left as loudly as they came. Dragging furniture, screaming, more screaming, slamming, screaming. Dewan said they were jumping up and down above his head. I hoped he and his fiancé were finally getting some rest and could live in their apartment again.

In the morning, Hope and I walked the trail together. Since my place was across the street from the park, she usually dropped me off on her way back home. We were finishing up our conversation when I saw the husband walking toward the building. He was wearing the same clothes from yesterday, the shorts and green shirt. Ahhh, moving. Then my neighbor and their two kids appeared. They were heading towards the building, towards us. I turned to Hope and said, "You have to stay with me, don't leave!"

As happens in practically every thriller, horror, and action movie, there was a resurgence of the antagonist at the end. Hope stayed with me as long as she could, suggesting that I walk her home, and when I couldn't because of my own schedule, I was left to enter the building with my neighbor inside. I grabbed my phone and started recording, holding it up like Jodie Foster entering the basement in Silence of the Lambs. Anticipation on high alert, I was looking left and right, wondering where the heck my neighbor was, then hustling up the stairs. I still had an order of protection filed against me, but I made it home without cause. One last hurrah of fear before they were gone.

The rest of the afternoon was quiet. I pulled my curtains back. The temperature was cool outside, perfect for open windows, breezes, and birds chirping. I started speaking out loud to Buster just to hear my voice, asking, "Can you hear how quiet it is?" He was probably enjoying the change as much as I was. Our oasis of a building was back. Though I knew it bothered me to hear them screaming all the time, I didn't fully appreciate just how depressed, tense, and generally all-around miserable I was until I felt the opposite way. It was nice to be home, a feeling I hadn't had in months. Buster and I took a little nap. I ate in my kitchen in silence. My shoulders were lower. I could hear my thoughts. I could feel myself breathing.

Friday, June 24, 2016

I woke up thinking maybe the hoju tattoo had something to do with my neighbor moving out. Wow, and wow.

Sunday, June 26, 2016

Day four of peace and quiet. The building had taken on a relaxed atmosphere. My neighbor Jim and his wife had come by the day before to drop off an extra small window screen they didn't need, and I gave them a tour of the apartment, showing them the repairs I had made. I walked past the super on my way home from teaching, and we high fived in passing. There were friendly hellos and doors being held open. The building felt like it could breathe again. I was giddy with how relaxed I felt. While I was still worried about going to court on July 6, part of me thought my neighbor moving out would make it less enticing for her to pursue a case against me. Would it be worth her time at this point? The eviction and arrest were still in the oven, baking, and not yet done.

As per Noah's request, I went online and paid rent. The payment would eventually make its way back to me. It was a game of sending a piece of paper from one account through the mail twice, so it ended up in a sister account, in escrow. Management could still pursue the eviction and claim my neighbor and her family were moved for their own safety. They weren't concerned about my safety, my frayed nerves from being arrested, or the panic attacks I'd been having while entering and leaving the building.

Monday, June 27, 2016

It was cool and breezy. The San Diego-type weekend weather had carried over to the weekday. I'd been waking early, getting Buster on the trail by 7:30 am, wanting to be awake. Later, while I was futzing around before needing to teach, my neighbor and her family came back, dragging a cart up the stairs while yelling. As they packed up some bits in their former apartment, the toddler was crying and the parents continued yelling. I started laughing, remembering how I'd endured five months of that, all day long. Then on my way out to teach, I heard them in the lobby. Their yelling acted like a GPS.

Walking down the stairs, I decided to put my sunglasses on. I didn't know why, but I thought that I would look less confrontational. In hindsight, I realized this was the strategy celebrities use to make themselves less recognizable. Instead of it having a don't-bother-me vibe, I had hoped it would come across as a I-don't-want-to-bother-you vibe. Maybe mirrored sunglasses would've worked better. At the bottom of the stairs I stopped cold. My neighbor was in the doorway trying to get a short wooden ladder and the cart, now full of home goods, through the door at the same time. She saw me. I saw her. Like an old western, two well-worn adversaries, meeting on a empty street, staring across from one another, looking as much into each other's eyes, as into the distance, sizing up the situation and possible outcomes. Fucking hell this woman was killing me.

I had thrown a reusable grocery bag in my messenger bag on the way out and quickly decided it needed to be folded perfectly, like a flag. I swung my messenger bag around to the front, grabbed the bag, and fluffed it out in the air a few times like a magician prior to making something disappear under a hanky. I smoothed out the wrinkles against my torso, and then carefully went about folding it in half the long way, then in half again. Then I made triangles until reaching near the end, where I tucked the last bit in, all folded. Normally, this takes me ten seconds, but I was making sure each triangle was perfect, edge to edge, buying time.

My neighbor cleared the doorway, but she wanted to keep it propped open. She tried the wooden ladder, and the door slid against it. That brown-framed single-glass door, it was one of those doors that refused to cooperate when you were trying to prop it open. Sure, it would stay put for four seconds when you put a brick down on the ground. But when you turned around it, it would push against the brick, sliding it out of the way, then closing. The doors in that building, whether they were being knocked on, "shoved" open, leaned against, or propped, didn't like anyone.

My neighbor discarded the wood ladder and tried putting the cart in front. If she wasn't the bitch who got me arrested and had an order of protection again me, I would be holding the door for her and trying to help. Instead, I was watching her from a safe distance. I was actually rooting for her versus the door and a little annoyed with myself for not feeling more anger towards her. I was pissed off, but I couldn't seem to muster the feeling beyond a pilot light. That's the problem with yoga; you don't hold onto things long enough for the fires to burn big. When my neighbors first moved out, my body started to release. I'd already begun letting go.

The door pushed against the cart, then one of the cart wheels got stuck in a little crack in the tile, and they both stopped. Wow, she even beat the door down, or open. With the door ajar, my neighbor moved to the side to let me pass. That was nice. Why was she being so nice? Did she feel remorse for her actions? Did she see how painfully I'd been trying to avoid any contact? Did she smell my fear and think what was the point of rubbing it in?

I walked through the doorway. On the steps between doors was a portable heater and some other possessions. At the bottom of the stairs, sitting on bags of stuff, was the daughter. I didn't know she was there all along. For a moment, briefly, I looked at her. We were looking at each other. She had beautiful eyes and above her eyes a smooth, clear forehead. That's where "the bump" was, the evidence of my having "shoved a door" open. That forehead, the site of pain for the both of us. I turned away from this adorable child, who I never harmed, and walked out. Would I see them again? Could I read my neighbor's body language as a sign that she wasn't going through with the assault charge? I remembered the summons, how this woman supposedly feared for her life and for the lives of her children. This woman didn't fear me. Maybe it was over.

Thursday, June 30, 2016

Noah emailed to thank me for updating him about my neighbors moving out. He asked again if I'd had any contact with them since. After they'd moved out of the building? He also asked if I knew why they had moved out, and I shared with him the same intel that the super gave me. I left out the part about the bathtub,

284

feeling like it would reflect poorly on the condition of the building where I was trying to stay, thus reflecting poorly on me by association. I updated him on my following his recommendation to open an escrow account and deposit returned checks there. I neglected to mention how nice it was to see my bank-account balance higher than it really should be.

Court was six days away. Waiting had followed the usual arc from "it seems so far off" to "it's coming up soon."

Saturday, July 2, 2016

Yesterday I'd felt depressed and slept most of the day. Now, I was determined to not get so much "rest." I walked the dog with Hope in the morning, got ready to teach, and threw a pair of jeans in my bag. While most women change into stretchy pants after work, I change out of them. I made a deal with myself to tool around the city. My first stop after class was at the beloved B&H Dairy for lunch. After that, I headed south, walking along aimlessly.

It was the Fourth of July weekend, the city empty, with most of its inhabitants at their weekend homes. The weather was a palatable mid-60s with blue skies. Sometimes, I would go through periods where I only used the city for errands. I'd strategize subway stops and commuting scenarios to maximize time that I didn't really need to save. I'd carry along a large messenger bag that always ended up too full in the end. Then by the time I got home, I was testy and exhausted, and didn't like the city, even though the city never told me to spend the afternoon picking up so much crap in one go-around.

Today, I wasn't going to buy enough blueberry jam to last four months. I wasn't going to run any errands, just walk. Four blocks into my walkabout I ran into a friend from the articles club, and we stopped and chatted on the sidewalk. She was still in shock after hearing about my arrest, and I was still digesting a cup of vegetable soup, four slices of buttered challah, and two cheese blintzes. Mentally, I had food coma, and as she was talking, I was spacing out with an internal dialog:

FRIEND: Hey!

ME: Hey!

FRIEND: I've told my friends and they can't believe the story either.

FOOD COMA: *Do they think I actually hit the kid?*

ME: It's hard to believe, and I lived it.

FRIEND: I mean, you're so tiny...

FOOD COMA: *Again with the tiny, I'm not tiny. Or am I really tiny and I have that body dysmorphia thing? I just ate enough food for two people.*

FRIEND: The idea of you pushing a door hard enough... (Here she pantomimed the act by moving her palms through the air in slow motion.)

FOOD COMA: *What's that thing called, didn't Michael Jackson have it...*

FRIEND: And it opens hard enough to hit a kid.

FOOD COMA: *Maybe it is just called body dysmorphia.*

ME: I know.

FRIEND: I was just at a friend's house and there were two kids and after three hours the boy had nothing on him, but the girl had scratches on her legs and a bruise on her knee and her hair was all messed up.

FOOD COMA: *I think they should keep a better eye on her brother, right?*

ME: I know, she could have had any number of bruises from just being a kid.

FOOD COMA: *Does she know which kid I'm talking about?*

FRIEND: When's your next court date?

FOOD COMA: *Funny, I'm kind of out and about trying not to think about it.*
ME: This Wednesday.
FRIEND: I don't know how you're holding together so well.
FOOD COMA: *Oh, I'm not, at all. I've been depressed, and it's been hard to leave the apartment.*
FRIEND: You look great.
FOOD COMA: *I've been getting a lot of sleep.*
ME: Thanks, yoga.
FRIEND: Is there anything I can do for you?
FOOD COMA: *Change the subject from child abuse, child endangerment, and my arrest.*
ME: No, your empathy and concern are great. I appreciate it.

We hugged and I moseyed along to a bookstore, McNulty's Tea & Coffee, and then home. It was a perfect afternoon to remember I lived in New York City. When I got back, there was a white envelope with a clear window in the mail. I opened the letter while walking up the stairs, and since my focus was on both things, I read "place" and then saw the word "lugar" and thought for a quick second, "Is court at Peter Luger's Steak House?" Then I realized "lugar" probably meant "place" in Spanish. One side of the letter was in English, and the other was in Spanish, but since I read left to right, I'd put them together. The location, place, or lugar was Manhattan Criminal Court at 100 Centre Street, Part B. I was due there in just over three days.

Later, I fell asleep on the sofa for an hour. I knew napping was better than a lot of other coping devices I could be using right now. But it had gotten annoying. I wasn't tired, I was just taking a break from the world, from my world. Then I took Buster out for a walk and ran into the super who told me both apartments, the ground-floor one and my neighbor's place, had been rented already. My neighbor's apartment? They'd put another family of five in there. When I heard that, I couldn't help but say, "Are you fucking kidding me?" I felt sympathy and frustration for Dewan and his fiancé below.

Sunday, July 3, 2017

It was early morning. I'd taken Buster on the trail, fed us, tidied up, and packed my bag for going to practice and then teaching. I was ready for what needed to be done, but I was sitting at my desk, legs folded into myself, curled up in the dark. It felt safe to sit there, not moving. I did a search online for Manhattan Criminal Court Part B and couldn't find anything helpful. I was once able to clean the tarnish off the very small copper parts inside a 1991 Saab master window switch control panel by using directions and photos I found online. It was a tricky project but the windows worked perfectly after. Yet I had no idea what was going to happen on Wednesday morning.

And I just wanted to lie down. I wanted to sleep until Wednesday morning, go to court, and find out what would happen then. I didn't want to spend more time worrying, thinking, and guessing. It was getting harder to distract myself. I felt like there was a huge wall around me, and nothing—books, movies, entertainment, or friends—was getting in. We naturally brace ourselves before a physical impact, throwing our hands up in protection. The same thing happens emotionally. I was shutting down, limiting the impact of a possibly bad experience. It was tiring. With sleep, I could time travel through the free hours, wake up, and have less time waiting. Practice would be the hardest thing I had to do today because of how much it asks, how much yoga asks, that we be present. After that, I could zone out in my commute and emotionally hide in my teaching. I could use the familiarity of my routine as a cloak.

Wednesday, June 4, 2016

Did I have any more right to innocence than anyone else who had appeared in court on false charges?

Tuesday, June 5, 2016

Snap. It was the day before court. There hadn't been any contact from my new lawyer Perry at Defender Peeps. I wanted to know they were going to be there tomorrow. Wasn't that the plan since Jack broke up with me? I called and left a message with Perry's assistant. On the Peeps site, he didn't have a photo. Mysterious. Since Noah was responding to everything, I sent him an email, and he affirmed I was on the calendar for tomorrow. Then I pictured a large white board with a large black marker square and then 31 squares inside that. I imagined one of the assistant's jobs was to fill out the squares with the current month and then add client's names in the boxes. For Wednesday, it would have my name and in parentheses it would read "idiot who knocked on door."

Monday night I had dinner downtown with friends visiting from Europe. We ate, we chatted, and they asked what I'd been up to. "Arrested," I told them. Just arrested, that was it, really. Both my self and my life had been seized. As I was telling them the story, I had their toddler on my lap, feeding him bits of my meal and wearing the other bits. What was life going to be like for my neighbor's daughter, living in that household?

After dinner, I remembered to text Nancy a picture of the court appearance letter so she had the deets. She graciously agreed to be my plus one again. And Nancy texted back:

NANCY: So, is it ok if I arrive by 9:30?

289

Knowing my friend's issues with punctuality, in addition to my own issues of negotiating meet-up times. I replied:

ME: When you say arrive by 9:30, do you mean downtown, in the courthouse or in the actual courtroom?

We'd been through this before. I felt like this was a situation that warranted very little hand holding. I also felt like you shouldn't haggle with your friend before their court appearance. It was 10:30 pm and I needed to relax. I was equally concerned about whether there would or wouldn't be resolution tomorrow regarding my neighbor's statement. What if the DA asked for more time? More waiting. Nancy and I started arguing via text about how I'd handled her question. I wanted my friend to come to court and be there for me, instead I was arguing with a therapist. I didn't feel like "seeing" how my text was received:

NANCY: Marcy, Why don't u just say, "Thanks, I'll see u tmrw." Is that so hard? I'm still working, and will be for awhile. So I'll see u tmrw
ME: You asked me a question. You didn't say I will be there at 9:30am or I will see you at 9:30am. And put yourself in my shoes...I have other concerns than your arrival

I ended our text exchange with "don't come," and then stopped looking at my phone. My thoughts were on that sworn statement and how I'd know in 11 hours. There was also the parallel world of my working and trying to maintain some normalcy: food delivery in the morning, teaching in the evening, plans later in the week. If only we could give life the one-minute sign.

Hanuman

↑
right
leg

splits ✓

- block under front butt cheek
- hips squared/ face forward,
  do not go so deep your
  hips turn sideways.

modify, back knee on mat,
hands on blocks, front
leg straight forward.

pressing down on them

- release with blocks, or fall over
  to the side

✗ pad the back knee if needed ✓

✗ Don't clench your butt, anyway, if
you're clenching, back out a bit,

you're not performing the pose ✓

291

Wednesday, July 6, 2016 Court

Sometimes the word "sleep" feels condescending. I had nightmares about a couple I knew who were divorcing. I kept dreaming the wife was getting rid of everything of theirs and the husband was crying. I dreamt it over and over again. I couldn't understand why she was letting go of everything, even the good things. In some dreams, I helped him salvage the stuff and held an estate sale. Apparently, I'm a pragmatic dreamer. Then I woke at 5:30 am to a bright summer light hitting the curtains like a flare. Buster's belly had been bad, so he hadn't slept well either. My nerves, in his tummy, poor little guy. He hopped off the bed, headed to the living room, and puked on the rug. I cleaned it up, decided I should run a load of laundry, took Buster out, then fell asleep on the sofa with the end of the wash cycle's beeping alarm thankfully waking me.

There wasn't any food until the delivery arrived, so I reluctantly took a bite of a Clif bar only to have the doorbell ring immediately with my order. I put away the food. Do the usual things, I thought. I hung my clothes to dry (they last longer that way, and water evaporates), put in another load, made an omelet, and packed a lunch. In my snotty yoga mind, I fancied myself as the only "alleged" person who would arrive to court with local organic carrots and a sandwich made from sprouted-wheat bread, almond butter and organic blueberry jam, wrapped in compost-friendly unbleached wax paper. My water bottle was filled, my journal and pen were packed, and my court-appearance document was in my bag. After the second load of laundry was finished and hung up to dry, I went about making myself look court presentable.

First, I glued my hair down with aloe-vera gel. I'd skipped a round of buzzing it down, wanting a softer vibe, wanting the grey spot at the top of my head to blend better. There was how I wanted to look, how I happened to end up looking, and there was how I appeared to others. I thought being aware of the last one was necessary for today. I'd been patting and patting my hair in place with gel, but when I pulled my hands away, I second-guessed this idea. Usually I allow my hair, the most disgruntled, tenured employee on my body, to do whatever it wants. Even at an inch short, it wanted to look like a field of grass blowing in violent winds. With the severity of too much gel and a part down the side, I had recreated a Lego hairpiece.

I gave up on my hair and got dressed. I put on black dress pants, a long-sleeve navy linen shirt buttoned to the top to hide a chest tattoo, and a black linen blazer. Then I headed to the long mirror on the living room closet door. Staring at my reflection, I was aware of how androgynous I appeared, especially since I'd chosen to wear a bralette this time. In formfitting yoga clothes I don't come across this way. Outwardly I was making a statement, while inwardly I was simply apathetic towards fashion. I choose clothing based on company ethics and freedom of movement. I'm wiggly. In this outfit, I didn't look like myself. I looked like I was going on a job interview for a job I didn't want. I don't do business casual. I can do artist. I can do yoga teacher. I can do personal home contractor in old coveralls. There isn't a version of me that pretends to be something I'm not: refined. In this outfit, my posture felt weird. In order to keep the blazer and shirt from moving in opposite directions, I couldn't do casual things, like raise my arms. If they stayed down, everything lay perfectly. I added black dress shoes. While I'd covered my tattoos for court, it was really too hot out to be dressed like this. Why did I even own these clothes and how did they get into my closet? When did I buy a black linen blazer, and when did I even start using the word blazer?

While walking to the subway, I felt awkward. I wouldn't mind looking absurd, like I was in a costume, but I wasn't technically in a costume. It was July, and I was covered in dark colors except for my hands and face. Before tattoos, I was just pale. Throughout my life, complete strangers would comment on this. There was the time, while on summer break from art school in Boston, a friend drove a couple of us to where her family rented a cabin on Cape Cod. There was a beach we'd go to that was considered "crowded" when there were just five other smaller groups nearby. At the New Jersey beaches I grew up going to, if you didn't get there by 11 am, there wasn't a spot. As in, no place to put down a blanket above the waterline.

On Cape Cod, one of the ladies came over from her camp to complain to us about the "crowds." It might have been code for "people not of my ilk." She was standing over us, with me there in a t-shirt and jean shorts (that bikini line). For a moment, she stopped talking to stare at me. *One of these is not like the others.* Then she asked, "Honey, do you have any sun protection on?" I said I did, but she wasn't convinced. "Honey," she continued, "do you know how pale you are?" I'd been asked this before, many times, in fact. As if, for my entire existence in my skin, the largest organ of the body, I had never passed a mirror, or looked down. On the fly, I decided to tell this woman I was a "before" model for a tanning salon back in Boston, and they superimposed someone else's head on my body. To tie a heartstring bow around my lie, and for style points, I added that this helped pay for tuition. Usually I'm a terrible liar, nervously laughing and giving myself away. I don't know how I delivered those lines so flawlessly, but she believed me, and it was a great vacation.

Once downtown, I exited the train at Franklin Street, in the most wonderful neighborhood, Tribeca. Then, sadly, I had to head immediately east to 100 Centre Street. I felt like a person going to work, but this wasn't how I felt going to work. This clothing was not uplifting. Teaching yoga is a great gig, even more so for the casual wear. Entering the courthouse through the usual banned-objects screening line, I again set off the medical detector. I was pulled to the side to do an imitation of da Vinci's famous anatomy drawing: legs wide and arms straight out. It was there that my outfit went awry. The pants decided to go where my waistline

294

actually is, about three inches from my tits. My shirt slid off to the right, and the jacket rose up so the collar was like a hood. After I was cleared to enter, I found a corner to put everything back in place. It looked like I was scolding the fabric: "Stay down, stop moving."

I took the elevator to the fourth floor and exited right, only because that's where a lot of people were loitering about. Without my reading glasses, I squinted to find Part B on a small sign. Appropriate for thematically feeling like I was walking the plank, I headed down a long hallway, to the end. Then I entered through a set of double doors, and to the right through another set. Like the DAT room, you entered facing the the judge's quarters. I plopped down on a pew, on the left side of the courtroom, one back from the middle row.

Part B was very similar to the DAT room, except the high windows were on the left wall. Along the right wall there was a secret door near the fencing that separated the judge's area from the pews. Through there lawyers appeared and disappeared. The DA's area was to the left of the judge, and to the right was where the court officers hung out. Most of the room was in 70s wood paneling. More dark brown everywhere. The pews were carved or black-markered with tags: "Dr. Brown," "Puck," "Large Marge," "B.S.Bobby." The morning started with a roll call, and names had numbers assigned to them. I was number 37. Did that mean 37 cases were to be heard ahead of mine? Or was it just a random number? A short while after I arrived, Nancy appeared and sat down beside me. We looked at one another, and she said something about not texting when it was late and both of us were tired. So began my second court appearance.

The judge came in. We rose, then sat. The first name was called. Someone announced that all cell phones had to be put away. Nancy and I dutifully complied. We were both prepared for the outage this round, me with my journal and pen, her with some paperwork. The stenographer arrived late, and the entire courtroom watched her set up. It was like waiting for the checkout lady to change her cash-register tape. Number 15 was called. Okay, did that mean they were starting at 15 and moving numerically forward, backwards, or randomly?

The pews, the dark-brown palette, and the non-sequential calling of names reminded me of temple. How during Friday-night services we might start from the back of the siddur prayer book, which was the beginning, but keep bouncing around, and maybe even finish where we began. This made it hard to figure out when services would be ending and I could eat pound cake washed down with grape juice.

Kids weren't allowed any toys during services. We had to simply sit and do nothing for what felt like hours. This would be helpful training for when I traveled through europe by bus in the 90s, sometimes taking 20 plus hour rides, before cell phones and wireless internet. Ninety-nine percent of successful travel is the ability to sit with yourself for long periods of time, and one percent is the ability to stay awake when you finally arrive. Sitting still as a kid was challenging. I wasn't out of control high energy with non-stop movement, more fussy from internally going out of my mind. To soothe my fidgeting, my mother let me hold her hand, and I obsessively rubbed my small fingers over her shiny smooth nail polish. I started writing as a kid to pass the time while waiting for adults.

I was wondering about Perry. Since I didn't know what he looked like, there was a bit of an "Ugly Duckling" thing happening every time a suit walked in. "Are you my lawyer?" Maybe Perry wasn't a "he." It could be anyone. They were on to the next person already. What would happen if my name was called and I didn't have counsel? This was going faster than the desk appearance ticket. Now they were calling numbers in the 30s.

The court doors opened, and bits of conversation slipped through. A man was saying, "That's the best-case scenario; here's the worst-case scenario." It was five after 10 am, and no lawyer had claimed me. Proceedings had stopped for some reason. My ass was starting to hurt on the wood. Would they mind if I took off my shoes and sat cross-legged? This was how our bodies were designed to sit; in sukhasana, or more commonly called "Indian style." The hip is a ball-and-socket joint. Everyone's is shaped differently with variations on bone size and angles. But no matter the person, when sitting crossed-legged, one shin in front of the other, the base of body forms a perfect tripod, distributing weight evenly. Sitting like this is easier on the spine. The weight of our legs and hamstrings don't pull on the lower back as they do when sitting in a chair. It also doesn't inhibit the function of the femoral artery, the second largest artery in the body, and the highway of blood distribution to the lower limbs. When we sit in chairs, with our legs at right angles in front of us, the head of the femur can pinch the femoral artery. Any blood flow constriction is bad, but what most people feel here is sleepy and restless.

I decided not to test the waters by sitting naturally, and instead changed my focus. I looked over to the young, well-dressed lawyers in the DA area. They were bored and constantly checking their cell phones. It seemed like there were too many of them for the workload. Number 34 was called, and Nancy hit my bag. "It's not me," I said, "I'm 37."

When lawyers entered the room, they walked straight down the left side to the fencing and grabbed a clipboard off the wall. I think they were signing in. There was usually a court officer manning that nook. The lawyer would whisper something to the officer, maybe a name or two, then receive files. Once the lawyers had the files, they would turn around to the pews and call out the names on the files, nodding at the response "here." Then the lawyers would walk along the fencing to the other side, where they would ask one of the DA grunts for more files. The hunting around for files in this area looked random. They were tucked in along the sides or in stacks. It didn't appear that there was a system. Once glanced over, those files got handed back to the DA staff.

There was a rash of defendants accepting pleas. They were agreeing to anger management classes with a fine, or days of community service with a fine. On top of the fine came a five percent court fee. Most fines were $120, which was steep for many of the defendants. Adding a cut on top was curious. I heard Nancy turning some papers over. She was making columns and looking at her calendar, doing patient billing. A name was called twice, and when the person didn't appear, the judge said, "involuntary return of warrant." Then his lawyer jumped up, and got his client from outside the courtroom.

Throughout the various proceedings, we didn't get to hear any of the details, just the style of crime, and which misdemeanor and which count it was. It became repetitive. All the drama boiled down to a title, with no story. Sometimes a DA grunt would say, "the people are not ready." More lawyers strolled in as if they were seniors and we "alleged" were freshmen. They didn't have to be on time. I peeked at my cell phone in case Perry had sent a message, but all I saw was a check-in from Hope. I took my phone and stepped out. There was an area between double-door entrances where lawyers took clients to talk. We were allowed to use cell phones there. I exchanged texts with Hope about was going on, which was nothing.

While I was texting, there was a woman speaking with her client. She had a tight perm of blonde curls with jet-black roots, and was wearing a grey skirt suit. She was as pale as I was, and I was intrigued about her decision to go faux blonde. Her client was explaining the incident that brought her to this moment. I could hear the phrases "why would I" and "all I was doing." This was the good stuff. This chance to vent was as close to "getting your day in court" as it was going to get. The woman's lawyer said "I hear you," and began a discussion about legal options. This wasn't the playground, and it wasn't about your version and then their version and then a time-out. It was just bureaucratic process, laws, and procedures.

There wouldn't be a moment, at this venue, where our stories got explained for the umpteenth time, and where finally, finally, a person would say, "You were wronged. Case dismissed, go home." Maybe there was an opportunity for it down the line, during the trial process. But right now, it seemed to be about pushing people to accept plea deals, one after the other. Outside the courtroom area, in the big hallway, there was a ruckus of people talking more animatedly. It was there that the emotional retells and the challenge of accepting fault as a means to resolution was processed more intensely. I think it was there that people realized justice is indeed blind, it isn't just a saying. Lawyers would walk their clients out to the big hallway for those kinds of conversations.

Back inside, Nancy was looking at spreadsheets of payments. On our side of the aisle, the crowd was thinning out. A youngish white man in a grey suit, white shirt, and green tie came in. He called out Steve somebody, made eye contact with his client, and then he called out my name. Welcome to the party Perry. I was all nerves. Hopefully, I would soon find out if they'd gotten a signed sworn statement. I watched Perry go to the DA desk. They were getting the files for him. Any minute now. He'd opened a file in one hand, and was flipping papers up in the other. He did this so quickly it looked like he was pretending to scan notes. Nancy was working. I had to pee, of course. Perry dropped the DA files off and motioned for me and the other guy to go outside. I made eye contact with Nancy, and left.

Perry walked out the first double doors and then turned around to talk. He told the other guy to wait and spoke with me first, introducing himself and handing me a business card. Then he got to the talking. My neighbor had signed a sworn statement. That soulless, remorseless, conniving exemplar of villainousness. That bitch. When we went out into the hallway to talk, I put my hands in my dress pants' pockets. This caused the bottom of my blazer to casually drape over my arms, as if I'd planned it. I really had adapted quickly to the business-casual look. I felt like we were colleagues discussing someone else's case.

Perry told me the DA's office was offering an harassment plea, no criminal record, and a small fine. I asked questions about the ramifications of taking the plea, even though he'd just told me everything, wanting to make sure I heard correctly that I would have no criminal record. Or maybe it wasn't that. Something about the plea was bothering me, and between the bad night's sleep and wearing dress pants and shoes, I couldn't figure it out. I was out of my element. I do all my thinking barefoot, in tights, without a pound of gel on my head.

I bought some time rephrasing my questions. Would it come up on a mortgage application? No. Affect a housing lottery? No. How about renting another apartment? No. Travel? No. Unless I was an immigrant, he didn't foresee an issue. Hmmm, maybe the problem was with the word "harassment." Where had I heard that word recently? Oh, for the love of a nagging bad feeling…I turned to Perry and asked, "Did you know my landlord is trying to evict me on this case, on the grounds of harassment?" He said he didn't know this, and asked if I'd spoken with one of the Defender Peeps' housing representatives. "Yes," I replied. "Noah." Perry got his cell phone out and said, "I've tried reaching him this morning about something else, and I don't think he's on his cell." You mean both of you are in the same office, have the same client, and aren't briefing one another? Seriously?

Perry began thinking out-loud, "If they're trying to evict you based on harassment, then you don't want to take the plea." *Ahead of you on that one, buddy.* Yeah, I wouldn't have a case then if I agreed now to harassment. While Perry was absorbed in thought, I asked if I could interrupt him, "Sure." I painted him a landscape, "This woman has four kids. There's no way she's showing up for a trial." Perry agreed, adding, "They never do, and the plea offer isn't going anywhere. Let's see if they run out of time and if the case is dismissed, which happens." He told me to wait in the courtroom, and headed off to speak with his other client.

As I walked back, I thought about explaining everything to Nancy so she would understand seeing me at the stand saying no to the plea deal. I headed back to the pew's side and dramatically flicked my head toward the door, motioning for her to follow me out. Once we were in the little area, I explained to her why I wasn't taking the harassment offer. I told her I wanted her to know before she heard it when I was up there. "That's good," Nancy said, "because otherwise, I would have raised my hand and said, 'Excuse me, I need to speak to the defendant for a moment.'" She exaggerated the word "excuse" with a high pitch, and I cracked up. I knew this woman, and if she thought I was going to do something egregiously doltish, and preventable, she would interrupt court proceedings.

We headed back in. When we sat back down, she whispered, "Pay $120 and lose your apartment, no thank you." It was a good point. It had me thinking about how tidy the harassment offer was in conjunction with the harassment eviction. Did the landlord offer my neighbor a different apartment if she agreed to sign the statement? It was a huge paranoid leap, but I still couldn't figure out why they moved them. I didn't buy the "they were being too demanding with repairs" excuse. There was a reason my landlord made the top 50 list of the worst landlords in New York City. Moving a tenant who complained too much to a better apartment was kind of fishy. It was too convenient, the plea and the "notice to cure." If I took the plea, I would probably lose my apartment. I wouldn't have a defense. And to think I caught it based on a gut feeling that something was off! How close I'd been to accepting the plea was unnerving. My sixth chakra, the area of intuition, saved the day. Trust this natural defense mechanism. Bad vibes prevent bad experiences.

When my name was called, I didn't accept the plea, and the next court date was set for September 15, 2016.

Childs Pose Twist

- knees wide
- arms forward to start

Feet together, NOT WIDE!

(face down)

switch sides, both arms forward for a moment (empty b)

left arm under right underarm 3-5 min

(face down)

head to left

- turn head to right

* end with hands on neck, elbows flat or on blocks, if there's time.

No Need to push butt against ~~butt~~ feet.

Gentle!

Sunday, July 10, 2016

As the week wore on, I taught, had a four-hour tattoo session on my back, and buzzed my hair back down. Ladies from the articles club checked in on me. Their concern had been really comforting. When I was updating those in the know, one friend said I'd "dodged a bullet" by not taking the plea because of intuition. I was less stressed than before, even though things were technically worse. My neighbor had signed a statement, putting her version of the story into factville. I wouldn't get a real signed statement. Instead, I would get that made-up statement the police furnished. I really didn't get to participate much in my criminal court case. At least worrying about whether or not she would was over. That got to me. Now I had no idea what was next. Was there going to be a trial? It seemed crazy to knock on a door and then end up in court for third-degree assault. It was like a prank that had gone on too long without me being able to call "uncle."

Monday, July 11, 2016

Catching up on paperwork, I checked my bank account and learned the last rent payment went through. The management company didn't mail it back to me. Interesting. It hadn't been deposited the week before that. It cleared after I didn't accept the harassment offer. Was that coincidence? I emailed Noah:

On July 11, 2016, 1:37 pm, Marcy Tropin wrote:

Hi Noah, Checking online it appears that my landlord has deposited July's rent. Whether or not that was a business error remains. I believe you said that means they have to start the eviction process over if it was a mistake? Also, I was in court this Wednesday for the criminal trail and met with Perry for the first time. By intuition and luck I didn't accept a plea offer of harassment. Had I done so it would have opened the door for the eviction. Hopefully moving forward, everyone can be on the same page. -Marcy

I thought I was justified in pointing out how I almost got myself evicted because my two lawyers didn't speak before my court hearing. I didn't feel comfortable completely letting it go. My apartment was my home, and as messed up as it had been to live there, it was where I lived. Noah replied later in the afternoon:

On July 11, 2016, 3:47 pm, Noah wrote:

Hi Marcy, Yes, there's a possibility we can argue that they've invalidated the Termination Notice if they accept your rent before they've served the "Notice of Petition." Could you take a screenshot showing when they deposited the check? Also, did they send you an invoice for July rent? It's good you didn't accept the plea. While I don't think it would have been fatal to your housing court case, it certainly wouldn't have helped. I will check with Perry about the possibility of resolving the criminal case with a dismissal, which would be the safest plea. Still no court papers from the landlord, correct? - Noah

The management company requested rent payments after the 10 of the month, even though rent was due on the first of the month. The notices were put in envelopes that weren't sealed, and the porter slid them under apartment doors. So yes, they were still requesting rent payments from me, but I didn't think this was exactly what Noah was looking for. Nonetheless, I photographed and emailed the request to him along with a screen capture of my cleared rent check.

On July 11, 2016, 4:22 pm, Marcy Tropin wrote:

Hi Noah, Attached please find proof of payment for July's rent as well as the request for payment for July from my landlord. The request for July's rent has two base rents. I would assume they are re-asking for June's rent, the one they sent back. I only paid July's. It would have gotten a little confusing to keep sending and receiving checks back. No other paperwork in the mail to date. Would love a dismissal!!! -Marcy

Perry mentioned something about dismissing the case, but it sounded more of an eventuality than a possibility. Could we pursue a dismissal? Shouldn't Perry have broached that on Wednesday? Where was Perry? After declining the plea on my behalf, he'd turned to me and said, "We'll talk." I began to walk away and then stepped back to shake his hand, needing some kind of goodbye formality. Would we talk?

Wednesday, July 13, 2016

Did I need to email Perry about the dismissal, or was Noah speaking to him about it? Would someone get back to me on the dismissal? Was the point of that to distract me from dropping the ball on the harassment plea? Despite my concerns, I was no longer as stressed or preoccupied as I had been before. I was oddly totally cool with everything. I'd moved on from shock and anger to resolved, with prejudice.

I thought about sending June's rent again. Once all the rent was out of the escrow account, I was hoping I wouldn't have to go into a bank branch to close it. I opened it online, but thought closing it might be an in-person thing. I didn't want to have to go through one more guy in a suit to get something done. This was of greater concern to me now than a possible trial. I'd been to court

305

before. When I turned 18, my mom and I changed our last name from my dad's, to one we'd made up. As part of the legal process, both of us had to swear to tell the whole truth, sit at the witness stand, and speak before a judge. My mother performed a melodramatic odium towards my father and started crying during her turn, and I answered all three of the court's questions with the efficient one-word negative of "no," and was out of there. I'd like to think the decision to change my name was a badass, Judy Chicago inspired, punk move. But it was merely a vanity thing.

The other time was appearing on behalf of my mother for an ambulance chase thing. I also had to deal with a crappy lawyer and an even crappier mediator for my bike-accident case in college. How did I prepare for being on the stand? By having survived years of extreme unpopularity as a child. Like the time I was at sleep-away camp and five girls from my bunk decided to corner me and make fun of my drinking root beer instead of cola. They didn't have a lot of material. I was good at sports and funny, with a slight loner thing going on. Having a lawyer try to rattle you is nothing compared to the unbridled insolence of children.

Friday, July 22, 2016

I began to think that maybe I should be a little worried about a possible criminal trial. I hadn't heard anything from my housing lawyer or criminal lawyer. Radio silence. I decided to email Perry about the possibility of a dismissal. This period between court appearances was going faster, though it was longer. People reached out here and there, asking how I was doing under such terrible circumstances. I responded from my air-conditioned, newly serene, and quiet apartment. Was it really so horrible? One of my clients, who didn't know about the arrest, started a joke with, "You haven't been to jail, have you?" And when I stood silently, not sure what to say, she picked up on the moment and stopped mid-joke, her voice changing to a concerned whisper,

"Oh, it's okay if you have." It could have been worse, it could get worse, and sometimes, I wasn't thinking about it.

Wednesday, July 27, 2016

I hadn't heard back from Perry. I checked online to see if the second go-around in sending June's rent had cleared. I kept thinking about what Noah said, that if they accidentally deposited a check they'd have to start the whole process over. I was wondering if they'd given up, as I hadn't received a new "notice to cure." With my neighbor moved out, it would be challenging to come up with new material after the first over-the-top ridiculous summons. Every one knows sequels suck.

Sending the rent and hoping it got deposited was a great idea. If the management company had given up trying to evict me, then shouldn't I take the harassment plea? Maybe I could take it at the next court appearance, which would be a strategically long period of time after my neighbor moved out. Then again, could they use it to try and evict me no matter what? There was also the issue of management finding out about the plea, as it seemed whatever happened in court didn't stay in court. Was it a bad idea in general to agree to harassment? These were the questions I could have asked Perry if he responded to emails.

Saturday, July 30, 2016

Management sent the rent check for June back in the mail, and it cracked me up. What were they doing? Going to start the eviction process all over again with my neighbor already moved out? It was stupid. And it wasn't intimidating. I thought they'd take my rent and move on to trying to evict the next tenant. Perry still hadn't responded to my email. I decided I might as well wait and see what happened on September 15. Why was I going to court then? Now it felt silly. I'd been thinking about possible next places to live, filling out housing lottery applications. Each application asked if I had a criminal record, and I wanted to answer "not yet." One day, I would move out of the place where I was arrested.

Sunday, July 31, 2016

I walked up home from the 145th Street subway stop because there was no local to 155th. It was Sunday, when the trains get to rest, but not the commuters. As I was heading out of the subway, I ran into a neighbor from around the corner, a journalist, and we got to talking. A popular topic of conversation in our hood was how to deal with the undiscriminating Highbridge Park masturbators. She didn't yell or film them like I did; she told them "good morning to you today" with a kind of 1950s housewife affection. Sometimes when I yelled, it startled them into turning around towards me, and then I would get flashed. Lately, I'd been skipping the yelling and going straight to pulling out my camera instead. I would pull mine out, and they would put theirs away.

The journalist purchased her apartment many years ago after having been a neighborhood renter. She was telling me how she really liked the grittiness and community feel of the area. I like how certain groups of people could choose to live in "gritty" neighborhoods. I agreed, there was a wonderful community feel. In our hood, people did their barbecuing in the front, not the back, and neighbors stopped by to join-in. There was bingo in the park, and often three generations of family hanging out together. Before we parted, I was telling her how Dewan said a woman was recently mugged at a bus stop. Standing in front of her building, she told me about how she was once mugged in the neighborhood. I decided to story-top her with the briefest version of my arrest. She was floored. Then I ran off to be home alone with my dog. No tea, no wine, no company. Was it careless of me not to take care of her reaction afterwards, even though it worked better for me, the person living the arrest?

Thursday, August 11, 2016

It was my birthday, and I booked a session for my back tattoo. I updated Emu on the case and eviction. We were going back and forth about who a jury would believe, and she said, "It's different when you add a kid." True. She also asked if I had a blonde wig I could wear to court. Then she stopped tattooing because she'd cracked herself up.

Monday, August 15, 2016

While on a cleaning tear around the apartment, I got an email from the building manager:

On August 15, 2016, 10:49 am, the b.m. wrote:

Hello Marcy, Hope you had a good weekend. I am sending you this email because we have not received rent in two months and you are in arrears for $…Please advise on when we can expect payment or unfortunately we will have to start a non-payment case. -Building Manager

Interesting. No note on the door like every one else got. Maybe it was because management kept mailing my rent checks back to me. This note had a different tone from her May email, when she let me know I should expect "court papers." I forwarded her message to Noah and asked him what to do. He replied immediately.

On August 15, 2016, 11:36 am, Noah wrote:

Hi Marcy, Interesting development. I thought they accepted and deposited July 2016 rent? Did they return the check along with that receipt you attached? Unless you dispute the amount of the arrears they are demanding, I recommend you send in a payment to avoid the nonpayment case. The fact that they are affirmatively soliciting rent from you is probably enough to vitiate the notice of termination in the (already flimsy) nuisance case. How's everything else going? Have you heard anything else from management or your neighbor? Hope you're also staying cool! Terrible out there. No AC in the office right now, but we persevere. -Noah

After a couple more exchanges, Noah called me. We talked about how I should respond to the email and whether or not I wanted to pay the late fee (nope). We discussed whether or not the building manager maybe forgot there was legal action against me. I doubted it. I explained how management usually started these things with the door notes. "So they're actioning everything?" Noah asked. I told him yes, they were. Wait, what does that mean? Noah mentioned that he'd had to call Perry because he was hard to reach by email. People aren't hard to reach by email unless they didn't have an email address. Perry was frustratingly hard to get a response from via email. He was probably receiving the communications. When I asked about the eviction, Noah said, "Right now, they've solicited rent so many times from you that they don't have a case."

The most important part of our exchange was that he didn't get my pop-culture reference and asked, "Was Barney Miller a sitcom?" Then I had to explain the Barney Miller show, which was indeed a sitcom, running from 1974 to 1982. It was set in a fictional New York City Greenwich Village police station before lead actors had to be perfectly beautiful specimens wearing sartorial delights their characters could never afford. This was back before shows taking place in the justice system made moral compass speeches ad nauseam. Before television had a contrived sense of immediacy. The show was thick with sardonic wit and acerbic comebacks. It also moved slowly. I loved it.

Growing up in New Jersey, there were two TV stations playing reruns after 11 pm, which was helpful for a kid falling asleep alone in a big house. One station had Taxi reruns, which I loved, but right after that, they played Twilight Zone episodes seemingly until daylight. As a kid (and probably even now) that "zone" was too frightening for me. I chose the Barney Miller station. Before I even cared about posture, I found the always-hunched-over Sgt. Fish and sloppy body language of his cohorts endearing. I was explaining this to my housing lawyer, and he totally got it, "Right, Public Defender, office without air conditioning..." and I added, "living the dream." He belly laughed. My work here was done.

I emailed the building manager:

On August 15, 2016, 12:15 pm, Marcy Tropin wrote:

Hi The Building Manager, I received both June's and August's rent back in the mail. I'm happy to resend them, but I think the amount is different than what you have? -Marcy

On August 15, 2016, 12:19 pm, the b.m. wrote:

Hhmmmm that is so weird I wonder why...The amount I have is because of late fees, but I will have them waived since they were sent back.

On August 15, 2016, 1:07 pm, Marcy Tropin wrote:

Done [followed by a screen shot of payment made online].

On August 15, 2016, 1:16 pm, the b.m. wrote:

Awesome thanks, the building manager

Yeah, namafuckingstay to you, lady. I let Noah know I paid the rent, and thanked him for his advice. It worked. Eviction resolved.

Thursday, August 18, 2016

While I went along with the building manager in pretending there hadn't been an eviction attempt, I would have liked an official word on their no longer trying. The best I would get was them accepting my rent and me not hearing anything. I could now move on, or stay put. It was my choice. With the eviction resolved and the neighbors out, there was just the third-degree assault to worry about.

On the subway I was telling Hope how anticlimactic it would be to just get a phone call that the case was dismissed. She said, "I'm rooting for that, an anticlimactic ending." *Oh yeah, me too.* I clarified this, saying it would feel like a "just kidding." Four months had passed since I was arrested. I was wondering how this case would be resolved emotionally. A dismissal would end the case, but I didn't think I would be going back to who I was before. I would be questioning what it was all about for a long time.

Saturday, September 3, 2016

Hope and I were walking the dogs on the trail and trying to figure out how a case gets dismissed. I was throwing out probables: whether or not my neighbor pursued it or was cooperative with the DA, whether or not the DA pursued it based on merit. Maybe factors like my not having any priors would come into play. I didn't know, really. Hope laughed at my saying "I don't have any priors." It wasn't a phrase she thought she'd hear in person. Add it to the list for both of us.

With court 12 days away, I was distracted and anxious about the case, and then I beat myself up for not doing more with my free time. It was hard to think about anything else. Perry never responded to any form of contact, which left me in the dark about what exactly would happen on the 15. I felt like I should be in the loop on the process, as I was one of the principals. Would a trial mean a jury? I wasn't comfortable keeping 12 people from work.

For freelancers like me, who don't have paid sick leave or vacation time, jury duty is a financial hardship. I always wanted an alternative, like community service. Let me tidy up a public park, or better yet, paint over poorly designed graffiti tags. I would be of greater service to the community there as opposed to serving as a juror with my short attention span and inability to sit still. As time went on, I thought I'd take the harassment plea instead of a trial. It didn't seem like a fair trade, though: knock on a door, get arrested, accept a plea bargain. I hadn't hung out with the notion of fairness since my arrest, or even since my neighbor moved in. I'd prefer a dismissal, I'd like a dismissal, I wanted a dismissal. I was tired, not from lack of sleep but from hypothetically pondering. I was worn out from "maybe."

Monday, September 12, 2016

For the past week, my belly had been distended and painful, like I was storing rocks in there. This was not a good look for my profession. I had traded focus for a tight chest. Sometimes, I would snap back to real time and find myself sitting on the sofa, scratching my head, staring off into space, neither present nor absent. Maybe I was getting up to do something or sitting down to read, and then it never happened. I'd heard 'dismissal' so many times from Noah that it seemed like it should have happened by now. Before the first court appearance, I thought all the things

313

being stretched out would have happened in one go: charges, offers, and the case beginning.

In the mail, I received the formal white letter in a windowed envelope from CJA, the criminal justice system, telling me to show up on Thursday or there would be a warrant issued for my arrest. They really should consider setting up email invite reminders instead.

Tuesday, September 13, 2016

In therapy, my shrink said that since my neighbor was crazy, it was likely that she would show up. I said I preferred she leaned the other way. There was no need to prepare me for the worst. I made a case for why my neighbor wouldn't show up: a gaggle of kids and court being all the way downtown. Then my shrink added that if my neighbor won, it would help her in a civil case in the event that she wanted to sue me. I started to become fond of AWOL Perry's "We'll talk." nonchalance. That was working for me. Let's talk about my crappy childhood instead.

Wednesday, September 14, 2016

I'd reached out to Noah, and while he got back to me immediately, he misunderstood my question about what to expect on the September 15:

On September 12, 2016, 7:54 pm, Noah wrote:

Hi Marcy, Yes you'll need to appear on 9/15 either way. Perry is handling the criminal case so you'd have to check in with him for status on that. -Noah

I got needy, and Noah told me to see other attorneys. This was the second lawyer who had dumped me via email. I felt badly for having reached out to him, like I'd done something wrong. Maybe it was him and not me. He did see other clients, after all.

I was moving around a lot, but I didn't think I was really doing anything. If there was a job requiring a person to sit down and get right back up 14 times in five minutes, I would have been able to make a career out of it. I rallied myself to do normal things. I emailed the ladies from articles club asking for some cheerleading for a possible criminal trial, and they responded in kind. I bought groceries. I took Buster out on the trail and found a mala-bead bracelet on the ground. I thought that was a good omen for tomorrow, though sad for the person who lost it. I checked the mail, and there was a legal-sized brown kraft envelope from management. Inside were papers so important that they could not be folded. I stomped up the stairs, wondering, "What are they doing now?" Inside was a lease-renewal form. This was not a healthy relationship, going to great lengths to breakup and then asking me to stay.

Since I was yoga'd out, I decided to go with Life Crisis Solutions and Tools Plan B: eat kids' cereal. To wash the cereal down I bought an expensive glass jug of milk from a farm that supposedly massaged the cows' bellies and let them watch reality TV. When medicating oneself with comfort food, it's best to go no holds barred. Though it wasn't great health wise, no one on their death bed will ever say, "I wish I'd eaten more kale." I tore through half the box in one sitting. While eating bowl after bowl, I was online searching "first day of criminal case" for fun. There was something about pre-trail motions. Wasn't that the last court date? Some results said cases are usually resolved prior to trial. None of this was familiar to me. I was enjoying the rare sugar high, feeling drunk on silly, rather than antsy with stress. I looked around my sparsely appointed apartment, imagining being sued by my neighbor. It wouldn't be a very good use of her time.

| Shin Up Wall | (like ankle to knee)

like to knee

Modify: bring bottom foot
in towards butt

+ add a block under your
~utt.

~ eventually back is against wall.

Such pwell

-hands on thigh or blocks

5MIN

←point foot

knee away from wall
to modify

-release by bringing hands down
back knee forward.

-no gain from pain, modify b
modify

↑
right
angle

↑
padding

Thursday, September 15, 2016 Court

Slept. Woke. Slept. Woke. Slept. Woke. At 7 am, I got up
to a cool mid-60s day out. Earlier in the week, it had been in the
nineties. It would be easier to cover my tattoos minus heat
exhaustion. After all waste-removal issues were resolved for my
dog and me, we snuggled on the sofa for a bit. At 8 am, I
reluctantly swapped pajamas for black dress pants, then tried on
three button-down shirts before settling on the navy linen number
I'd worn the last time to court. Then I got this great idea to snazz it
up by reaching way back into the closet for a real bra again. In July
I wore a bralette, but I was too premenstrual for one this round. I
was also too bloated for my pants and had a nice muffin top going
on. Between anxiety, stress, and hormones, I was holding water
like a chamois cloth.

When I put the bra on, my right boob wasn't as bloated as
my left and barely filled the cup. This made my right shoulder
tense up to keep the strap from sliding off no matter how much I
tried to synch it down. I looked in the mirror. My face was
swollen. There was a south star volcano, one singular threatening
blemish, that had crescendoed into an angry red bump on my chin.
It looked like someone had held onto my nose and pulled my face
forward and down, then attempted to drain it of vital liquids
through a hole in my jaw. I topped things off with my long black
cardigan. In the mirror, it looked as though someone had dressed
me for hospital visiting hours. If this thing kept going on, I should
probably get an outfit for court that I actually liked wearing.

I glued my hair down, doing the Lego part on the left, and
re-noticed how pale I was. I left the bathroom and walked through
the living room, past my dog on the sofa, where he had been
watching me go back and forth, back and forth. I gave him a kiss
and said, "wish me luck, buddy." I grabbed my bag, tossing in a
pen, notebook, reading material, banana, water bottle, and Clif bar.
Then I threw it over my shoulder messenger style, across my chest,

and left. I'd sold the dress shoes after my last court appearance and only had black boots to match. They were a little heavy and out of place, but so was I. With my size-nine, hobbit-worthy feet and short hair, I looked like a middle-aged Tank Girl. Walking to the subway, all I wanted to do was get back home and into well-worn cottons. It hadn't been an hour yet, and already, the bra was fighting me.

Walking through Tribeca to Centre Street, the early morning's fall light was golden gorgeous, especially how it was hitting old buildings. I was eating my banana, strolling along. It was the first time my court date was on a Thursday. There was kind of a different crowd out and about—quieter, respectful, better put together. At the courthouse, there was a long line for security. I nervously drank all my water, momentarily confusing the scene with TSA. Then a guy cut in front of me in line and I wanted to say to him, "Maybe this behavior is the reason why you're here?" Then again, maybe it was my inability to take any shit that was the reason I was there.

Once inside, I found out it was the same courtroom as last time, second floor, down the long hallway. I entered a little past 9:30 am, and things had already started. Nancy wasn't coming. I was there on my own, which was a lot more nerve wracking or nerve wrecking. We'd had a disagreement back in August, and she'd been MIA all week, even though I knew she knew I'd be in court today. I wondered when Perry would show up.

Hope texted and advised me to look out for my neighbor. My back started to hurt ten minutes after I started sitting on the pews. I was hungry again. I didn't want to be there. I just knocked on a door. I didn't assault anyone. We were instructed that all cell phones were to be put away. It was a woman judge. She was engaging, and involved. Court officers rotated their positions around the courtroom, keeping their attentions sharp and boredom at bay. A motion to dismiss was denied. Had my lawyer filed a motion to dismiss? Another woman was taken to a different courtroom. I desperately wanted to readjust my rogue right boob in the bra.

A couple sat down in front of me. There was a tall lady with long black hair pulled back into a thick braid. She had perfect, smooth white skin, and was wearing a sleeveless 60s patterned dress. The guy she was with was wrinkled sun-red, with long salty-red hair, pulled into a low ponytail at the back. He was shorter than her, than me. His grey-and-white pinstriped suit was baggy on him, especially in the shoulders. His beard was a dried-out fuzzy brown. His hands were covered with handmade tattoos, one of them the poke-needle kind, all of them faded to a blue-green. They reminded me of actors I couldn't place, particularly the guy.

"Your case will be dismissed...sealed in six months...two days community service. Good luck to you." No way, it was the "Good Luck To You" judge from my DAT. Seeing a judge twice now made me feel like a regular. Like court was my local dive and the bartender knew my drink. Sitting there alone, I kept thinking that Nancy could have texted a "good luck." We weren't technically at odds. The couple in front had come in with a cup of coffee each, and an officer told them to take their drinks outside. I like how coffee drinkers take the beverage everywhere. I wouldn't have minded a fruit smoothie myself. The lady took their coffees and said she had to use the bathroom before leaving the guy. He took his black Stetson-style hat off his lap and put it to the side next to him, as if holding her seat, though the pew was otherwise empty.

The judge said "good morning" to each defendant and lawyer at the start of a new case. At the end of one, she said, "Good luck to you, young man." Most people had lawyers who were the same ethnicity as them. The lady came back. She kept fussing over the guy, moving stray hairs behind his ear, consoling him. Judging by how anxious the guy was, I assumed it was his case they were there for. He shuffled a bit, and his black-framed glasses fell out the back of the pew. Neither of them noticed, even though the glasses made a clank on the tiled floor, hitting the ground at my feet. I leaned forward, picked them up, tapped on the lady's shoulder, and handed them back. They thanked me. It was the most interesting thing that had happened so far, except maybe when I unbuttoned my shirt and reached in there to adjust the girls. My chest was really unhappy with my decision to jail it. The couple went back to their world and worries. Like I had something stuck in my teeth, I still couldn't place why these people were so familiar to me. Watching them have each other in this gloomy room, in an area of the city no one goes to unless forced or paid, I was sad about Nancy. It was hard being here alone externally, and being without her support internally.

I started to remember a dream I had last night where I went to get my hair cut at a salon owned by Annie Lennox. The place was all white, all bright white. Lennox wore a white flowing lab coat that was similar to the ones worn at salons in the waking world. The kind of smock stylists wear to let you know the establishment is high end, and that they use the fancy products with strong chemicals. Lennox cut my hair as I watched from outside looking in through the glass storefront window. She was cutting my hair in a way that would make it grow out perfectly. We all thought this was brilliant, and I said it was worth the money. In real life, my hair grows out like a mullet, then an evergreen, then a mullet, then an evergreen, until all the different areas meet to form a shape similar to that of Gilda Radner's Saturday Night Live character Roseannadanna: a trapezoid. I'd been thinking of letting it do that, like waving a white flag, I surrender! Go English garden yourself, you wiry-thin badass stuff up there.

It was 10:04 am. The next guy's case was dismissed, with the record sealed in six months. What did sealed in six months mean? I realized each time I'd heard the phrase it conjured up images of things rotting in old food containers. The guy went up without a lawyer, letting himself in through the chain link divider.

He was maybe in his mid-20s, wearing blue jeans and a pink "Thrasher" t-shirt that was a couple of sizes too small, like a little girl's shirt. How come he got to go up to the big-people table without a guardian?

I wanted to take my boots off, open my own shirt two buttons, roll up my sleeves, and do some seated poses on the pew. I did some subtle stuff instead, crossing my left leg over my right and twisting, then switching sides, putting a leg on a thigh and leaning forward. There wasn't enough time this morning for me to practice. Many cases were dismissed and sealed or given sentences of community service. A couple rows down, closer to the action, one pew's back was carved with the words "fuck everybody." Three cops came in, went behind the wood fencing, and stood in a row at attention, arms behind their backs. Against the wall near the judge, the secret door opened, and they headed in. For a flash, I could see the jail cells inside, with their off-white colored bars reaching all the way to the ceiling. It was hard to imagine, with how casual things were going out here in the courtroom, that human beings were being held back there. Moments later, the three officers came out the secret door, and left.

Another officer came into the room. We were being heavily guarded today. A woman diagonally across from me had stretched her legs out, slid off her shoes, crossed her ankles, and rested her bare feet on the shoes. Behind her, a man in black socks and black flip-flops picked a ball of hair off the toe of one of his socks, flicked it somewhere, and then stretched his legs out. There was a wide breadth of approaches to appearance and demeanor amongst the "alleged" congregants.

I looked around as the courtroom filled. My neighbor wasn't there. Was she supposed to be there? It seemed like it was only defendants. I imagined it would be a very different vibe if every side was present. Perry had walked in. Today he was wearing a light-green suit with maybe a pink tie. I could't get a good look because his back was to me. My belly did a flip. My chest tightened. Any second now, I would go from observer to participant.

Perry showed a name to a DA grunt. They talked. A young DA guy with pale freckly skin and red hair hunted for the file. I don't know when youth became an affront to me, but there was no way that guy was out of his teens. I like anyone handling my business to be older than I am. This is especially the case with my primary-care physician. I want her to have used the parts I'm asking about—and to have had access to information about them—longer than I have. You wouldn't want to buy a car from someone who'd never driven. It was taking this squirt a long time to find the file, looking through multiple areas and piles. The alphabet usually works, last name first. Why weren't they using that over there? You can't do an internet search in the material world. It's best to stick with known systems. Like usual, I needed to pee.

A man had sat down behind me and was anxiously tapping his foot. I told myself to breathe. Perry was taking some notes. The guy behind me got up, saying "fuck" under his breath. He walked over to the DA's area. Earlier he had pled guilty to a fourth-degree misdemeanor of marijuana possession. He was found with four ounces at 6 am on Park Avenue, somewhere just above the hundredth block. I think he was waiting for an important piece of paper and wanted to know the status.

Perry called someone else's name. Hmmmm. Now he had two files, maybe three. Where was the other person? He made eye contact with me and at the same time tipped a file in the air to let me know he saw me. This saved me from having to hear my name being called out loud. I was very happy about that. Often, when I hear my name called, it isn't my name at all. When I order food, I use M.J. for Marcy Jill. I used to use Marcy, but then I'd get hangry whenever someone named Mary wasn't picking up their order. I changed my waiting name to "M.J." when I was in a hospital reception area about to be admitted for being depressed and suicidal.

Back in 1992, while attending art school in Boston, I started going to therapy after I saw a friend of mine come out of a little room near the welding and ceramic studios where I practically lived. He told me he went to counseling sessions in there, adding that therapy was free because our small art school was associated with a University, and explained that this was how the PhD candidates satisfied an hours requirement. I signed up out of curiosity and intuition. Then I spent nearly two years explaining various childhood scenarios and asking, "Was that normal?" My therapist would repeatedly say, "No." I got depressed in there, then I got really depressed and didn't want to be alive anymore.

At the time, I was working at the music store HMV in Harvard Square. From Friday through Sunday, I was the customer service department. If you returned anything to HMV over the weekend in the spring of 1994, it was to me. I worked from opening to close those three days, over thirty hours. Aside from talk therapy, what really pushed me over the edge mentally was the movie Dennis the Menace. For months, it played silently, over and over again, on all the screens in the store. The entire sales area, one large open floorpan, had been decorated with television sets to advertise new-on-video movies. It was a lot of screens. I didn't hear a word of the movie, but I watched it hundreds of times. Without sound, it was a strangely violent movie. There was a little boy named Dennis who terrorized his neighbor, played by Walter Matthau. While a DJ nuanced the music selection from a glass room at the back of the store, he never played any other movie. It was on an endless loop.

My therapist at school would do the talk stuff, and a psychiatrist on the University campus would do the meds. By year two, I'd tried six different antidepressants, and each one either didn't work or had side effects that were too debilitating. By June of '94, I had amassed a pile of pills, and was thinking of taking them all at once. During this time, my therapist was trying to get me to voluntarily admit myself to a program. Otherwise, she was going to have to involuntarily admit me, and I would lose the ability to chose a hospital, leave or make any decisions for myself. This was a very tricky and conflicting situation for me: I was vacillating between not wanting to lose her trust and not wanting to be alive.

One night, coming home from work, I exited the "T" (subway) and walked my usual route along the Back Bay Fens. If I followed the crosswalks I had to wait for multiple lights. Instead, I often chose to do one crazy sprint after cars had passed, jaywalking where it was convenient for me. That night, I didn't wait for the cars to pass. I closed my eyes and stepped out into traffic. Drivers would be nearing the end of a turn, without much time to see me. Instead of feeling an impact, I heard the sound of screeching brakes, horns, and yelling out windows. I opened my eyes and ran. I scared myself. I made that decision, to try and end my life, without making the decision. I did it without thinking. I saw how I couldn't trust myself, and decided to enter a hospital. After contacting my therapist, I was instructed to go to a place where you were told which programs had free beds. Armed with a dear friend and with some advice about which programs to avoid, ready to battle my depression by surrendering to the weight of it, I sat in the reception area hearing Mary Trippin, Mary Trippin, Mary Trippin, until I realized it was me they were calling. It was then I decided, along with getting mentally healthy, that I would use "M.J." for callbacks.

Instead of meeting outside the courtroom, Perry came over, sat down next to me, and explained what was going on. We talked as if he'd been sitting there all along, like we were picking up from a previous conversation. His tone was low, serious and directed. It sounded like he was using a big-boy voice, as though I'd been convicted of a more serious crime—murder—and it pulled me in. I wasn't taking notes while he was speaking, so I had the triple task of listening, processing, and committing everything to memory. This was hard. Normally I couldn't do one of those alone very well.

Perry had filed a motion to get my statement that the police officers made up removed because they shouldn't have interrogated me, and they never read me my Miranda rights. I told Perry I never said those things anyway. He was unmoved. I asked him if he heard that a lot. He told me it didn't really matter if my statement was true or not; it just needed to be out, and the judge should grant that in a hearing. I guessed motions needed hearings. It would have been great if there was an interpreter behind Perry, like a person signing, except holding up cards with explanations so I could follow what he was saying in real time. After the hearing, the judge would set a court date for trial. Okay, at least now I knew why I was there, but not why Perry didn't respond to emails or phone calls.

I asked about a jury. Perry told me that in New York State, I wouldn't get a jury for a B-level misdemeanor. So much for the right to a trial by jury and the Sixth Amendment. Guess I hadn't needed to stress about taking 12 people away from work. There was a window for when the trial had to take place, and it was 45 days from today. There were some pinochle-type rules about which days counted and which didn't. Weekends didn't. Only a month and a half counted because the DA had a hard time getting my neighbor's signature. That was a good sign, that she didn't want to sign. Or, that she was being difficult. It was more likely that she was difficult, surprise, surprise.

The day-counting thing was so wishy-washy I felt like Perry was making it up as he went along. It was a backyard baseball game. The neighbor's yard was an out, but if you knocked one off the big oak by the neighbor's yard it was a home run. Second base was a sprinkler. If you hit a gutter along the roof, it was a double, if the ball rolled off the roof and was caught, it was an out, and if the ball fell into the gutter, well, then the game was over. My arrest happened in April, and it was now September, but less than 30 days had counted toward my case.

While Perry was telling me this, I was thinking of football, seeing an absolutely beautiful pass arcing through 30 yards of air to a one-handed catch. But then a player nowhere near the action was caught pinching another guy's butt, and the ball gets pulled back ten yards for holding. The holding calls are such bullshit. But it's all bullshit, really. Rules and Constitutional Amendments that didn't seem to exist in real life: from the lease and its "warrant of habitability" to the police needing a warrant before entering my apartment. I'd counted all the days since my arrest. I lived through each and every single one of them worrying about this case, my future, my life. They had meant something to me. But for the court, my neighbor, and the police, they hadn't counted.

Perry didn't think my neighbor would show up. I reminded him that we both didn't think she would show. It was just my shrink who did. Every one else voted no. Perry said the case couldn't be dismissed because there was no grounds for dismissal. He added that the judge decided what was considered reasonable doubt. I looked back over to the judge. She had pleasant manners, but was no pushover. Perry told me to bring in other people who might have seen what happened, or who knew of my neighbors' behavior. It didn't seem like he was familiar with the case. I was alone in a hallway, the cameras weren't working, and no one was going on a field trip to Centre Street on my behalf. Possibly Dewan would, but boy, would that be a huge favor. He'd have to take time off from work.

The DA was still offering me harassment as a plea, which Perry didn't think was generous. Maybe they would make a better offer at trial. I told Perry that if my neighbor showed up and I accepted the harassment charge, that would give her grounds to follow through with a civil trial. I wondered if the DA would really go through the trouble of trying me if I didn't take the plea. Wait, was this going to trial for real? A trial by a judge? Was I understanding this all correctly? It was a long and drawn-out process. Perry told me a trial wouldn't start until October, maybe November. In my head, I was asking him "Didn't you tell me today was the trial, without answering emails or phone calls to help me prepare...and are you now saying it's in two more months? In November?" More time waiting. Perry got up and told me to stay where I was, adding, "It'll happen soon." It was ominous phrasing.

I was to wait until we were called up, and Perry would request that my fake Police statement be removed. The familiar lady and guy were still sitting in front of me. She was holding up a small round compact to her face, looking in the mirror while powdering her cheeks. Tap tap here, tap tap there. Turning her head left and right, tilting her chin up and down for better angles. I'd never understood rubbing chemicals into one's skin. Men don't do this, why did women?

Looking around, no one in the pews seemed preoccupied with how they looked, or how anyone else looked. We all just wanted to get out of there. I was fantastically ill-humored after being reminded of that fake statement, and I was grouchy having been informed the case was going to go on even longer before it officially started. It was disappointing that Noah had been misinformed about a dismissal. It had gotten my hopes up. There was never a chance for dismissal. Was I being too naïve, or had Noah either not been able to get a clear answer from Perry, or never bothered even asking? I sat there digesting our conversation, fuming. Look at all the paperwork and fuss for just knocking on a door.

It was 10:50 am. The courtroom was getting busier. I looked over at Perry. He had a naturally serious, downward-smile, resting face. I wondered what he looked like when he did smile. He was a muscular man, maybe a gym rat. Suddenly, I connected my intense irritability with how my lower abdomen was feeling. I had started my cycle early. I didn't have a tampon or ibuprofen in my bag, and this didn't look like the venue or audience where I could go poking around for an "extra." I also couldn't leave because Perry had said, "It'll happen soon," though maybe he meant the blood hemorrhaging from my vagina. I had about 40 minutes until the pain would be so bad that I wouldn't be able to stand up. How was it possible that this happened every month, for over three decades, and I still failed to plan ahead for it on occasion? Maybe there would be a break for lunch, and I could run to a drugstore.

Perry was sitting in the front pew, where the lawyers got to play with their phones. Maybe I could sneak a text to him, but say something like I had a headache and needed to find aspirin. For all their obsession with lady parts, men do not like any menstrual talk. Not that it would be appropriate, but it was what it was. Perry had thick, graying hair, he wore politician style: fluffy with a deep side part. I wondered how much older I was than him. I wondered if he cared that I didn't shove the door open. He wore a wedding ring. It was interesting how this was his workday, that he did this day in and day out. I didn't want to be part of his world for another minute.

I couldn't get Perry's attention. I just sat there hoping my name would be called soon. Behind me, lawyers were talking, asking, "Do you have one or two cases on today?" "Two." "Two? You want to pick up another one?" What were we, like trading cards? Perry took a call, and left through the secret side door. The door's brown veneer was smudged black along the edge, where years of hands and oils had quietly left the courtroom. I'd thought that today, there would be forward movement. Now I felt stupid about sending that email to the articles club ladies asking for support with my trial.

When Perry left, I noticed his tie wasn't pink. Instead, it had orange and brown angled stripes. Since most of the courtroom was a shade of bowel release, it was exciting when someone came in with a little color on them. Sometimes, it felt like I was in a place of worship, and sometimes it felt like I was in a friend's basement in the 70s. Maybe the lady in front had something in her bag, and I could lean over and quietly ask her. Her Guy friend, Roger somebody, was being called up the podium. He brought his hat, his security blanket, an adult binky. Roger stood holding it by his side, spinning the brim in one hand, while his lady friend looked on, her head tilted to the left in concern. I kept sliding forward in the pew, then noticing my crappy posture and pushing myself back up to sit tall. I was miserable.

I couldn't hear what Roger's lawyer was saying even though the podium had a microphone. I was only getting a phrase here and there. And in this situation, it wasn't okay to yell out, "Can't hear in the back!" The word "superseding" was used. There was superseding information. A court officer took papers from Roger's lawyer, held in a manila file folder like all other important papers, and gave it to the judge and then to a DA grunt. Roger's lady friend flipped her long braid behind her as she closed up some bags and nervously organized. He was going to be out of town from October through December for work. The odd block of time, like a shooting schedule, refueled my quandary about where I'd seen him before. The judge okayed a delay after it was confirmed he'd already purchased plane tickets. With that resolved, Roger began to leave. At the same time, the judge addressed his lawyer, and Roger turned back around. He was told multiple times to step out until he understood. Go back to your seat, Roger. It was 11:08 am, and I wanted to eat, take an over-the-counter pain killer, cork up my issue, and go home, though not in that order.

My name was called. I'd readied my messenger bag by pulling its strap shorter so it was more like a shoulder bag. I threw my notebook and pen inside, and stood up. When I did, my pants had static clung to the tubes of my socks. I had to pull my pants' legs down from my calves. Every second it took, the whole court was waiting. I grabbed my bag in my hand, and walked up the aisle with it bouncing against my leg. At the fencing, Perry unhooked the chain, let me in, and hooked it closed behind him. I placed my bag on the floor by my feet thinking it would be rude to use the podium and table in front. Then I noticed I was accidentally standing amore-close to Perry and kicked my bag some to scoot over a bit. Before that, it was like we were about to say vows. The judge said "Good morning," and Perry responded in kind. Now that I was in the judge's paddock area, I could see this wasn't really an inclusive salutation, and I remained silent, holding my hands behind my back.

There was some talk using terms I'd never heard. The VDF was due on September 15. Wait, wasn't that today? They exchanged some more decisions that had to do with my life, but I had no idea what was going on. Now dates were being decided for the next court appearance. The Judge suggested October 25, 26, or 27, but none of those worked for the DA. The judge suggested Monday, November 7. That worked for the DA. I reached down to get my bag, slowly, so my pants didn't ride up, and placed it in front of me, taking out my phone. Perry was checking his. November 7 didn't work for him. The judge suggested Wednesday the 9. Perry countered with the 15. Was anyone there concerned with or interested in my schedule? I was not excited that the dates kept getting further and further away. Perry backtracked and agreed to November 7. This was a day when I taught in the evening, but I assumed things would start in the morning. I looked towards the judge to see if she wanted to confer with me as well. When nothing happened, I began putting the date of November 7 in my phone's calendar.

While I was doing that, the judge confirmed that the order of protection was still in order. There was a pause, silence. I looked up from my phone, and realized they needed me for this. This is the problem I have with television and movies. Everyone knows when they're supposed to talk, and that rarely happens in real life. Apparently, it was my line: "Yes, your honor." With that, I was given a piece of paper with the next court-appearance date, and turned to Perry who looked me in the eye and said, "Don't worry about this." *Okeydokey Perry.* We shook hands, and I left the courtroom.

They were done with me. I was done. I headed to the elevators and put on my baseball cap, my security blanket. As I walked out of 100 Centre Street and into the city, I thought how it will be cold in November.

Baddha Konasana at the wall
w/ elbow stretch

hand on elbows + forearms
30a stretch'd

- feet together
- knees bent
- arms out, against wall
  try to slide hands to
  touch, while folding
  forward.

- feet close → harder
- head towards feet , or fin

5 MIN

input
elbows

☆ eventually bend
you down
↓

332

Saturday, September 17, 2016

It was late in the afternoon, and I was readying for work, making a smoothie and putting everything that needed to be in my bag near my bag when Nancy called. Already prepared on the table were slices of raw cheese and organic blue chips so I could pace myself and not get a head freeze. Buster was sitting nearby in his perfect-statue pose, hoping for a bite of cheese, looking at the cutting board, then at me, then back at the cutting board. Subtle. I was hungry but answered anyway, and it sounded like I was on speakerphone. Nancy and I hadn't spoken in awhile. I was in court on Thursday, and she had chosen a way to communicate that she knew I didn't care for. We'd been through this many times before. While my voice was coming through perfectly through her car's speakers, I was hearing both inside car noises and outside car noises.

This was not how you called someone to maybe get an update on their criminal trial and learn whether they'd been found guilty of third-degree assault. Though I knew I was on speakerphone, I asked whether I was anyway. My passive-aggressive way of letting her know it annoyed me. "Yes," Nancy said, adding her husband was with her and they were stuck in traffic. *Are you killing time?* "We can hear you," she declared victoriously, and as usual showing no concern for whether this was happening the other way around. On my plate, I had food, hunger, a silly dog, and jerky friends. It felt like Nancy's call was fueled by the relief she'd figured out something to pass the time with while sitting in traffic, rather than inspired by genuine concern. "We're dying to know how it went on Thursday," she said, her tone more appropriate for "How'd the date go last night?" than "Did you get the test results back?" It was so cheerful, so fucking cheerful. I said I was eating lunch, which I wanted to be true, and asked if I could I call back at 3 pm. All agreed, and the call ended. I never called back, and took a sadness that I didn't have time to unpack with me to work.

After teaching class, I headed with Goldie and another student to Goldie's apartment on the Upper West Side. We planned on eating ice cream on her fifth-floor balcony garden in another one of those crazy awesome NYC apartments. It was a beautiful night. We settled in with pints, bowls, and big spoons, and caught up. It was another conversation where I expressed how embarrassed I was to be feeling so much stress. Each time I'd said this, the response was that what I was going through was indeed stressful, and it was appropriate to be feeling that way. Then I told them about how Nancy and I were going through some friendship bumps, trying to break some patterns, not necessarily fighting, and how she never texted or called on Thursday, the day of my last court appearance. I also relayed the car exchange, and my student said, "If you're so dying to know, why not call on Thursday? Why wait till Saturday?" It was a good point, and it made me sadder.

Goldie had worked in fashion since forever and wanted to revisit my court appearance, making sure I wore clothes that fit and flat shoes and hid my tattoos. Then they talked about how they loved tattoos, but blah, blah, blah. I'd already been to court a bunch of times, and it seemed like the dress code was fairly loose, but I didn't say anything. Sometimes, it's hard to flip the switch from teaching a group class and telling 30 plus people what to do, to being told what to do.

Thursday, September 22, 2016

I could go a couple of days without thinking about a criminal trial, putting it in a corner of my thoughts for a time-out. But then, it would come running out into the middle, screaming and causing trouble again. Instead of snuggling between me and the sofa for stress naps, Buster had taken to having me against the sofa while he was perched on the outside. He would lie there facing the front door. My anxiety had a spice of fear now, and he must have been picking up that I was scared. Because he was a small nugget of a dog, his protection was more endearing than anything else.

Still distracted, I went to open an e-book and ended up searching for "third-degree assault" instead. I was reading about what would happen if I was found guilty, and how I could be forced to pay restitution of up to $15,000. Then there were the life limitations of having a criminal record: no student loans, no bank financing, issues with job applications, and limitations on traveling abroad. The ramifications for knocking on a door were so far-reaching that I started to cry, then closed my eyes. Sleep was the only way to turn it off, to avoid the thinking. I was going to waste the next six weeks, and I couldn't fight against it.

Wednesday, September 28, 2016

I was updating my shrink on the case. In attempting a retell, I kept contradicting myself, or the information I'd been given was contradictory. Perry said there wouldn't be a jury because this was a class-B misdemeanor. But third-degree assault was a felony. Perry believed my neighbor wouldn't show up, and then said the case would be dismissed. Yet, I'd heard the district attorney could still pursue the case regardless. Maybe I was missing facts in the retell. Facts are aesthetically different from details. Details are great for storytelling, but facts aren't usually the best stuff. Which day, what time of day, those can cause more of a distraction, pushing people out rather than pulling them in. Maybe I couldn't recall exactly what my lawyer said, but I could report there was an odd bump on his chin and his hands moved a lot while he stayed still. I'd been engaged with the courtroom itself, with its symbolic nod to the interior decorating of religious venues, with how different defendants would bide their time in the pews, with the nonchalance of lawyers, and with my uncomfortable clothing. I thought about recreating the experience as a performance, having people rotate each character, from judge to court officer to lawyer to the alleged. Doing it in one long, constant, choreographed moment, where the transfers continued as the dialog continued. With outfits, postures, and attitudes being swapped from one side of the law to the other.

Before becoming a yoga teacher I was trained as a visual artist. So while I struggled with verbal cognition and was slow to process language, I could say with authority that the light streaming in from those high windows was perfect for filming. I was going to try and stay true to who I was, and how I saw the world, throughout this nightmare process. Yeah, I didn't know why I wouldn't get a jury, but I needed to do the things that kept me focused on being me.

Now that I was at peak confusion and a trial date had been set, I had been thinking about reaching out to Frankie in Cleveland again and asking for her help in understanding what was going on. While she was a busy new mom, maybe she needed a baby brain break. Since Perry was unreachable, I needed outside counsel to my counsel. It didn't feel like things were going well. It was still hard to process how knocking on a door created such a mess. I felt like I was getting comfortable being tired and worn out from not knowing what was happening with the case. Even if nothing happened in court, at all, I would always have been arrested. It was months ago, and it was yesterday in my thoughts. It was the pink puffer, the black sweatpants, the spot just outside the kitchen, and the feeling I still couldn't shake of having my arms behind my back and my wrists tightly locked together. The best I hoped for is that my arrest would somehow fade into the background one day. During moments of hypothetical fears, I had the desire to flee the country and leave Buster with a friend. Calling Frankie might be a better idea.

Thursday, September 29, 2016

I reached out to Frankie via text:

ME: Hey!! How are you!? My case is going to trial in November and I'm stressed and confused about what's going on. Could we please set up a time to chat on the phone where I can pick your brain??! -Marcy

FRANKIE: Hey! Sorry to hear the case is still happening. My days are pretty tough to predict right now, but maybe tomorrow evening? That way [my husband] is around to take care of [the baby]

FRANKIE: Also, I can usually text more easily if you have more immediate questions

ME: Hi. Totally get your schedule right now!! I'll try to figure out easy text questions...After schlepping groceries home. Which I'm sure you miss!!!

FRANKIE: Hahaha. Ohh NYC grocery shopping, how I don't miss thee at all

ME: First, your daughter is adorable. Your family is adorable. Your new life is enviable. Now let's move on to mine and 3rd degree assault!!

ME: DA offered me only harassment and fine. Didn't take it bc landlord was trying to evict me on harassment. (Woohoo). Landlord dropped that. No jury for 3rd degree assault? And DA still isn't making a better offer. Do they still proceed if she doesn't show up?

FRANKIE: Haha thank you! Yes let's move onto more pressing matters. Ok first things first: my opinion is that the harassment violation offer is BS but standard from the DA on an assault case. 3rd degree assault is a B misdemeanor which means you do NOT have a right to a jury trial, so you will be tried before a judge

FRANKIE: Without knowing anything about the case I can't see how they could possibly go forward without her unless they have other witnesses

FRANKIE: Any indication that she isn't cooperative?

FRANKIE: Also, who is your attorney?

FRANKIE: Do you have any witnesses who will testify about the complainant if she does come forward? Based on what you've told me other people know she's batshit. She didn't sound like someone who would show up for court, which is great for you. A lot of times if the case actually gets sent out to trial the DA will make a better offer, but if their witness is never going to show up then it would eventually get dismissed (although that can take time)

ME: It took them a long time to get her to sign the statement. That's my only intel. My attorney is Perry from Defender Peeps

FRANKIE: Ok, Defender Peeps? I know people there. They are a great org

ME: Yes. DP

ME: The neighbor below will sign a statement about her

FRANKIE: Ok, and your lawyer has all this info I assume?

ME: Nope. He hasn't contacted me once!

FRANKIE: Ok well you really need to reach out to him with this info

FRANKIE: Have you tried reaching him?

FRANKIE: They have investigators who will interview witnesses

ME: Do you think it's bc he's busy w/ other cases in front?

ME: Ah. I didn't know that. He does not respond to emails

FRANKIE: I'm sure he has a ton of cases, but he really needs all this info just in case it does go to trial. It may be that 99% of these cases go nowhere because the complainant doesn't show up and he's acting accordingly, but you should try calling him. Often a voice mail is more likely to get a response

FRANKIE: I'd just leave a message conveying that you have some questions about the case and some information that would be helpful and that you're stressed about the case and would just like to get a better idea of what's going to happen

FRANKIE: Aaah ok. Just got some intel why he doesn't respond

ME: Ok. I'll email and call. Are you saying the trial date isn't really the trial date? That's the issue I ran into last week in that I never know why I'm going to court

FRANKIE: Sounds like he may have some intense personal stuff going on. I would call the main number and ask to speak to his supervisor and just say you're a little worried about the case.

ME: Really!?

FRANKIE: Yeah these cases drag on and on and just get rescheduled over and over for many reasons: no court parts available for trial, witness not available, etc

ME: The last court thing he submitted motions to exclude the made-up police statement

FRANKIE: Sure but if you haven't heard back soon I would call a supervisor. Sounds like there's a chance your case would be reassigned

FRANKIE: Oh ok, well was there a decision on the motion or he just submitted? If just submitted the case would be on for decision on the motion, not trial

ME: Oh boy

FRANKIE: I really think you should talk to a supervisor to get a clearer picture of what is going on procedurally and to tell them about your witness etc

ME: Won't they refer me back to Perry?

ME: I just don't want to rock the boat of free defense

FRANKIE: No, don't worry about that. I would just say, I'm just a little worried bc I haven't had much communication and I just wanted to talk to someone about my case

FRANKIE: I'm sure they're aware of his personal situation, so I doubt it would rock any boats. I actually know his supervisor

FRANKIE: I'm getting this info from my other legal aid friend who is in the know. It's a small defender world

ME: When did we decide he has a personal situation? You have inside intel!!

FRANKIE: Haha I get it but this is your life and based on the info I have I don't think it will be a problem

FRANKIE: Maybe don't say you know that he has stuff going on...I'm like deep throat over here. You've got an inside source.

ME: Wow. You've relieved some stress and made things more interesting. Thank You!!

ME: Can I give you a better nickname?

FRANKIE: Haha yes please

ME: You know. Texting doesn't lend itself to nicknames. Feel free to drop something in the hat...

FRANKIE: Haha, mom brain also doesn't lend itself. I'll think on it...

ME: MomBrain it is!!

FRANKIE: Well there you go

While we were texting, Frankie was also exchanging texts with a friend on the inside. My lawyer's distance wasn't a professional stance; it was due to personal issues. That was helpful to know. At first I didn't want to poke around the Defenders Peeps office saying I should be receiving more communication in case I wasn't entitled to it. Usually, when I ask for a supervisor, it's on the phone with customer service, we've hit a wall, and I need the baton passed to the next person on the other side of that wall. Now I'd gotten the okay to contact Perry's supervisor.

To prep for another blind phone call, and possible voice mail message, I went online to the DP website to see if Perry's

supervisor had a photo. This fifth-chakra block of mine, the area of communication, was something I needed to tend to once the case was over. Whenever that happened. I kept my voicemail message simple, using words I could easily pronounce, saying I had questions about my case, and asking his supervisor to please call back at her earliest convenience. If this sounding-out issue was an actual thing, hopefully it was called something with one syllable. Malapropisms is an unjustly challenging word for people who make those types of mistakes.

It did feel like I was ratting Perry out. I knew what it was like to receive negative feedback because some of my regular students liked to read to me other students' complaints for laughs. Usually theirs, not mine. I didn't have access to the feedback because I wasn't a member of the class package company students used. There, in the world of anonymous complaining, were some keen observations about my notorious disdain, and eventual ban, of water bottles. I did this because my classes were taught mostly in the dark, and I'd trip over or accidentally kick the bottles into other students. Beyond the codependency and separation anxiety for over-priced containers, holding quantities of liquid no student needed to drink during a one hour restorative class, were some helpful and constructive insights.

There was the woman who hated my class and then quoted me when I accidentally said, "cats are assholes." *It's amazing I've had such a long career.* One student complained she didn't get enough spots in my class. When I relayed this to a yoga teacher friend of mine she said, "If you want more spots honey, do a private." I wanted to let these people know: it's just a yoga class. That even the best meals eventually end up in the toilet. That they shouldn't dwell on ephemeral life experiences. And to stop writing reviews about them.

After reviewing my text exchange with Frankie, I started having a different perspective on speaking with Perry's supervisor. Should I tell her how I almost took the harassment plea because he and Noah hadn't spoken? I could have been evicted because of that. Frankie told me I'd probably be assigned new counsel. I'd be the one breaking up with a lawyer this time. Then I got excited about the possibility of Defender Peeps sending an investigator to the building for some sleuthing.

Friday, September 30, 2016

I was trying to think of people in similar anticlimactic, yet ongoing and committed, paradigms. Like those end-of-the-world cult members who prepared for it to be all over on, say, January 30, and how they must have felt on January 31. The case went on and on after each court appearance. I needed to figure out how to go on while it was going on and on, instead of waiting for it to be over.

Perry's supervisor, Diana, called me back. It sounded like she had read my file and knew everything. Who were these people with excellent reading-comprehension skills and retention? I politely explained that I had no idea what was happening, and how it was causing me anxiety. This came out a little rehearsed, as I'd been thinking about an opening. It was maybe not too convincing to say I was having anxiety about something without showing a hint of anxiety.

Diana proceeded to effortlessly and patiently explain all that had transpired since my arrest. It was wonderful. I was listening to the CliffsNotes version of my life going back to April. Here was all the essential information, not the kind of stuff I'd been paying attention to, like how depressing medium brown is, and how creepy the Centre Street elevators were. This was the scene in an action movie when the antagonist goes on and on about their plot to take over the world, mostly to make sure the audience is caught up, while the protagonist is being slowly lowered into a venomous snake pit.

Diana explained that the desk appearance ticket was to hear my arraignment, to read out the official charges. This was when the case officially started. She explained supporting deposition, and how the prosecutor needed it. They had to furnish that by the next court appearance on July 6. That was needed when the police officers' statement wasn't enough to prove the case at a trial because the officer wasn't a witness. This is when I found out that my neighbor had signed her statement.

On September 15, motions were filed for a hearing about the evidence the police officers took. That evidence could be property or statements, and would be used to argue that they shouldn't have arrested me in the first place because they didn't have probable cause. This was a common argument, and made to ensure that if the case went to trial, there also wouldn't be evidence against me. Then I chimed in that I never made that statement, and Diana affirmed, "or that you never made that statement." Finally, someone was hearing me on that one.

Diana explained these so-called statements. They stemmed from when officers casually asked what happened, and people blabbed and blabbed and blabbed and then that became their statement. Defender Peeps would need to know when the "statement" was taken from me: at my door, before they handcuffed me, or afterward. The Miranda rights came into play as well. Also on September 15, the judge ordered a voluntary disclosure form (VDF) to be submitted by September 29. They were already supposed to have been submitted. The police didn't have to show all the evidence they had (huh?), but they did have to show some info, such as any photos or medical records from the incident and records of a 911 call if there was one.

I asked about my charges, explaining how I'd read that third-degree assault is a class A felony but was told it was a class B misdemeanor. Diana clarified that the prosecutors would pursue a class A felony if they were seeking jail time and class B if it was unlikely they were seeking jail time. What I was being charged

343

with had been reduced to attempted assault in the third degree. There was no jail time being sought! Diana noted that September 29 had passed yesterday, and—I heard a rustling of papers in the background—the VDF hadn't been submitted. This was a good thing. It meant the DA's office was not paying attention to the case. When she said this, I had an image of a stack of files, three feet high, on the corner of a desk, and mine sandwiched somewhere near the bottom. Diana said the DA had 90 days to try me, but not 90 sequential days. Some days counted, and some days didn't. *Ah jeez, here we go again.* The judge showed favoritism towards the prosecutor in terms of counting days. From May 18 through July 6, approximately seven weeks, that counted. From September 15 to November 7 wouldn't count. If on November 7 the prosecutor wasn't ready, the clock would start again.

Diana told me not to worry because in all likelihood, they wouldn't be ready. However, if they did produce all of the disclosure forms, then Defender Peeps would find something else to string out the clock with. I asked if that was the active strategy. "Yes, it is," Diana said, "even though you might want a trial..." I immediately interrupted, "I don't want a trial." The Peeps' goal was to get the case dismissed because time had run out. This was similar to timed sports: have a lead and run the clock down. I was excited and relieved that there was a strategy. Diana said this was what they did for most of their clients, trying to get cases dismissed, then they're sealed six months after, rather than settling or going to trial. She told me to expect at least two more court dates to help accrue time.

Walk-through over, Diana asked about other people in the building who might have kept records and had issues with my neighbor. I told her about Dewan, and explained that he lived in the apartment below the neighbor who had me arrested, and kept meticulous records. When I relayed that my neighbor had been moved out by the management company, Diana's voice became conspiratorially low. "Ohhhhh," she said. "Do you know where they moved her?" It was nice to provide some interesting tidbit to the conversation, because she'd had me riveted since "hi."

It's not every day you can speak to someone over the phone who tells you what the fuck's been going on with your life with such insight. This wasn't like therapy. This was a play-by-play, and it was awesome. Diana said my neighbor moving out could look bad, in that the company did it for her safety, or good, in that she'd been such a hassle. I'd thought about both those scenarios, too. Diana was thinking out loud, like she was hatching a plan, "Maybe the prosecutor doesn't know how to find her now." She was sounding self-satisfied, and I loved it.

Diana asked if I knew how the management company kept records of tenant complaints and the process they used to resolve issues. I explained how I went from the super to the building manager to 311, to no avail. Then I added that the management company would be fantastically unhelpful in providing any information they had about my neighbor. "Not if they are subpoenaed," Diana replied. *Snnnap*. I also mentioned that I had sent an email of concern about my neighbor yelling at her children before I was arrested, and she requested that I forward it.

When I asked Diana about what would happen on November 7, I didn't write down her answer. I think at this point in the conversation she reiterated that we would be running out the clock. I was on board with this plan. I didn't know that there was a course of action before. It was exciting! There was a plan! I liked having a plan. I just wished they would have explained the strategy to me going all the way back before my July 6 court date, when I was having a nervous breakdown.

Before we ended the call, I told Diana I didn't want my conversation with her to rock the boat in any way. She responded with a solution in a third of a second, saying, "I'll tell Perry you called, he wasn't in the office, and we chatted." Another great strategy. I got off the phone feeling overjoyed. I just had to wait out the clock. They were going to find reasons to wait out the clock. We wouldn't let the prosecutors know they hadn't submitted paperwork, and my case would keep getting lower and lower in the pile. Before my chat with Diana, time was a burden. Now, it was how my case was going to get resolved.

While Diana and I were on the phone, I was trying to take notes and give the impression of someone with excellent listening skills. But it was hard to participate in the conversation and transcribe it at the same time. I'd start jotting down a sentence at the end when I realized it was important, then shove the beginning in front somewhere on the page. I was trying to hold the phone to my ear, keep my notebook open, and write. But with only two hands, I used my left hand to hold the phone, my left elbow to hold the notebook open, and my right hand to furiously make marks, some of which were barely legible. To let Diana know I heard her on certain points, I'd make a noise that was supposed to be the equivalent of "I see," "I'm listening," or "Got it." But it sounded like grunting, prehistoric grunting, from the time before language. Maybe a noise with origins dating back to the first challenging bowel movement. After one of those grunts, I zoned out and asked myself, "What the hell is that noise you're making?" At that point, it was too late for me to listen, take notes, and find a new noise. So I had to stick with it.

Wednesday, October 19, 2016

I changed the music on my cell phone from dark, sad, angsty stuff about being wronged, angry, or fed up to lighter fair. The conversation with Diana had changed my outlook. Knowing there was a strategy, I stopped thinking as much about it. The burden of worry lessened. I did question why Perry kept telling me the next court appearance was a trial, and why all the speculating over whether or not my neighbor would show up. About 48 hours after Diana and I spoke, I pissed out about five pounds of water retention stress, giving me a lightness in spirit and in body.

Energetically, it no longer felt like my nervous system was being dragged behind train. They had a plan. Perry never called back or checked in. I guessed we'd see one another in November.

The daymares and thinking about horrible outcomes started to fade. Though I still had flashbacks of being arrested. And I thought about the people who were innocent and died in jail or in custody, not just externally, but internally, their spirits taken from them. Sometimes, you can't get past the disbelief of your situation, and move on to survival, because the injustice is too crushing. You go from your home, your car, and your life to a whole other world as if it's normal. If the police see you as a criminal and you don't see yourself that way, it works against you. The decision isn't jointly made. Only their opinion matters.

Resisting arrest is the light between red and green. It can be a seven-second grace period, or last two seconds. And it's not you counting. At my closet door, processing the moment, surrounded by the police, what travelled through my nervous system like lightening was the what-ifs. While I shouldn't have felt fear in the presence of officers, I was terrified, for my and my dog's safety. It still scared me, the delicate flash of time when the police entered my apartment and I was able to make a good decision without any time to think. And I still thought about the moment outside the bathroom, knowing that in seconds everything was going to change, watching a yellow light turn red.

Friday, November 4, 2016

When I was updating friends these past couple of weeks, relaying the conversation I had with Diana, people kept asking why Defender Peeps couldn't have told me their strategy from the start. How different it might have been, had I known. All that worrying and stress. One of my favorite responses from a friend was, "That's still going on?"—like my arrest was a cold I'd caught months ago. Yeah, it was still going on, I still had a scratchy throat, a little cough, and some third-degree assault to clear up.

SUPINE TRIANGLE AT WALL

(the pose I was doing before getting unrolled)

- one foot at wall, one leg on bolster

- do both sides   (10 MIN)

- slide leg on bolster up

- head turns away from leg.

locked in stereo

- don't tense leg to hold it in place

- DO BOTH SIDES !!
  > < ≥
   palms up →

head to
left

bolster →
slides down,
puts check
against it

WALL

Monday, November 7, 2016

I was up early thanks to daylight savings time. Unlike the other court dates, this time I didn't stress about my appearance or what was in my bag. I strolled around the place, grabbing what I needed. There were some cords lying around from going out on Friday, and I threw those on, adding my enviable linen blue top, and the only sweater I own. It was chilly out, so I got to wear a wool coat and scarf. I enjoy a coat; it's like a sartorial blanket. My hair was in chia pet mode, a baby jewfro, with sideburns like feathered wings that no amount of gel could tame. I'd spent most of the morning reading on the sofa with Buster lying across my chest. The intense anxiety I'd experienced before going to court in the past was replaced by a mild case of apathy.

Even my commute was "whatever." Instead of making two train transfers to position myself at the subway station closest to the courthouse, I stayed on the express and got off at Canal Street. I'd commuted to Centre Street enough times now that the area had become familiar, and I thought I could vary my route. This allowed me to enjoy having a seat all the way down from Washington Heights, even though all I would be doing in the courtroom was sitting.

I got out of the subway and tooled around, casually weaving my way east. Fall is a great time to walk around New York City: the throngs of tourists have thinned out, it isn't hot, and the light has a dazzling glow. As I moseyed through the winding streets, I got lost and ended up navigating my way to the courthouse by watching a blue dot (satellite me) move along my phone's map. When I arrived, there were security lines out both entrances, wrapping around the block. It reminded me of waiting for concert tickets way back in the day. Once I was on line, the next person behind me was a guy holding a toddler. I implored him to go to the front, advising, "Say you need to change the diaper." He didn't believe they'd let him cut, but I got the people around us to rally with me and we all promised to let the guy back in line if it didn't work out.

It was 48 degrees out. Everyone was complaining about the cold, the long lines, the waiting in long lines in the cold. Why were the lines so long? It wasn't like there was a roller coaster on the other side. The new guy behind me was handsome in a works-outdoors kind of way. I asked him "What did you do?" jokingly, and he told me he got arrested for pasting signs. "Was it your own art or advertising?" I inquired. "Advertising," he replied. He asked me what I did. I looked him in the eyes by tilting my head up and said, "I beat the shit out of someone." You know, if you've never, ever, said something like that out loud, it's kind of fun. "I knocked on a neighbor's door," I confessed, "and she had me arrested."

Once we were through the entrance doors of 100 Centre Street, the line split into two with an officer pointing and yelling at people to go to the shorter line, not realizing every time he did this, he was the one creating the shorter line. After our stuff went through the X-ray conveyer belt, the officer overseeing that checkpoint had to grab the empty bins for the smaller items: keys, cell phones, belts, anything with metal. When he got the bins at the finish, he banged them upside down together to make sure nothing had been left behind. He turned them over, bang bang, and placed them at the beginning for the next person. It seemed like a visual confirmation would do just as well. When we got inside, the sound of the bins tapping metronomed our shuffling through security. I entered like I worked there, an old hag at this screening thing. All told, it took 30 minutes to get into the courtroom, which I preferred to waiting in the pews.

It was about 10 am. I tried to warm up my stiff hands while settling in, opening and closing them, and rubbing them together. I was shaking off the cold and the dystopian vibe of security, but the courtroom that morning had such a heavy fog of communal regret I almost wanted to be back outside at the buildings entrance. In my previous life, before being handcuffed

351

and taken away, I'd think of impersonal safety screening as the thing you did before catching a plane or attending a show. There was no payoff here though. Manhattan Criminal Court was no joke. Maybe you came into the courtroom protected by an arrogant sense of denial, but with minimal distraction, this was where you got to sit, and think, whether you wanted to or not. Every time I arrived to court, I was re-humbled by the realization that other people would be making decisions about my future.

It was the "good luck to you" lady judge. Perry wasn't there yet. Surprise, surprise. I guessed he didn't get an incentivizing letter in the mail regarding a no-show warrant. I wanted to eat my Clif bar, but I didn't want to get yelled at for eating in the courtroom. I tried to open it quietly while it was still in my bag, breaking off a third, looking left and right, and shoving the thing into my mouth. I really shouldn't have been there, in court. I couldn't even sneak a piece of food without sweating it out. I just didn't have the constitution for a career in crime.

I heard a new bastardization of my name being called out by some one who wasn't Perry. Did I have a new lawyer? This guy was tall with a mustache and receding blonde hair that was thin and close-cropped, wearing a dark grey two-piece suit. We were now into fall fabric weights. His jacket was uncreased, and stayed flat with movement. A version of my name was called out again, and when I raised my hand, the new guy nodded. The new lawyer had been there the whole time. That was a good sign. He was looking through two files after calling another name. This was exciting: maybe I wouldn't have to be here for hours.

I was watching the new lawyer like a hunter, observing his movements, waiting. He motioned for us to speak outside, and I was up and through the doors first. In the pseudo-private hall between the double doors, he was fidgety and engaged. He made a habit of putting his left hand in his pocket and hunching over me when he was listening. Then he would take his hand out and step back to talk, looking at the ceiling. After two instances of this I wanted to tell him the answers weren't up there. When I first met with Jack for my desk appearance ticket, I was all nerves. But now I was standing with my hands on my hips and my head cocked.

My first impression of this new lawyer was that he was wet behind the ears, that he had that first-day feeling of watching what you were doing while doing it. He told me Perry was on family medical leave. Goodness. Now that this wasn't about me, I really hoped everything was okay. My new lawyer said we were going to go up there and tell them we weren't ready, and then talk some more. He kind of had no idea what was going on and suggested I take the harassment offer before we went back in. I inhaled and said, "Let me catch ya up so we're on the same page." Then I explained the landlord thing and how I wanted to waste 90 days. In the frustration of the moment I didn't find my new lawyer and his Bambi legal legs, all that endearing. *I'm going for a dismissal, buddy, I don't know what you're going for.* Now we were on the same page. With that, he handed me his business card with his cell phone written on it. Wow, I never got Perry's cell number. He also told me the clock had stopped. I know. Time has never stopped for me or the slow and steady atrophying of my body, but in terms of this case, it had. I went back inside to sit in the pews and brood.

My name was called, and I fumbled to put away my notebook and pen and grab my coat all at the same time. It reminded me of the time I took surfing lessons. My instructor was from a place where surfing is a regular kid activity. She was laid-back and had overdeveloped deltoids, the shoulder-pad muscles, so large it was as though someone had put a short stack of pancakes on top of each arm. Our first lesson started off in the sand, with me on the board jumping into positions very similar to yoga poses. I really thought that gave me an advantage.

Then we headed out into the ocean to wait for waves. We'd lie bellies down on our boards, chitchatting in the sun and on the gentle motioning waves. I was positioned facing the beach and she was facing out to sea, watching. When she saw a wave coming, our conversation went from super mellow to her screaming, "Paddle! Paddle! Paddle!" Startled, I'd then have to start using my arms like I was digging holes in the water and, eventually, perfectly time going through those yoga poses all the way up to standing. Except every single time, I'd rush the moves and wipe out, ending up under the water looking up at my board. After a couple of rounds of this, I realized what the issue was and paddled back out to her. "You know," I said, "I just don't respond well to being yelled at." Having my name called over a microphone by a judge never failed to startle me.

Around the time of my arrest I'd been diagnosed as having PTSD (post-traumatic stress disorder). As it turned out, my delicate nervous system wasn't a genetic gift, or my fault. I started therapy the summer before my arrest, after a failed attempt with ADHD (attention deficit hyperactivity disorder) medication. I went in just wanting a drug so I could keep my ass in a chair and write. When that didn't work, therapy was offered, and I balked at it. The last time I'd gone into therapy, I fell down an emotional dark hole and ended up spending 11 days in a hospital because I was a threat to myself. *No thanks!* I resisted.

I spent that August taking Buster on the trail, stomping up and down a hill in the middle, arguing the merits of therapy to myself. It intuitively seemed like a good idea, but it was also something I didn't want to take on at all. I was interested in creative pursuits, not being a patient again. There was a Pandora's box that I'd resolved long ago to keep closed. Even so, it often felt like I was spending my life healing from the first 18 years of it, whether in therapy, on the mat, with bodyworkers, or simply catching up to where I should be in emotional maturity. Maybe other people wanted to spend their lives living out of that box, but not me, even though it often felt like I didn't have a choice. This new shrink was also offering to discount her fee by a heck of a lot. It would be silly not to try.

As therapy progressed I learned I had been misdiagnosed with ADHD (with a pay-to-play, script-for-hire, doctor). During one session, my shrink was explaining "euthymia" to me. It's the horizon line: normal, not depressed, groovy. Above that is "hyperthymia": the sun, being super happy. Then there's "dysthymia" way down below euthymia: depression, probably that hole I was climbing out of in '94. Using her left forearm as the euthymia line, my shrink waved below it with her right hand, saying, "...and this is where you live."

Aside from outside forces, maybe this was why I moved around a lot. If you don't know you're depressed, it's easy to blame other factors. Probably what I really didn't like was where I was living internally, below that line. My shrink said I was suffering from PTSD and its side effects: depression and anxiety. My sound sensitivity was probably another side effect. This was a lot to hear and take in when originally my goal was to get a pill so I could to sit still long enough to finish a screenplay. It was around then that my shrink wrote the note I had in my wallet at the time of my arrest, excusing me from creative pursuits until I was ready.

I had a hard time with the PTSD diagnosis. I thought it should be reserved for those returning from battle, our war veterans. It seemed disingenuous to be grouped amongst real sufferers. I didn't want a patch to wear for my childhood, and I didn't want to wave a flag. I just wanted to be free of any limitations, emotional or mental, that those early years had imprinted. I began to read about PTSD which helped to humanize the medical term. I had to get past being labeled as having a mental illness.

When I was diagnosed with depression in '94, it was a weight. It was the thing that held me down. But what if I chose to view depression as a quirk. Everything has quirks. What if most people were like Dodge trucks, going for miles and miles without needing much maintenance, and depression was like a 1987 Volvo station wagon: the electric complicated and temperamental to weather, the engine requiring a long time to warm up, and sometimes, inexplicably, with no visible cause, not wanting to start at all. Depression as a vintage car. After awhile, I started to think of having PTSD as similar to having any other disability, like nearsightedness. I didn't want to use the phrase "I suffer from depression and anxiety." I decided I'd prefer to say I managed it, like wearing prescription glasses.

My messenger bag sloppy over my shoulder, my coat positioned over the hand with the hoju, adjusting my shirt to make sure my chest tattoo didn't show, I passed through the chain in the courtroom fence, and again stood at the podium. As usual, the judge said good morning, and this time, I said good morning back. I was a little tired of having a supporting role with so few lines. I had done nothing wrong and felt empowered by this knowledge rather than defeated. There was a new whiff of indifference to my standing before the courtroom and its hierarchies of justice. *I'm going to wait this thing out, motherfuckers.* Diana passed along her confidence and knowledge, and I carried the still-strong vapors of our conversation with me.

There were some terms exchanged that I didn't catch, and then the DA said they couldn't find the witness. This made me happy. It was like they accidentally showed their hand. Was my neighbor supposed to be here today? I'd forgotten to worry about it. And why was I there anyways? Right, a trial, that stale carrot. There's not going to be a trial. I'm not falling for that again. Stop testing me. Stop pretending I don't exist as you make decisions regarding my welfare. I'm standing here, right here. I'm not a procedure, I'm not a statute, I'm a person. What the hell is this process? I come to court and nothing happens except maybe years are shaved off my life and a bit of taxpayer money is wasted so three groups can exchange papers and make new appearance dates. I never shoved a door open and hit a kid, the woman lied, let it go, let me go.

The first matter of business was that the DA hadn't given my lawyer's office the VDF (voluntary disclosure form). I thought that was the same form due in September the day before I'd spoken to Diana. Did that mean that time had accrued? The judge was annoyed by this and said it was now due by November 22, adding, "second request" like a warning shot. But hadn't she made a "second request" the last time I was in court? At least the VDF not being submitted worked to my favor. Stay low on that pile!

While this was going on my new lawyer Bambi reached over and grabbed two forms from piles of papers printed in duplicate. He started scribbling on them fast. Being in court, being in the world, is a lot like a surf lesson: nothing happens, you're hanging out, enjoying life, the view, and then, "Paddle, Paddle, Paddle!" The second order of business was the order of protection. Did the DA want this extended because it expired on November 17? Yes, they did. I wanted to blurt out, "She doesn't even live in the building anymore!" But I just stood there. I was instructed to wait and sign the new order of protection. My lawyer asked about it including incidental contact. The DA grunt flipped through pages and confirmed it didn't. Good catch Bambi! The judge then asked the DA to add this.

A new court appearance date was set for Tuesday, January 3. When the judge said this, I happened to be making eye contact with her, and my eyes widened. "Does that work?" she asked. Tuesday was the one weekday I had an early afternoon class, and couldn't change my schedule. I turned to my lawyer and he asked me if that worked for me. I liked that I was being included in my own schedule this round. I said, "Thank you," and then, "No." I kept saying "Thank you" to everything. I leaned in and whispered to Bambi, telling him that any other day, I could make it work. The pause in proceedings annoyed the judge. "Wednesday?" the new lawyer called out, and everyone agreed on Wednesday, January 4. Before heading back to the pew, I was reminded to wait to sign the new order of protection. There wasn't a code of conduct about saving seats, and I was thrown off by not being able to return to where I was previously. I'd taken a liking to the pews on the right side of the courtroom. I plopped down on the other side, feeling out of place. The person behind me was tap-kicking my pew nervously. I kept my stuff in my arms, hoping to get up soon.

The new lawyer was working with his second client. By this time my pen had run out of ink, and I had nothing to do but sit and listen to the proceedings, and the tapping. Just as it was beginning to feel interminable, the new lawyer motioned for his clients to meet him outside. I entered the hall as the new lawyer and his first client were speaking. The guy was retelling the whole story of his arrest. The new lawyer seemed disinterested. A couple of times, the guy made punching moves in the air. This desperation to get a legal authority figure to hear your story was a scratch that couldn't be itched. If you were there in court, your version didn't make the cut. Their conversation ended with the new lawyer saying, "Well, let's see what they come back with." The resolution that the client was looking for—that we were all looking for— required time travel.

The new lawyer came up to me, talking fast. At the 80-day mark, he was going to ask for a dismissal. Fine by me! He explained that we weren't high on the DA's list, and that was why they hadn't turned over the VDF. Adding that we didn't want to ask for it. Yes, don't bother the DA. Don't wake the kraken. When the new lawyer began talking, he began walking, through the double doors, out into the long hallway, with me in tow. We were both walking away from the courtroom. Halfway down the hall, he stopped and said, "I'm going this way," and we parted. If I could have given him advice, it would have been not to treat his clients like groupies.

It seemed like the new lawyer was purposefully walking me out and I kept going. I headed to the elevators, which took up two sides of a short corridor with a set of windows at the end. I liked seeing those windows. They reminded me of the outside

world. I was looking at the view, waiting for the arrival beep of the elevator, when I remembered I was supposed to sign the new order of protection. I headed back to the courtroom to see if I could find the new lawyer, but he wasn't there, and I didn't feel like going to the front to ask around. I turned around and left. I didn't want to be in that courtroom. I headed back to the elevators.

Once downstairs I texted the new lawyer thinking that wasn't a lot of time between receiving his mobile number and using it. I waited at the entrance doors in case he replied back. This way, I wouldn't have to go through security again. I was leaning on a door, the whole physical and emotional package of my being in one slumping gesture. I wanted very badly to leave. After a couple of minutes I took off. I walked a block, checked my phone, saw nothing, kept walking, checked the phone again, and then hopped on the subway. Hopefully not signing wasn't a big deal. They couldn't even find my neighbor.

At home, unwinding with the dog, I received a text hours later:

NEW LAWYER: Sorry. My phone was charging in the office. Did you wait and sign?
ME: Unfortunately, I took our walking out and not hearing back as a sign it was okay to leave.

The following morning I receive a text back:

NEW LAWYER: Ok. Don't worry about it.

Okay then, I won't. Cause. She. Doesn't. Live. Here. And frankly, I'm not a threat to her and never was.

| Reverse Supine Triangle |

(10 MIN)

- leg at wall is over body
- come out of by bending knees, lie on floor, for a couple f minutes, straight.

left hand

turned away (from) wall →

Right leg

Left leg

right hand

WALL

- as close to hand as possible
- double check alignment
torso

Tuesday, November 29, 2016

I texted Frankie a thank you:

ME: You're awesome!!
FRANKIE: Please elaborate! (I'd love to hear more about how I'm awesome)
ME: Anytime! I forgot to thank you for the text convo we had some time ago. I did end up speaking to my lawyer's supervisor, who was amazing. She explained their strategy: "waste" 90 court days, go for dismissal. And was great. I kind of wished I'd known to ask about a strategy or was told up front so every time I appeared in court I wasn't undoing 20 years of yoga...so thanks for telling me to do that and the hand holding, while you're a new mom!!! You're awesome
FRANKIE: Haha, I'm so so glad you reached out and got more info. It's such a stressful process, but sometimes when you're in the muck of it all the time you forget what a weight it is on people experiencing it for the first time (and with little to no info).
FRANKIE : Is the case still going?
ME: It is ongoing. I have a new lawyer. The DA keeps forgetting to hand over the VDF, and they can't find the witness (she moved) so it's looking like they could care less about me (knock wood) and I just need to keep showing up
FRANKIE: That all sounds like great news (except the part where it's not over). Now you have gotten a glimpse into the massive time suck that is our system of justice!
ME: It's fucking ridiculous. It's an endurance of patience
FRANKIE: Yeah, it's so fucking ridiculous how easy it is for some lying piece of shit to tie you up in the system...for sooo long

FRANKIE: The DAs really have no interest in truth, they have an interest in whether they can keep making you come back until you take a plea that they can add to their quota. For real. It's a fucked up system
ME: That's a helpful insight. I refuse to take the harassment plea. Once I found out it's about coming and waiting I was like, I can do that, I'm a yogini, I can sit and do nothing
FRANKIE: Oh yeah, certainly don't take the plea. They don't have shit without a witness
ME: When I first went to court, dressed nicely, I was taken aback at how blasé and impatient people were. And casually dressed. But now I understand it might be their tenth time showing up. And missing work. Btw, you seem to have a new lingo. Very kind of 'Wired' inspired. Is that a Cleveland thing?
FRANKIE: Yeah. It's hard to have a lot of respect for a system that shows you no respect in return
FRANKIE: Haha, no...I'm just letting my curse words fly because I try not to use them all day
FRANKIE: And the whole system makes me angry when I think about it
ME: I have this theory that there's always some crap on your plate stinking up everything else. Once that crap is cleaned up we get maybe three months off and then a new load comes
FRANKIE: Well hopefully you'll get a real long break after this.
ME: Kind of like having a baby?
FRANKIE: Haha yeah. Once you get used to one phase it's on to the next and back to having no idea what you're doing
ME: Just keep her alive. That's all. Variations on that

Tuesday, January 3, 2017

I'd received my court letter in the mail for tomorrow's appearance. In the past these notices felt like reminders to not be happy, "Remember! You were arrested!!" Now it felt like an urgent notice to renew a magazine subscription, three months in advance, special offer included. I was to be there at 9:30 am, Part B. If I did not come to court a warrant would be issued for my arrest. Yeah, yeah, yeah. I couldn't even remember what this appearance was for. Was the made-up police statement already striked, stricken, had a stroke? Mostly, I was focused on the end-of days-rain we'd had for 48 hours straight and what I'd wear to court in a downpour. I was also trying to remember to have a pen with ink in it in my bag. There was still the what-if factor, like the DA finding my neighbor. Even though it was getting easier to show up to court, that didn't mean the results would be determined by my comfort level. As I was walking upstairs with the mail I saw a three-day notice to vacate on the apartment door below mine. Management had a new eviction to occupy their time. I was no longer the harassing darling of the building.

Halasana at Wall (Plow)

- lie with head to wall
- slide away so arms are straight
    & fingertips just barely touch wall
- legs over head, touch wall effect
- arms behind back
- interlace fingers, clasp palms
    roll arms underneath
- walk feet down wall

if you can
it's is not painful ⇒

5-7 min

* don't pull chin down

Breathe
Breathe } OR
Breathe } DIE!

364

Wednesday, January 4, 2017

I'd slept poorly. The steam pipe in the bedroom made banging noises in the winter. It was like a ghost rattling chains in the basement. I'd also had crazy stress dreams. In one, in order to enter my apartment building, I had to go through an old lady's place, but only during certain hours. At some point in the dream, I couldn't remember what I did with my car, probably because I didn't currently own a car. I kept walking back to the place where I thought it was double parked and then drawing a blank. I even hired a cab to drive me around the neighborhood looking for it. I might have had a more restful night had I paced back and forth in the living room while banging my head with a spoon. The morning was filled with long blinks, and me saying "right" out loud to snap myself into getting going.

I'd given up on dressing for court and pulled on black jeans that were hanging on the back of the bathroom door. They needed another wear before being deemed truly worthy of the laundry pile. Though it had been raining for days and days, today it was dry and 51 degrees out. I grabbed a pink plaid button-down shirt, and threw my one sweater on top. It was a perfect wool coat, scarf, and boot day. I was cozy toasty and comfortable. It looked like I was going to a museum. Maybe all those other defendants I'd been judgmental about—the ones rocking casual attire—started off like I did, pseudo dressing like lawyers. Maybe as their court appearances wore on, so did their comfort levels, and interest. I couldn't recall if this was my fourth or fifth court appearance. But I decided that if I did hit double digits, I was going in old yoga clothes.

My hair was in the phase where people at work excitedly ask, "Are you growing your hair out?" Sometimes it seemed like girlie girls were always waiting, chomping at the bit, as if all along I'd secretly desired their tutelage. The grey spot at the top was finally blending in and catching less glare in overhead lighting.

Last week a student of mine said I looked young. I wondered how old she thought I was. Usually when someone says you look young, it's an intended compliment based on your being old. You don't tell a 20-year-old you think they look young. They are young. I guessed she thought I was at the age where it's a compliment? When did that happen? I was 43. Shouldn't I be hearing that in my 60s?

There was a line again for security, and again no cupcakes or ramen at the end. It wasn't as cold out as it had been in November. On the walk over, I read a historical building sign about the Mudd Club on White Street. I loved those signs. This was where this cool thing happened, this was where this author resided, or this gallery was, or where the original location was for so-and-so.

I was not in the mood for being in line for court. I already did my time waiting in those security lines. The woman behind me was on the phone with customer service. She had ordered something for delivery, then cancelled the delivery, and now wanted a refund. She was annoyed and speaking loudly, so I stepped out of the line to the left for some space, but because she was standing behind me, she too stepped to the left. I was her thread. With not much to do, I listened in. She'd made the purchase this morning before court. Wow, I'd barely gotten up and managed to get here. The item was a safe. She'd woken up early and bought a safe? She was giving out her address on East 23rd Street. Now we all knew where she lived, that she obviously wasn't at home, and didn't have a safe, but had a need for one. This really wasn't the place to be giving out those kinds of details. Every single person in that line was there to defend themselves against an alleged crime. As they say, "Know your audience."

Every time I came down here I was reminded of how much better off I'd be living in a small town, preferably by a large body of water, far from any neighbors I could hear. I was also reminded of my species' lack of manners. It was 9:30 am, and no one was happy in this line. There was a somber, resolved, head-low thing going on. Make a quiet phone call, lady.

On the way in I made the metal detectors beep and was sent to be scanned by the magical metal-detecting wand. Eight months before this, the way the officers weren't chatty made the process feel official and intense. But today it felt comical. I started rambling on to amuse myself, "Hey, good morning, how are you, not as cold out today, that belt looks heavy…" It was really nice to be in jeans and not in business-casual dress pants. Those pants just never lay right: they rode up a ton and stuck to my socks. Unlike trousers, jeans are friendly. They're like dogs, they like to go wherever you're going.

The courtroom was kind of empty when I arrived. I didn't think I saw my new lawyer. It was just past 9:45 am. The "good luck to you" judge was seated. Now that I'd gotten there, and I was committed to being there, I was hungry and my muscles wanted to do yoga, especially for my back. This was my body's response to court: let's get out of here and do absolutely anything else. I was in my usual pew to the right side of the isle, one row back from center. Right away, sitting in the courtroom with nothing to do, I got antsy. The lawyers at the front were walking back and forth, back and forth, watching their phones, the sound of their dress shoes clicking on the floor. The person in front of me smelled like long cigarettes. I practiced blind contour drawing on some of the people in the pews, but it felt like it could piss someone off, so I gave it up quickly. The back of the pew was carved with the words "Sweet Thunder," "Edith-N-Jude," and "bunnee."

This was so fucking boring. I never wanted to be there again. Ever. With more lawyers coming and going, I realized I couldn't remember what the new lawyer looked like. He was tall, though lots of people seemed tall to me. A defendant named Jacob had just sat down after appearing before the judge. He was wearing dark-wash skinny blue jeans rolled above the ankles and pointy black patent leather shiny Doc Marten loafers without socks. His skin was pale with acne scars on his cheeks and near his mouth. He wore his curly hair a little long on top and short everywhere else, like the lead singer for Simply Red back in the 80s. Or like the haircut I had when I was arrested.

My name was called, and I did my rushed, bolting-up-to-stand routine. I was still in the moment after first arriving, looking like I was ready to leave. I had my coat unbuttoned but on, my messenger bag strap still draped across my chest, and my scarf wrapped one loop around my neck. Would they let me leave if I looked like I wanted to leave? I stepped into the aisle, carrying my pen and notebook for security, scarf ends flapping around where the messenger bag strap wasn't holding them down, and looked around for my new lawyer. *Bambi!?* As I got closer to the fence and its ridiculous chain closure, I realized it was just me going up to the podium. For a second, in my sleepy head, I thought, "Maybe I can wing this."

The judge was watching me with bemusement as I slowly walked down the aisle and told me it was okay to proceed in. I took the chain from the person coming out and had the hardest time hooking it back on. With my pen and notebook in one hand, and the top of the chain requiring two hands, one to pull the large spring down and then another to place the hook around a small eye, it took me a couple of tries. The instant I finished and turned to walk towards the podium, the judge started speaking to me, "Ma'am, I've called you without your lawyer because your case is being dismissed." I felt my eyes widen so much my eyebrows met my hairline. I watched the judge as she phrased something to the DA. When she looked back to me I mouthed a "Thank you." After the DA made a note in my file the judge addressed the courtroom to formally announce my case was dismissed with a hit of the gavel. Then she added, "Good luck to you."

CRIMINAL COURT OF THE CITY OF NEW YORK
COUNTY OF NEW YORK

THE PEOPLE OF THE STATE OF NEW YORK

-against-

Marcy Tropin (F 42),

Defendant.

MISDEMEANOR

Police Officer ████████████████ of the 33rd Precinct, states as follows:

The defendant is charged with:

PL 120.00(2)   Assault in the Third Degree
                      (defendant #1: 1 count)

On or about April 11, 2016 at about 3:30 P.M., inside 535 Edgecombe Avenue in the County and State of New York, the defendant recklessly caused physical injury to another person.

The factual basis for this charge is as follows:

I am informed by ████████████████, of an address known to the District Attorney's Office, that during a verbal dispute with the defendant, the defendant pushed ████ apartment door open, striking ████████ in the head. I am further informed by ████ that ████ is her one-year-old daughter. I observed ████████ head and observed a red bump with bruising and swelling.

False statements made in this written instrument are punishable as a class A misdemeanor pursuant to section 210.45 of the Penal Law, and as other crimes.

_____   4/26/16   1640
Police Officer ████████████   Date   Time

371

REST

HOURS

legs up wall

SAVASANA
- lying on mat
- or rug
- hardwood floor

hangs off 5
block tall
block flat
push tank

legs on bolster
bolster on block
- wrap legs tightly in a blanket/s.

BLANKET/S

(MUSH YOURSELF)

Acknowledgements

The author would like to thank the following:

Chenault Conway, Molly M. Ginty, Georgia Grant, Heidi Korthase, Bridget McDevitt, Carol Pitts, Bonnie Schertz, Zoe Slatoff, Rudy D. Smith, Renate S., Jill Sutton, Stephanie Tamez, Deborah G. Taylor, Susan Thorson, Carrie Trippe, "Nancy," the Articles Club Ladies.

And Buster.